TREATING SUBSTANCE ABUSE

THE GUILFORD SUBSTANCE ABUSE SERIES
Howard T. Blane and Thomas R. Kosten, *Editors*

Recent Volumes

TREATING SUBSTANCE ABUSE
Theory and Technique

Edited by

FREDERICK ROTGERS
DANIEL S. KELLER
JON MORGENSTERN

THE GUILFORD PRESS
New York London

©1996 The Guilford Press
A Division of Guilford Publications, Inc.
72 Spring Street, New York, NY 10012

Printed in the United States of America

This book is printed on acid-free paper.

Last digit is print number: 9 8 7 6 5 4

Library of Congress Cataloging-in-Publication Data

Treating substance abuse : theory and technique / [edited by]
Frederick Rotgers, Daniel S. Keller, Jon Morgenstern.
    p.   cm. — (The Guilford substance abuse series)
  Includes bibliographical references and index.
  ISBN 1-57230-025-6
  1. Substance abuse—Treatment. I. Rotgers, Frederick.
II. Keller, Daniel S. III. Morgenstern, Jon. IV. Series.
  [DNLM: 1. Substance Abuse—therapy. 2 Substance Abuse—
psychology. 3. Alcoholism—psychology. 4. Alcoholism—therapy.
WM 270 T7818 1996
RC564.T7347 1996
616.8606—dc20
DNLM/DLC   95-25144
                                                CIP

Contributors

Alison Bell, R.N., Nurse Specialist, Alcohol and Other Drugs, Faculty of Nursing, Sydney University, Sydney, New South Wales, Australia

Kathleen M. Carroll, Ph.D., Assistant Professor of Psychiatry, Yale University School of Medicine, Substance Abuse Center, New Haven, Connecticut

Elizabeth E. Epstein, Ph.D., Assistant Research Professor, Center of Alcohol Studies, Rutgers University, Piscataway, New Jersey

Daniel S. Keller, Ph.D., Research Assistant Professor, Department of Psychiatry, Division of Alcoholism and Drug Abuse, New York University School of Medicine, New York, New York

Jeremy Leeds, Ph.D., Assistant Professor, Department of Applied Psychology, School of Education, New York University, New York, New York

Barbara A. McCrady, Ph.D., Director, Division of Clinical Services, Center of Alcohol Studies, Rutgers University, Piscataway, New Jersey

James R. McKay, Ph.D., Assistant Professor of Psychology in Psychiatry, Department of Psychiatry, University of Pennsylvania School of Medicine, Philadelphia, Pennsylvania

Thomas J. Morgan, Psy.D., Research Associate, Center of Alcohol Studies, Rutgers University, Piscataway, New Jersey

Jon Morgenstern, Ph.D., Assistant Research Professor, Center of Alcohol Studies, Rutgers University, Piscataway, New Jersey

Joseph Nowinski, Ph.D., Clinical Psychologist, HumanCare Specialists, North Windham, Connecticut

Stephen Rollnick, Ph.D., Consultant Clinical Psychologist, Department of General Practice, University of Wales School of Medicine, Cardiff, Wales, United Kingdom

Frederick Rotgers, Psy.D., Assistant Research Professor, Center of Alcohol Studies, Rutgers University, Piscataway, New Jersey

Bill Saunders, M. Phil., Associate Professor, School of Psychology, Curtin University of Technology, Perth, Western Australia

Tania Towers, B.App.Sc., Postgrad. Dip. Psych., M. Psych., Research Assistant, School of Psychology, Curtin University, Perth, Western Australia

Celia Wilkinson, B.Sc., M.Sc., Lecturer, Health Studies, Edith Cowan University, Perth, Western Australia

John Wallace, Ph.D., Director of Education, Research, and Evaluation, ADCARE Hospital, Worcester, Massachusetts

Contents

Introduction

FREDERICK ROTGERS
DANIEL S. KELLER
JON MORGENSTERN

Psychoactive substance use disorders (PSUDs) affect a staggering proportion of the population of the United States and other Western nations. Recent epidemiologic data obtained as part of the Epidemiologic Catchment Area study of the National Institute of Mental Health indicate that nearly 20% (or about 48 million people) of the general population of the United States qualified for a PSUD diagnosis at some point during their lifetime (Regier et al., 1990). The same researchers found that persons suffering from psychiatric disorder who come for mental health treatment had twice the risk of having a drinking problem, and four times the risk of having a drug problem compared to the general population. Nearly a third (29%) of persons seeking mental health treatment will also suffer from a PSUD at some point in their life.

The impact of the problem of PSUDs goes beyond the large numbers of persons with those disorders who enter mental health treatment. A wide-ranging economic analysis of addictions treatment prepared for the President's Commission on Model State Drug Laws (Langenbucher, McCrady, Brick, & Esterly, 1993) estimated that the cost of PSUDs to U.S. society, both for direct services to persons suffering from PSUDs, and for services to their families, lies between $150 billion and $200 billion annually. Given these estimates of the prevalence and costs of PSUDs the provision of adequate treatment services to persons suffering from these disorders is of extreme importance.

Until the mid-1970s, with few exceptions, treatment for persons

1

suffering from PSUDs was largely uniform. Persons with drinking problems, or problems with drugs other than opiates, were typically referred
to inpatient programs, where they would receive 28 days of detoxification
and psychoeducational information about alcohol and drugs and be
introduced to 12-Step-based self-help groups. In addition to these activities, counseling was provided that attempted to encourage the client to
surrender him/herself to a higher power and dedicate his/her life to the
achievement of abstinence from alcohol and drugs. Persons with opiate
use problems were often referred to even longer inpatient programs run
by ex-addicts according to a therapeutic community model. Other opiate-
using clients were referred to methadone maintenance programs. For
many years substance abuse treatment was conducted largely according
to these three models (12-Step, therapeutic community, or methadone
maintenance) with little difference across programs espousing similar
philosophies and little attempt to tailor treatment services to specific client
needs.

Today, substance abuse treatment is a field in transition, a transition
driven in large part by a paradox. The paradox stems from two observations
clinicians and researchers make routinely: that the old traditional substance
abuse treatments worked for many clients, yet for many other clients
traditional treatments appear to have little, if any, long-term benefit. As
practitioners, researchers, and observers of the field, we believe that these
and other significant issues are driving a reassessment of the philosophies,
techniques, and delivery of substance abuse treatment services in the United
States and abroad. In this introduction we set the stage for the chapters that
follow by attempting to characterize some of those issues. We begin with an
outline of what we see as the most important forces driving change in the
field, followed by an outline of this book and what we have tried to achieve
in it. We hope that this chapter will set the stage for a more sophisticated
integration of the information contained in the book and will prompt our
readers to begin to think in terms of not only how to treat particular clients
but how an individual client's treatment can be conceptualized within the
framework of substance abuse treatment as a whole. We begin with our
assessment of the current status of the field.

WHY WE PRODUCED THIS BOOK:
A RESPONSE TO FORCES OF CHANGE

Over the past 20 years, as the United States has waged a "war" against
substance use, there has begun to be increasing uneasiness among sub-

stance abuse treatment providers with the unstable, and often poor, outcomes that result from mainstream treatments—treatments that traditionally have been expensive in both time and money (see Holder, Longabaugh, Miller, & Rubonis, 1991, for a comparison of various costs of different types of treatment). Despite the best efforts of treatment providers to help people with alcohol and drug problems to resolve those problems, and concerted efforts by proponents of traditional models of addiction and substance abuse treatment to destigmatize substance abuse and dependence, the vast majority of persons with alcohol and drug problems do not seek treatment at all. Estimates of the ratio of treated to untreated persons with PSUDs range from 1:3 to 1:13 (Sobell, Sobell, Toneatto, & Leo, 1993).

Those persons suffering from PSUDs who do enter treatment often apparently fail to benefit from that treatment in the long term, with relapse being a much more frequent treatment outcome than providers would like, and as many as 30–40% or more of treated clients, depending on a variety of other variables, resuming substance use within the first year following treatment. Outcome research continues to find high relapse rates despite increasing attempts to keep clients in contact with treatment personnel for longer periods of aftercare. With the advent of managed health care delivery, third-party payers have become reluctant to fund extensive substance abuse treatment because of these sorts of data, despite other clear evidence of the benefits of providing such treatment (Langenbucher et al., 1993). Recent data from one private inpatient program with which one of the editors (FR) is associated showed a drop in mean length of stay for uncomplicated substance abuse inpatients from 19 days to 11 days between 1993 and 1994 alone, a nearly 50% decline in length of stay in 1 year! Economic forces of the sort that produced this drastic decline in hospital stay length in one facility are now beginning to push practitioners toward use of briefer interventions and greater accountability for outcomes.

Traditional approaches to substance abuse treatment have tended to advocate a relatively uniform approach for all clients, with a heavy emphasis on working the 12 steps of programs such as Alcoholics Anonymous or Narcotics Anonymous as the preferred method for all comers. Although many treatment providers and researchers have begun to recognize that substance abusers are an extraordinarily heterogeneous group from a variety of perspectives, most treatment programs in the United States still offer only a limited range of treatment options, typically based on 12-Step thinking.

Disillusionment and discontent with traditional treatment adjuncts and philosophies have also begun to appear among clients themselves, and an ever increasing number of self-help alternatives to traditional 12-Step support groups have been developed within the last 10 years (McCrady & Delaney, 1995). These alternatives have typically focused on tailoring the recovery process to these client characteristics that make it difficult for clients to accept and identify with traditional 12-Step approaches. For example, Rational Recovery (Trimpey, 1992) was developed as a clear reaction against what was perceived by its founders as a heavy emphasis on religious spirituality and powerlessness in 12-Step thinking, rather than an emphasis that Rational Recovery's founder and followers prefer on empowerment of the substance abuser to cope with his/her substance abuse problem.

While the field of substance abuse treatment has begun to move toward a greater diversity of treatment approaches, in the field of psychotherapy and behavior change generally (of which substance abuse counseling and treatment clearly form a subset), there has been a contrasting movement toward integration of traditionally disparate approaches to behavior change. Models such as Lazarus's (1981) multimodal therapy and Prochaska and DiClemente's (1982) stages of change have been proposed as ways of understanding and conceptualizing the process of behavior change and developing treatment packages that are tailored to individual client needs. More and more therapists have begun to utilize techniques from a variety of theoretical orientations to help clients cope with the problems that brought them to therapy in the first place.

We attempt to respond to this movement by incorporating insights from the psychotherapy research and practice literature along with current research findings and theory specific to substance abuse treatment in a volume that will help practitioners, both novice and experienced, keep pace with the rapid changes occurring in the field. We believe the time is ripe to bring together clear, concise expositions of current prominent theoretical and technical models of substance abuse treatment in one place. This belief has several bases:

1. No such book exists in the field at the present time.
2. As health care reform proceeds in the United States and consumers of treatment services become more sophisticated, there will be increasing pressure for treatment providers to be well versed in a variety of approaches, particularly ones that have some measure of scientific support for their efficacy. The "Johnny one-note" approach to substance abuse treatment that has characterized the field will increasingly be replaced by "different strokes for different folks."
3. It is our belief that successful practice must be firmly grounded in an understanding of both theory and technique and how they

interrelate to guide treatment. All too often, in our experience as teachers of both novice and experienced practitioners, there appears to be a woeful lack of understanding of why certain techniques are used and an absence of any guiding philosophy to structure treatment. We have also found this to be true in two empirical studies of treatment providers (Morgenstern & McCrady, 1992; Rotgers & Morgenstern, 1994). This lack of a clear-cut rationale for what many clinicians do with their clients creates disturbing opportunities for treatment to be inadequately provided, thereby leading to poorer outcomes than clients are entitled to expect.

TREATMENT OUTCOME RESEARCH AND THE DEVELOPMENT OF NEW TECHNOLOGIES

Since the late 1970s there has been an increased interest among treatment researchers in demonstrating the efficacy of various approaches to treatment of substance abuse. Although some traditional approaches to recovery have been difficult to study scientifically (however, a recent conference on research into Alcoholics Anonymous [McCrady & Miller, 1993] suggests that new approaches are being developed to address this problem), many others have been the subject of scientific scrutiny (Emrick, Tonigan, Montgomery, & Little, 1993). In addition, a variety of new, often empirically driven approaches have appeared, some of which have been integrated in various ways into traditional treatments.

Approaches such as relapse prevention, originally outlined by Marlatt (Marlatt & Gordon, 1985) and others working within a cognitive-behavioral theoretical framework, have been widely adopted and adapted by practitioners working within a 12-Step perspective (e.g., Gorski, 1989). Advances in neurobiology have led to an increasingly promising investigation of pharmacotherapeutic approaches to substance abuse treatment in addition to the traditional methadone maintenance therapy for opiate addicts and disulfiram (Antabuse) treatment for alcoholics.

Therapists working within both family systems and behavioral frameworks have developed new procedures for working not only with the substance abuser but with his/her family and social networks (O'Farrell & Cowles, 1989; Sisson & Azrin, 1989). Some models (e.g., Galanter, 1993) attempt to integrate traditional 12-Step approaches with an emphasis on family and social network involvement in treatment.

Finally, and perhaps most successfully from the standpoint of the scientific evidence of efficacy, behavior therapists working within a variety of learning theory models have developed treatment techniques and methods designed to address some of the most intractable aspects of substance abuse, for example, motivating substance users to begin behavior change efforts (Miller & Rollnick, 1991) and helping recovering users cope with craving and urges to use (Childress et al., 1993). In addition, a number of treatment researchers have begun to gather data suggesting that behavioral approaches work well with particular client types, thus providing evidence that matching clients to treatments may be possible.

The notion of matching clients to treatments is an old one in the substance abuse field, having been proposed by figures such as E. M. Jellinek as early as the 1940s. Currently, heavily funded research efforts are under way in an attempt to develop algorithms that will enable client–treatment matching by practitioners based on a thorough assessment of client characteristics. The most ambitious study of this kind is Project MATCH, a multisite project (Project MATCH Research Group, 1993) that has been funded by the National Institute on Alcohol Abuse and Alcoholism to study client response to three divergent treatment technologies and to attempt to identify client characteristics that may be predictive of favorable outcome with each treatment.

Studies such as Project MATCH are based on several of the changes in thinking about substance abusers noted earlier, but most specifically on the idea that substance abusers are a heterogeneous population who diverge on a variety of characteristics. Current treatment outcome research has also begun to recognize that substance abuse and dependence must be viewed in a developmental fashion, and that one treatment episode may not produce a complete "cure" the first time behavior change is attempted. This research grows out of a recognition that slips and relapses appear to be a common occurrence among persons who are ultimately successful in reducing or eliminating substance use.

Beginning with work by Schacter (1982) it has become increasingly clear that many people with substance abuse problems, even ones who are clearly substance dependent, resolve those problems on their own without treatment of any kind and without the use of support groups such as Alcoholics Anonymous or Narcotics Anonymous. The recognition that there are "natural" recovery processes at work in the resolution of many substance abuse problems has been a driving notion behind Prochaska and DiClemente's work with the stages-of-change model (Prochaska, DiClemente, & Norcross, 1992) Increased attention is being devoted to understanding and harnessing these natural change processes to help substance abusers who do seek treatment.

HOW THIS BOOK IS ORGANIZED:
WHAT IS INCLUDED AND WHY

In order to help new and experienced practitioners to better prepare for the significant increase in emphasis on matching clients to treatment, which we foresee will occur, we have assembled a group of authors who are experts in, and strong proponents of, five major approaches to treatment theory and technique that are available to nonphysicians: (1) 12-Step, (2) psychodynamic, (3) marital/family therapy, (4) behavioral, and (5) motivational enhancement. These approaches were selected for a variety of reasons.

Approaches based on the Alcoholics Anonymous 12-Step model (Wallace, Chapter 1, and Nowinski, Chapter 2) are clearly dominant in substance abuse treatment in the United States, and will likely continue to be influential for years to come. This influence may very well be enhanced by the fact that researchers are now beginning to devise ways of assessing the efficacy of both formal treatments based on 12-Step thinking and 12-Step self-help groups such as Alcoholics Anonymous (McCrady & Miller, 1993). As anecdotal evidence of efficacy is replaced by scientific evidence and the client characteristics associated with greatest success with 12-Step approaches are identified, we believe that these approaches will be strengthened greatly.

Although psychodynamic thinkers have traditionally ignored substance abusers, viewing substance abuse as either untreatable within a psychodynamic framework or as merely symptomatic of other problems, a number of innovative approaches to substance abuse have begun to develop within the psychodynamically oriented treatment community (Leeds & Morgenstern, Chapter 3, and Keller, Chapter 4). These new approaches have the particular attraction of being useful ways of enhancing the efficacy and implementation of other treatment approaches. Although traditionally not a mainstream line of thought in the substance abuse field, we believe that psychodynamic thinking has much to offer clinicians and present it here for that reason.

Marital/family approaches (McCrady & Epstein, Chapter 5, and McKay, Chapter 6) to substance abuse treatment have a long and diverse history and in recent years have begun to garner a great deal of scientific support for their efficacy. In addition to strong empirical support, these approaches have the advantage of providing a means of integrating apparently disparate aspects of the client's life into a coherent treatment and support network that can help produce and maintain changes in substance use.

Behavioral approaches (Rotgers, Chapter 7, and Morgan, Chapter

8), while not widely used clinically, have amassed the greatest scientific evidence supporting their efficacy of any of the approaches presented in this book. Behavioral theory is ideally suited to client–treatment matching because it is inherently individually oriented, with each client's treatment being potentially different in scope and process from every other client's. This ready ability of behaviorally based clinicians to tailor treatment to client needs is an important characteristic that we believe makes behavioral approaches worthy of much wider use.

Motivational enhancement approaches (Saunders, Wilkinson, & Towers, Chapter 9, and Bell & Rollnick, Chapter 10) are newcomers to the substance abuse treatment armamentarium. Based on research from social psychology and on the process by which people change, motivational enhancement approaches attempt to mobilize clients to change behavior from less healthful to more health-promoting patterns. To some extent a reaction against traditional confrontational approaches to treatment that have focused on aggressively breaking through client "denial", motivational enhancement approaches provide a promising means for removing barriers to treatment entry, enhancing treatment compliance, and promoting more successful long-range outcomes.

In addition to chapters on these five approaches, we have included a chapter focusing on psychopharmacologic approaches to substance abuse treatment (Carroll, Chapter 11). Although used only by physicians at present, psychopharmacologic approaches to substance abuse treatment are among the most extensively studied and promising methods currently available. Should the promise of medications to suppress urges to use drugs or alcohol be fulfilled, nonphysician clinicians and physicians alike will need to understand how those medications are integrated into psychosocial treatments. In our view, even if a so-called magic pill is discovered, it will not provide the complete answer for all substance abusers, and psychosocial treatments will continue to occupy a prominent place in the treatment armamentarium. In fact, recent research (O'Malley et al., 1992) has found that psychosocial and psychopharmacologic treatments can enhance each other's efficacy, suggesting that a combination treatment will likely become the norm in the future.

The book is organized into paired chapters covering each treatment approach, with the exception of psychopharmacologic approaches which are represented by a single chapter. Each pair of chapters is composed of a chapter focusing solely on the theory behind the approach being considered and one focusing on translation of the theory into clinical practice. The chapter on psychopharmacology is stand-alone, primarily because we felt that the theory underlying this approach was far too complex and broad to be usefully encapsulated in a short chapter, and secondarily because we believe that most of our readers will likely not be involved directly in the implementation of that approach.

We asked our authors to address a number of specific questions that we believe are critical to the conduct of substance abuse treatments. Authors of theory chapters were asked to state the basic assumptions of their approach as clearly and concisely as possible and to address a number of other questions in their chapters. These questions focused on how the theory under consideration addresses the etiology, maintenance, and change of PSUDs, the role of environmental factors in the etiology, maintenance, and change of PSUDs; the theory's view of the the heterogeneity–homogeneity of persons with PSUDs, and the extent to which the theory proposes that different types of clients be treated differently (e.g., depending on drug of choice, demographic variables, and family history); and the critical tasks that must be accomplished in order for treatment conducted according to the author's theory to be successful. Finally, authors were asked to provide a brief statement of the degree of empirical support for their theoretical position.

Authors of technique chapters were specifically asked to translate the theoretical position they adopt into therapist actions and strategies during treatment. Questions were asked about sequencing of treatment activities, how "denial" and "resistance" are addressed, what the role of self-help groups is from that treatment perspective, how treatment termination is decided on, how modality of treatment (individual, group, marital, family) is selected, and how slips or relapses are addressed in treatment. Use of case study material was encouraged.

Our authors are experienced clinicians, deeply versed in the nuances of the approaches they espouse, and we have asked them to be advocates for their approaches. Many of our authors are clinical researchers as well and have been deeply committed to empirical study of their approaches as well as to their use clinically. While it is impossible to exclude each author's own unique vision completely from his/her chapter, we have attempted to have our authors produce chapters that portray each approach and its derivative techniques in a broad way that is characteristic of how that approach works in practice. Our authors are authorities on, not originators of, the positions they espouse.

Several implicit themes become apparent as one reads through the chapters. The first, and most striking, is the diversity of approaches represented here. This is particularly surprising given the homogeneity of approaches that existed in the field as few as 20 years ago. A second theme that emerges is the significant extent to which cross-fertilization of ideas and techniques characterizes these approaches, despite differing theoretical and technical bases. Third, it becomes clear that each of these approaches carries with it both limitations and advantages, and that none of these approaches will work uniformly well for all clients despite what its proponents might argue. These latter two implicit themes combine to form a third: that the wave of the future in substance abuse treatment appears to be some form of client–treatment matching for optimal outcomes.

Through this volume, we have addressed a broad audience. It is aimed at advanced undergraduates, beginning graduate students, and candidates for certification as substance abuse counselors who are learning to do substance abuse treatment for the first time. We also believe that experienced substance abuse clinicians who have been trained in a single approach but who wish to become familiar with other approaches will find the book a useful starting point without having to wade through a huge professional or scientific literature to do so. Finally, general psychotherapists and general medical practitioners will find this book helpful in approaching issues of substance abuse with clients who may be in treatment for other disorders, again avoiding the necessity of having to go directly to the professional or scientific literature to do so. For those who do wish to delve into the professional literature on particular approaches we have included references with each chapter to serve as a guide to the most prominent publications within each treatment approach.

We recognize that this book is not comprehensive, nor do we intend it to be. Rather, it is a focused introduction to treatment theories and techniques that we believe will form the core of any adequate substance abuse treatment program for the foreseeable future.

REFERENCES

Childress, A. R., Hole, A. V., Ehrman, R. N., Robbins, S. J., McLellan, A. T., & O'Brien, C. P. (1993). Cue reactivity and cue reactivity interventions in drug dependence. In L. S. Onken, J. D. Blaine, & J. J. Boren (Eds.), *Behavioral treatments for drug abuse and dependence* (NIDA Research Monograph 137). Washington, DC: U.S. Government Printing Office.

Emrick, C. D., Tonigan, J. S., Montgomery, H., & Little, L. (1993). Alcoholics Anonymous: What is currently known? In B. S. McCrady & W. R. Miller (Eds.), *Research on Alcoholics Anonymous: Opportunities and alternatives.* New Brunswick, NJ: Rutgers Center of Alcohol Studies.

Galanter, M. (1993). *Network therapy for alcohol and drug abuse: A new approach in practice.* New York: Basic Books.

Gorski, T. T. (1989). *Passages through recovery: An action plan for preventing relapse.* Center City, MN: Hazelden.

Holder, H. D., Longabaugh, R., Miller, W. R., & Rubonis, A. V. (1991). The cost effectiveness of treatment for alcoholism: A first approximation. *Journal of Studies on Alcohol, 52,* 517–540.

Langenbucher, J. W., McCrady, B. S., Brick, J., & Esterly, R. (1993). *Socioeconomic evaluations of addictions treatment.* Washington, DC: President's Commission on Model State Drug Laws.

Lazarus, A. A. (1981). *The practice of multimodal therapy.* New York: McGraw-Hill.

Marlatt, G. A., & Gordon, J. R. (Eds.). (1985). *Relapse prevention: Maintenance strategies in the treatment of addictive behaviors.* New York: Guilford Press.

McCrady, B. S., & Delaney, S. I. (1995). Self-help groups. In R. K. Hester & W. R. Miller (Eds.), *Handbook of alcoholism treatment approaches: Effective Alternatives* (2nd ed.). Needham Heights, MA: Allyn & Bacon.

McCrady, B. S., & Miller, W. R. (Eds.). (1993). *Research on Alcoholics Anonymous: Opportunities and alternatives.* New Brunswick, NJ: Rutgers Center of Alcohol Studies.

Miller, W. R., & Rollnick, S. (1991). *Motivational interviewing: Preparing people to change addictive behavior.* New York: Guilford Press.

Morgenstern, J., & McCrady, B. S. (1992). Curative factors in alcohol and drug treatment: Behavioral and disease model perspectives. *British Journal of Addiction, 87,* 901–912.

O'Farrell, T. J., & Cowles, K. S. (1989). Marital and family therapy. In R. K. Hester & W. R. Miller (Eds.), *Handbook of alcoholism treatment approaches: Effective alternatives.* New York: Pergamon Press.

O'Malley, S. S., Jaffe, A. J., Chang, G., Schottenfeld, R. S., Meyer, R. E., & Rounsaville, B. (1992). Naltrexone and coping skills therapy for alcohol dependence: A controlled study. *Archives of General Psychiatry, 49,* 881–887.

Prochaska, J. O., & DiClemente, C. C. (1982). Transtheoretical therapy: Toward a more integrative model of change. *Psychotherapy: Theory, Research and Practice, 20,* 161–173.

Prochaska, J. O., DiClemente, C. C., & Norcross, J. C. (1992). In search of how people change: Applications to addictive behaviors. *American Psychologist, 47,* 1102–1114.

Project MATCH Research Group. (1993). Project MATCH: Rationale and methods for a multisite clinical trial matching patients to alcoholism treatment. *Alcoholism: Clinical and Experimental Research, 17,* 1130–1145.

Regier, D. A., Farmer, M. E., Rae, D. S., Locke, B. Z, Keith, S. J., Judd, L. L., & Goodwin, F. K. (1990). Comorbidity of mental disorders with alcohol and other drug abuse: Results from the Epidemiologic Catchment Area (ECA) study. *Journal of the American Medical Association, 264,* 2511–2518.

Rotgers, F., & Morgenstern, J. (1994). *Processes comprising successful substance abuse treatment: A survey of counselors.* Unpublished manuscript, Rutgers Center of Alcohol Studies, New Brunswick, NJ.

Schacter, S. (1982). Recidivism and self-cure of smoking and obesity. *American Psychologist, 37,* 436–444.

Sisson, R., & Azrin, N. (1989). The community reinforcement approach. In R. K.

Hester & W. R. Miller (Eds.), *Handbook of alcoholism treatment approaches: Effective alternatives.* New York: Pergamon Press.
Sobell, L. C., Sobell, M. B., Toneatto, T., & Leo, G. I. (1993). What triggers the resolution of alcohol problems without treatment? *Alcoholism: Clinical and Experimental Research, 17,* 217–224.
Trimpey, J. (1992). *The small book: A revolutionary alternative for overcoming alcohol and drug dependence* (3rd ed.). New York: Delacorte Press.

CHAPTER 1

Theory of 12-Step-Oriented Treatment

JOHN WALLACE

Precise definitions of 12-Step theory and its derivative, 12-Step technique of treatment, are difficult to achieve. The literature of Alcoholics Anonymous (AA), from which all 12-Step programs have been derived, does not lend itself to unambiguous interpretation. Moreover, treatment programs that utilize the 12-Steps of AA in some manner or another are characterized by considerable heterogeneity. These programs vary in how the steps and concepts of AA are construed and applied and also in the additional theories and techniques they employ. The writings of those theorists who have been categorized as 12-Step theorists reveal so many differences in concepts, utilization of particular databases, and emphases that efforts to describe this body of work more often than not result in stereotypes rather than sensitive and accurate descriptions (e.g., Peele, 1985). A further complication is that some authorities sympathetic to both AA and formal treatment approaches would argue that the very term "12-Step treatment" is a misnomer or oxymoron because AA is not a treatment program and those treatment programs that do nothing but teach the steps and traditions of AA are not treatment programs either. AA is best thought of as a "fellowship" or, perhaps, a social movement; it does not conduct assessments, arrive at diagnoses, dispense medications, write treatment plans, provide case management, and do group and individual therapy. And treatment programs that do not do at least some of these functions cannot be considered treatment programs either.

Despite these caveats, it is possible to discern some common characteristics among those programs that are sympathetic to AA and make some use of AA concepts while employing other concepts and procedures as well. This chapter focuses on these common characteristics.

Throughout this chapter, then, the term "12-Step treatment" refers to certain core concepts, implicit assumptions, informal hypotheses, and explicit ideas that constitute one recognizable approach to addictions treatment and recovery. I make no claim to be a spokesperson for AA or any other 12-Step program. The material presented here is best construed as one observer's view on this complex matter and not as a final, definitive statement on what AA is or what 12-Step treatment theory is.

CONCEPT OF ADDICTION

The 12-Step approach to the origins, maintenance, and modification of addictive behaviors has for some time constituted an informal biopsychosocialspiritual model of addiction (Wallace, 1989a). Although 12-Step talk is the language of laypersons and not that of professional psychologists or other scientists, it is a rich, comprehensive language with many references to the physical, psychological, social, and spiritual aspects of human beings. When, for example, newcomers to AA are told that they have a disease that prevents them from being able to predict and control their drinking in a consistent manner, a biomedical concept has been advocated. But when an AA sponsor tells a newcomer to avoid former drinking companions and drinking situations, the sponsor is making a clear statement about the importance of interpersonal and socioenvironmental factors in recovery. And when members of an AA group share experiences and advice about such psychological matters as depression, anger, loneliness, self-pity, jealousy, resentments, and sexuality, they are obviously involved in a form of folk psychotherapy.

From its inception, AA seemed to offer at least a two-dimensional concept of addiction in its formal literature. William Silkworth (Alcoholics Anonymous, 1976), for example, in the classic work, *Alcoholics Anonymous,* called attention to both biological and psychological factors in alcoholism. For Silkworth, alcoholism was the result of an allergy to alcohol (physical) coupled with an obsession with the substance (psychological). Bill Wilson (1953), the founder of AA, spoke of alcoholism as an "illness" but wrote extensively on the psychodynamic aspects of drinking problems. Within recent years, theorists sympathetic to 12-Step programs have contributed formal biopsychosocial models (e.g., Wallace, 1985, 1989c). In short, both the history of AA and modern thinking reveal implicit and explicit concern with multidimensional models of addiction.

DISEASE MODELS

Although both advocates and opponents of biological factors have argued heatedly in favor of or in opposition to a disease concept of alcoholism and other addictions, these arguments have been characterized on both sides by lack of rigorous definitions, misleading generalities, neglect of an abundant body of biological research, and polemic rather than scientific discourse (e.g., Peele, 1988, 1989, 1990). Few of the participants in these proceedings appear to have realized that many disease concepts or models are available and that debate might more profitably center around which of these models more accurately describe addictive phenomena and best fit available data.

In what sense can alcoholism and other drug addictions be considered diseases? Perhaps the simplest answer to this question involves the many biomedical consequences of alcoholism and drug addiction. Alcoholics and addicts are often seriously ill people as a direct result of drug intake. Whether or not one believes in biological etiological factors is simply irrelevant in many practical treatment contexts. Dangerous withdrawal symptoms, overdoses, cardiac conditions, liver disease, pancreatic disease, and so forth must be treated medically despite one's ideology about the origins of these problems. Moreover, the presence of these most serious medical sequelae of alcohol and other drug ingestion clearly indicates that further attempts at drinking or drug taking by the patient must be vigorously opposed by clinicians responsible for the patient's care. In effect, this first and probably least controversial of the disease models can be termed the "medical consequences model."

A considerably more complicated disease model can be termed the "biopsychosocialspiritual consequences/maintenance model." This disease model is multidimensional and hence much richer than the narrow medical consequences model. Interacting biological, psychological, social, and spiritual factors are at issue here rather than medical problems. Furthermore, rather than focusing on the important but extraordinarily complex question of etiology, the biopsychosocialspiritual consequences/maintenance disease model permits both theorists and clinicians to attend to the critical factors involved in changing addictive behaviors by addressing the multiple factors that maintain them once begun. As will be explained shortly, this model asserts that excessive alcohol and other drug use leads to profound biological, psychological, social, and spiritual negative consequences. The distress associated with these multidimensional negative consequences leads to further excessive drug use, which, in turn, leads to more negative consequences and more distress. Hence, a vicious cycle is established that maintains excessive drug and alcohol use.

Each of the dimensions of the biopsychosocial model is discussed separately in the following sections.

The Biological Dimension

As a considerable body of research in this century has shown, the brain is an electrochemical information processing system. Important neuromodulators, neurotransmitters, and neurohormones have been identified and processes involved in presynaptic and postsynaptic neurotransmission of information have been studied extensively. In effect, the human brain is a sea of chemicals. Alcohol and other drugs enter this chemical environment of the brain and produce profound changes. These changes in the chemistry of the brain are associated with important positive and negative cognitive, affective, and behavior changes. It is probable that the reinforcement value of various drugs lies in their capacities to effect acute changes in brain chemistry. Hence, a drug such as cocaine produces initial feelings of alertness, euphoria, arousal, and energization, probably because of its impact upon dopaminergic, serotonergic, and noradrenergic synapses. But whereas the initial or acute effects of cocaine are to enhance dopaminergic and other neurotransmitter transmission, the drug's longer-term or chronic effects are to disrupt such neurotransmission through negative impact upon levels of these important neurochemicals (Dackis & Gold, 1985). As the levels of dopamine and other neurotransmitters fall as a result of continued cocaine use, associated negative changes in mood, affect, cognition, and behavior take place as well. Euphoria gives way to depression; alertness and arousal yield to difficulties in attentional processes and fatigue; feelings of well-being are replaced by irritation and agitation. Cognitive pathology in the form of delusions and hallucinations may suddenly appear and cause the chronic cocaine user further extreme discomfort. But despite these negative outcomes of chronic use, the cocaine addict remains attracted to the chemical in seeming defiance of all that is reasonable and rational. The paradox, however, is readily resolved when we realize that the addict is caught in a vicious cycle: initial positive reinforcement with initial drug use, which leads to abnormal changes in brain chemistry with chronic use which, in turn, lead to negative mood, affective, and cognitive states. These negative psychological states motivate further drug-seeking behavior because the addict remembers the highly reinforcing, positive psychological states associated with neurotransmitter release and enhancement upon initial use. Similar vicious biopsychological states occur with chronic use of drugs other than cocaine. Alcohol, for example, produces many changes by impacting diffusely upon numerous brain processes and structures. Alcohol in large quantities produces both acute and chronic effects on cell membranes (Goldstein, 1983; Hunt, 1985), neurotransmitter systems (Tarter & Van Thiel, 1985), calcium channels, and brain enzymes (Wallace, 1989b). With regard to the latter, research has shown abnormal adenylate cyclase activity for as long as 4 years after alcohol consumption has ceased (Tabakoff et al., 1988). These many changes in brain structure and processes lead to vicious cycles in which drinking leads to more negative consequences and, in turn, motivates more drug-seeking behavior.

The Psychological Dimension

Chronic excessive use of psychoactive substances may produce important changes in brain chemistry and processes and these changes are linked to further significant alterations in mood and affect. Chronic consumption of large quantities of alcohol may, for example, lead to depression and anxiety. Patients admitted to alcoholism treatment facilities routinely show depressive and anxiety symptoms on admission. By the third to fourth week of treatment, however, these symptoms disappear in the vast majority of patients (Brown, Irwin, & Schuckit, 1991; Brown & Schuckit, 1988). In effect, symptoms of depression and anxiety are often pharmacologically induced in alcoholic patients, who may enter into vicious cycles in which drinking both creates and alleviates (temporarily) these uncomfortable states. Some psychological negative consequences, however, are not linked directly to the pharmacologic impact of alcohol and other drugs but are a product of general life happenings of the addicted person. Alcoholics, for example, frequently show serious deficiencies in self-esteem. Although some of these problems in self-regarding attitudes may have preceded active alcoholism, it is probable that negative self-esteem in alcoholics is largely an outcome of such things as shame and embarrassment associated with public drunken comportment, arrests for drunken driving, remorse, guilt or harm done to others while intoxicated, loss of employment, rejection by spouses or lovers, and so forth. Further, many alcoholics show an identity problem. This problem in identity and self-understanding is often the direct outcome of the repeated conflict between the morals and core values of the sober personality at odds with the actions of the intoxicated person. The psychological negative consequences of alcoholism and addiction include low self-esteem; anger; grandiosity; resentments toward others; repressive defenses including denial, rationalization, assimilative projection, minimization of difficulties, avoidance of feelings, and resistance to feedback from others about self; hostility; excessive self-pity and sensitivity; lack of self-confidence; low frustration tolerance; and fears of various kinds. All alcoholics and addicts do not, of course, show every one of these psychological problems, but they do occur with such frequency among addicted populations that clinicians should expect them and plan therapeutic activities that address them. The important point here, however, is not that alcoholics and addicts show a universal set of negative psychological sequelae of chronic drug intake. Rather, it is that psychological negative consequences may also enter into negative cycles that paradoxically maintain the patterns of heavy psychoactive substance use that gave rise to them. In effect, chronic heavy alcohol and other drug consumption is linked to events that eventuate in many psychological problems. The discomfort associated with these psychological problems leads to further drug-seeking behavior and consumption, which in turn leads to an intensification of personal difficulties. And so it goes.

The Social Dimension

Alcoholics and other drug addicts who continue to drink and use drugs must contend with mounting social problems as well as the intense discomfort of the physical and psychological negative outcomes discussed above. Usually the first thing to deteriorate is the complex web of intimate personal relationships that sustain and nurture healthy continued growth and functioning. The marriages of alcoholic and drug-addicted individuals typically become filled with pain, frustration, and anger turning into smoldering resentments, fear, shattered expectations, guilt, sorrow, bitterness, self-pity, depression, and pervasive feelings of hopelessness and helplessness. In the face of this intense emotional stress and discomfort that characterize the majority of addicted relationships, alcoholics and other addicts often feel that they have no other choice but to seek relief by continuing to use the substances that led to their marital problems in the first place. Addicted people as a further consequence of their drinking and drug use do not have well-developed skills for addressing relationship problems, resolving marital conflicts, and nurturing intimate relationships. In effect, they have overlearned the strategy of dealing with the pain of relationship problems by drinking and taking drugs. Moreover, the partners of addicted people also have overlearned maladaptive strategies for coping with relationship problems in marriage. Often obsessed with the need to control an uncontrollable situation, they develop patterns of reacting and responding to their partners' addictive behaviors and actions while intoxicated that usually make matters worse. The wives, husbands, and lovers of addicted people are not the only intimates caught up in the turmoil of addiction. The children of alcoholics and addicts also react to the stress, pain, conflict, and emotional upheaval of the alcoholic and drug-addicted marriage. These children may show many emotional and social problems of their own, including excessive fears, acting out at home and in the community, school and learning difficulties, fighting, delinquency, truancy, early sexual experimentation, lack of self-confidence, and drinking and drug use problems of their own (Wallace, 1987). These problems in parenting and child rearing usher further stress and disorder into a marital system that is already overwhelmed. Unfortunately, additional marital/family stress leads to further drinking and drug use and intensification of family dysfunction and maladaptive problem solution efforts. Obviously, family treatment of some form or another is a necessary part of primary treatment of addiction and occupies a central role in most modern treatment programs that utilize the steps and concepts of AA.

Marital/family difficulties are not the only negative consequences of drinking and drug use that maintain addictive behavior. Alcoholics and addicts show a host of other difficulties that may involve one or more of the following: employment and career troubles, legal and financial problems, disturbed friendships, arrests, incarcerations, community rejection and other forms of social stigma, decline in social status, role identity confusion, role ambiguity and ambivalence, and loss of social position. The pain and stress associated with these unhappy social outcomes usually result in further deterioration of the alcoholic and addict and further drinking and drug use. Obviously, without vigorous intervention and treatment services, this downward spiral into chronic alcoholism and drug addiction is not likely to be reversed. Although some alcoholics and addicts who have gone deeply into addiction have managed to turn their lives around without intervention and treatment, this does not appear to be the case for the majority of those unfortunate persons whose illnesses have become chronic.

The Spiritual Dimension

Spirituality is the fourth and final dimension in the biopsychosocialspiritual consequences/maintenance disease model. More will be said shortly about the focus on spirituality in 12-Step theory; however, mention must be made here of the impact of alcoholic drinking and drug addiction upon the spiritual life of a person. For many people, heavy drinking and drug use culminate in intense feelings of alienation, apartness, emptiness, meaninglessness, and lack of purpose in living. Moral values may have been compromised in the erratic acting out of intoxicated behaviors, urges, cognitions, and motivations. Knowledge about self and conviction about personal goals, objectives, and direction appear to become more and more uncertain and confused as addiction deepens. In a sense, alcoholics and addicts of other kinds seem to be ships without rudders cast adrift on turbulent seas. More than one alcoholic has described the terrible sense of inner emptiness and meaninglessness that characterized periods of active alcoholism. Despair is often the outcome of alcoholism and also the stimulus for further drinking. Nothing fills the inner void of alcoholics and addicts like alcohol and drugs do. Never mind that alcohol and drugs ushered in the desperation of spiritual emptiness, alienation, and suffering in the first place. Alcohol and drugs can quickly "fix" these painful states of being. The "fix," of course, is always temporary and usually followed by even greater spiritual distress, but active alcoholics and addicts do not care about delayed punishments. The immediate reinforcement of relief from painful states of being drives addicted people to continue to make choices not in their best interests.

THE PREDISPOSITION DISEASE MODELS

In contrast to the two consequences disease models discussed above, the "predisposition disease model" assumes that alcoholics and other drug-addicted people were set up for addiction by biological differences that preceded the onset of drinking or drug use. From this point of view, genetically transmitted biological risk factors predispose some individuals to addiction once exposure to alcohol and other substances has taken place. In actuality, there are several predisposition models and each of these shows variations. The first of these types of predisposition models could be called the genetic determination predisposition model. In this model, environment is considered irrelevant in determining alcoholism and drug addiction. These problems are considered to be determined entirely by genes. All that is required in a genetic determination model is the gene for a specific disorder. Alcoholism, for example, is thought to be the result of an "alcoholism gene." Cocaine dependence is associated with a gene for "cocainism." And heroin addiction is the consequence of a specific gene for this type of addiction. Recent research on genes for alcoholism and cocaine addiction is illustrative of the type of research generated by this model.

A second predisposition disease model is the "genetic influence disease model." This model makes no assumptions about genes for specific disorders and assumes that multiple biological risk factors interacting with psychosocial environmental factors determine addiction. In effect, neither genetics nor environment operating alone is sufficient to produce alcoholism or drug addiction; alcoholism and drug addiction require the joint presence of both biological and psychosocial environmental factors (Tarter & Edwards, 1986).

A third predisposition model is a "mixed genetic determination/influence model." In this model, different types of alcoholism and other types of addiction exist and different etiologic theories are necessary to explain each type. Cloninger's (1983) distinction between Type I and Type II alcoholism is an example of this approach. According to Cloninger, Type I alcoholism is explained by a genetic influence disease model as both genetic influence and environmental influence are necessary to produce the illness. Type II alcoholism, however, does not require the presence of environmental risk factors and is considered to be determined entirely by genetic factors operating independently of environment.

Predisposing biological risk factors that have been proposed include the following: defects in one or more neurotransmitter or neuromodulator systems, deficiencies in enzymes involved in neurotransmission, arousal system dysregulation, irregularities in cell membrane processes and structures, and abnormalities concerning various brain condensation products formed when alcohol is consumed (Wallace, 1989b).

THEORETICAL IMPLICATIONS
OF DISEASE MODELS FOR TREATMENT

Regardless of the specific disease model chosen, theorists who advocate the importance of biological factors in the origins and maintenance of addictive behaviors appear to show similarities in their approaches to applications in treatment. These similarities are discussed separately in the following sections.

Powerlessness

As the first step of AA asserts, an admission of one's powerlessness over alcohol or some other chemical must take place before progress can be expected. In 12-Step theory, the individual need not admit to being an alcoholic or drug addict or to being powerless in general. All that is required is an admission that one's use of psychoactive chemicals is no longer under one's personal control. The person's chemical use has become uncontrolled and/or the person's behavior while using chemicals has become uncontrolled. From this point of view, people who cannot consistently predict and control when, where, and how much they drink and drug and/or cannot guarantee their actions once they start to drink or use drugs are perceived as powerless over alcohol or some other chemical. As with other matters, theorists differ in how they approach the issue of loss of control and powerlessness. Some theorists take an all-or-none position and seem to imply that the loss of control is total and that the individual is not only powerless over alcohol or some other chemical but powerless over all aspects of his/her life. Other theorists seem to take a more moderate and balanced position and regard loss of control and powerlessness as matters of degree rather than absolutes. Impaired control and unpredictability of one's behavior once alcohol or drug use has begun are seen as critical. In other words, these more moderate theorists recognize that at various stages in the person's drinking history, considerable control over alcohol may have been evident and may, in fact, still be present. The key here, however, is that the person cannot exercise *consistent control* over chemical use and cannot consistently predict and control his/her behavior once chemical use has begun on any given occasion. Moreover, the reason that the individual has impaired control and cannot consistently control his/her drinking and/or behavior while drinking or using drugs is that the individual is suffering from a disease not unlike other diseases in which choice, will, and moral conviction do not, for the most part, make much difference.

Recognition, Identification, and Acceptance

Before an admission of powerlessness can be made, other changes in the cognitive system must be achieved. Typically, addicted people make tactical use of a variety of defenses that may prevent many of them from seeing even the most devastating negative consequences of alcohol and drug use. Denial, rationalization, minimization, and other forms of repressive defenses make it difficult for the addicted person to see his/her life clearly and to take steps to change. Many of these defenses probably have their roots in shame, guilt, remorse, fear, and strong motivation to continue drinking and drug use. Whatever their origins, these defenses must be overcome and awareness must take the place of the mindlessness and lack of clarity that result from heavy alcohol and other drug consumption. The person must recognize the many negative biopsychosocial consequences that drinking and drug use have caused in his/her life. As treatment progresses, the person is brought to see how many of his/her problems are directly attributable to the disease of alcoholism and/or other drug addiction. In the early stages of treatment and recovery, teaching of a disease concept of some form or another is helpful to the patient in managing otherwise overwhelming feelings of guilt, shame, anger, and remorse that may accompany the uncovering process as defenses fall away. *Identification* with others with similar problems of alcoholism and chemical dependency is useful to the patient and is encouraged. Identification with others also helps to reduce guilt, shame, anger, anxiety, and remorse. Moreover, it eases entry into supportive fellowships such as AA, where the many benefits of community can be made available to recovering people. Emotional support; a sense of belonging; a means to deal with loneliness, alienation, and isolation; shared problem solving; exposure to sober and clean role models; and enhanced motivation to avoid drug and alcohol use are but a few of the many benefits of identification with others who suffer from the same diseases. Finally, *acceptance* of some disease concept and all that it implies for one's future behaviors with regard to alcohol and other drugs is critical. It is not enough simply to know the elements of a disease concept—even a complicated, neurochemical concept—one must also apply the concept to self and accept fully its implications for self. Perhaps the most significant outcome of acceptance of a disease model is the decision to remain abstinent from alcohol and other drugs of addiction.

THE CENTRAL ROLE OF ABSTINENCE

All disease models of alcoholism and other drug addiction stress the central role of abstinence if recovery is to be achieved and maintained. Members of 12-Step programs such as AA reject controlled intoxification as a recovery goal for themselves for two simple but important reasons. First, although they personally tried many ways to control their drinking and behavior while drinking, virtually all report eventual failure. Second, virtually none of the members of AA and other 12-Step programs report firsthand knowledge of alcoholics and addicts in their home communities who have learned how to be successful at controlled intoxication. What members of 12-Step recovery programs see in their own communities are many attempts at controlled intoxication by others and eventual universal failure. Twelve-Step theorists report similar observations in both community and clinical contexts. Clinicians who work out of a 12-Step orientation report no success at sustained controlled intoxication among those patients they have treated and/or followed. Again, as with general community observations by laypeople, professionally trained clinicians see virtually no sustained, long-term controlled intoxification behaviors among alcoholics and other addicted populations. Moreover, some theorists sympathetic to 12-Step theory who have extensive research backgrounds have challenged the optimistic claims by certain controlled drinking researchers and enthusiasts as grossly exaggerated and incapable of standing up to rigorous scientific analyses (e.g., Wallace, 1990, 1993). Also, attempts to replicate or substantiate previous optimistic findings on controlled drinking have failed (Pendery, Maltzman, & West, 1982; Rychtarik, Foy, Scott, Lokey, & Prue, 1987), whereas new research on alcoholics has demonstrated stable moderate drinking to be a rare outcome among treated alcoholics (Helzer et al., 1985).

Despite the absence of lay ethnographic observations on successful sustained controlled intoxication by alcoholics and other addicts and despite the absence of a scientifically acceptable body of evidence in favor of controlled intoxication, some critics of 12-Step theory have continued to dismiss the insistence on abstinence and to urge instead the widespread adoption of controlled intoxication treatment goals (Peele, 1983; Searles, 1993). The position of these critics, who, for the most part, are psychologists, is difficult to comprehend because psychology as a rigorous scientific discipline insists on conclusions drawn from carefully conducted and methodologically sound studies. Furthermore, the issue of controlled intoxication treatment goals for alcoholics and addicts is not a trivial one. Because alcoholics who continue to drink are at sharply increased risk for many biopsychosocial consequences including death; disease; traumatic injury; legal, financial, marital, and employment difficulties; and psychological/psychiatric problems, advocacy of controlled intoxication treatment goals for alcoholics and addicts raises many professional and ethical questions, and especially so in the absence of a convincing body of scientific evidence in favor of such goals.

From a 12-Step theory perspective, little progress can be expected in treatment and recovery if alcoholics and addicts continue to attempt to drink alcohol and use unauthorized drugs. There are several reasons why this is the case. First, the pharmacologic actions of drugs such as alcohol and cocaine increase the likelihood of compulsive use rather than decrease such use in addicted people. Changes in brain chemistry with continued use probably serve as important internal cues for compulsive use. Also, alcoholics and other addicts often appear to possess poor impulse control, low frustration tolerance, weakly controlled anger, impatience, and various cognitive impairments (Tarter, Alterman, & Edwards, 1987). Because alcohol and certain other drugs appear to exacerbate these difficulties, it seems most appropriate for alcoholics and addicts to avoid these chemicals altogether. In order to stay clean and sober, addicts and alcoholics need all their wits about them, not less. Second, the continued use of psychoactive substances keeps addicted people caught in the mind-set of solving problems with chemicals rather than through searching for personal, emotional, cognitive, interpersonal, and spiritual growth and development. And as alcohol and other drugs trigger urges and cognitions about continued use, alcoholics and addicts who attempt to drink and use with control seem to end up even more obsessed with the substances. In many cases, even those small numbers of alcoholics who managed through incredible effort to achieve some controlled drinking gave it up in favor of abstinence because of the reported misery and unhappiness of being continually obsessed with the "next drink" and the enormous amount of work required in holding their drinking down to a set quota of a few drinks a day.

Not only do attempts to drink and use drugs keep alcoholics and addicts caught up in chemical solutions to problems of living, they separate addicted people from clean and sober friends and 12-Step fellowship programs. It is difficult to feel a part of AA if your brain is thoroughly soaked in marijuana and you are sitting in a roomful of clean and sober people rejoicing in their sobriety. In contrast to 12-Step fellowship programs, there has been no enduring support group devoted to the pursuit of moderate intoxication for alcoholics, moderate cocaine use for cocaine addicts, moderate cigarette smoking for nicotine addicts, and so forth. Although there have been attempts to establish some of these, none has yet been proven to stand the test of time as have AA, Narcotics Anonymous, and other abstinence-oriented programs.

SPIRITUALITY AND THE PROBLEM OF POWERLESSNESS

Once addicted people have admitted their powerlessness over alcohol and/or other drugs, they find themselves faced with a new dilemma. If they cannot personally control their behavior with regard to these chemicals, who will do it for them? The 12-Step answer to this dilemma is at first blush disarmingly simple, but it is far more complicated on further analysis. According to the second and third steps of AA, addicted people are urged to believe in and turn their will and their lives over to a power greater than themselves. This emphasis on spirituality has been a boon to many and a stumbling block to others. Some critics have seized upon the similarities between AA and religion and have rejected the AA claim that it is a spiritual program and not a religious one. This emphasis by critics on similarities, however, ignores the many differences between AA and organized religions. An orange is round and so is the world, but an orange is not the world. Similarities do not prove identities. Of course, the literature of AA and the talk of some of its members contain double messages and ambiguities that encourage misperception. But, in the final analysis, despite similarities and double messages, AA and its offspring 12-Step theory cannot be considered to constitute religions. The steps of AA, for example, are not requirements but suggestions for recovery and, as such, cannot constitute dogma. Although it does have a founder in the person of Bill Wilson, AA has no central religious figure or leader who is worshipped and adored, as do Christianity, Buddhism, Hinduism, and Judaism.

In approaching the distinction between religion and spirituality, the thoughts of the transpersonal psychologist Ken Wilber (1993) may prove helpful. Wilber draws a distinction between what he terms "exoteric" religions and a form of spirituality he terms "esoteric." In Wilber's words:

> Exoteric or "outer" religion is mythic religion, religion that is terribly concrete and literal, that really believes, for example, that Moses parted the Red Sea, that Christ was born from a virgin, that the world was created in six days, that manna once literally rained down from heaven, and so on. Exoteric religions the world over consist of those type of beliefs. The Hindus believe that the earth, since it needs to be supported, is sitting on an elephant which since it needs to be supported, is sitting on a tortoise which in turn is sitting on a serpent. . . . Lao Tzu was nine hundred years old when he was born, Krishna made love to four thousand cow maidens, Brahma was born from a crack in a cosmic egg, and so on. That's exoteric religion, a series of belief structures that attempt to explain the mysteries of the world in mythic terms rather than direct experiential or evidential terms. . . . Esoteric spirituality, on the other hand, is "inner or hidden." The reason that esoteric . . . is hidden is not that it is secret or anything, but that it is a matter of direct experience and personal awareness. Esoteric (spirituality) asks that you believe nothing on faith, or obediently swallow any dogma. Rather, esoteric (spirituality) is a set of personal experiments that you conduct scientifically in the laboratory of your own awareness. Like all good science, it is based on direct experience, not mere belief or wish, and it is publicly checked or validated by a peer group of those who have also performed the experiment. (p. 176)

In a very real sense, 12-Step theory embraces a point of view that closely approximates Wilber's esoteric mysticism. Members of AA perform an experiment (in this case, the experiment is to try to follow the suggested 12 steps of the program) and then observe over time through direct experience the consequences of having done so. But what of this notion of a power greater than self in which one may believe and to whom one gives one's will and one's life? How may the concept of a higher power be approached without resorting to conventional religiosity? Twelve-Step fellowship programs neatly dodge thorny problems here simply by defining the AA group as a power greater than self. There is a certain cunning in this position because the problem is not that addicted people need to find a conventional god but that they need to give another approach a try. In AA terms, they need to "get out of the driver's seat." Left to their own devices, many addicted people fail again and again but still keep returning to the belief in their own willpower as the means to conquer their addictions. By turning over their will and their lives to others at the beginning of their recoveries, addicted people become open to new cognitions, alternative behavioral strategies for dealing with their problems, and fresh approaches to dealing with their chemical addictions.

While the group as a power greater than self can serve many addicted people well in the beginning stages of recovery, it is also useful in 12-Step theory to introduce patients to other ways of construing a "God of their own understanding." Some people, of course, do enter recovery programs with well-developed religious convictions and prefer to continue with these. Others, however, have virtually no understanding of how to proceed in these matters or are openly hostile to anything that even remotely resembles religiosity. Resistance to spirituality may constitute a reasoned intellectual position or may flow directly from highly negative childhood experiences with organized religions. In either case, addicted people may benefit from consideration of alternative ways of construing these matters. As the theologian Paul Tillich (1952) asserted, God is a person's ultimate concern in life. From this perspective, almost anything can become a god or higher power. People have made gods of money, sexuality, fame, prestige, social position, and so forth. In the case of addicted people, alcohol and drugs often achieve this power of ultimate concerns and, as such, take precedence over all other aspects of the addict's life. Marriage, family, friendships, jobs, careers, health, and well-being often take a backseat to the addict's drive to seek out his/her drug of choice and "get high." In effect, drugs and alcohol become powers greater than self, directing forces that drive all aspects of the addict's feelings, cognitions, and behaviors. In a real sense, the addict's problem is not to find a higher power, because he/she already has one. The trick is for the addict to switch from a destructive higher power to a constructive and beneficial one. As sobriety lengthens, the person may consider nondeistic directing forces for his/her life other than the recovery group. Examples of these higher powers are love, knowledge, creativity, and justice. Ordering one's life and seeking direction in terms of abstract principles rather than concrete religious figures is one way to develop a nondeistic spirituality for oneself. This is not without historical precedent. Many great men and women in history found comfort, strength, and direction in principles rather than in the mythic structures of exoteric religions. And for many alcoholics and addicts, a strong, even passionate commitment to some power or principle greater than self seems necessary if the powerful allure of psychoactive chemicals and the addict life-style is to be overcome.

In the final analysis, the 12-Step theory emphasis on turning one's will and life over to the care of a power greater than self is an attempt to deal with the grandiosity, extreme self-centeredness, egotistical concerns, inability to delay gratification, faulty decision-making processes, and urgent needs of many active alcoholics and addicts. "Do it my way," "Me first!," "I'm right and you're wrong," "Look at it from my point of view," and "I want it and I want it right now!" could very well be the theme songs of many active alcoholics and addicts. Spiritual growth and development as defined above are means to overcome extreme self-centeredness and to achieve significant and necessary changes in the structure of the self and in one's way of being in the world.

AWARENESS, SELF-EXAMINATION, AND SELF-CRITICISM

Because of the alcoholic's and addict's use of repressive defenses and general mindlessness when drinking and using drugs, 12-Step theory emphasizes the importance of achieving and utilizing knowledge about self. In 12-Step fellowship programs, the writing of a personal inventory and then sharing this inventory with at least one other person is one means through which personal shortcomings as well as strengths can be realized. In 12-Step treatment programs, the strong emphasis on group therapy and individual counseling is devoted to the same end. Although 12-Step-oriented therapists differ in counseling techniques and theoretical orientations, most seem to work toward increasing the patient's awareness of his/her motivations; typical ways of dealing with stress, anger, rejection, and fears; and the consequences of an active alcoholic or addict lifestyle. Awareness of one's feelings and the need to share these feelings in a safe, supportive, and caring interpersonal context are stressed.

Twelve-Step therapists also stress awareness of emotional states, attitudes, and actions that may signal the beginning of an active relapse process. According to many 12-Step theorists, the alcoholic or addict is never completely "fixed." Individuals are encouraged to think of themselves as always in recovery and never as recovered. Some theorists, however, reject this point of view and argue that addicted people can recover completely from addictive disease, as do persons with illnesses of other types. Whatever the theorist's position on this issue of "recovering" versus "recovered," virtually all theorists and clinicians stress the importance of continued self-scrutiny and self-examination in avoiding relapse.

Along with continued self-scrutiny, individuals are encouraged to engage in self-criticism as well. Several steps of the AA fellowship program speak directly to these matters. It is suggested to members that they make a list of all the people they harmed during their period of active addiction and wherever possible, make amends to them. Making amends is thought to have several desirable outcomes. First, making amends for past wrongdoing toward others enables the alcoholic or addict to deal with excessive guilt, remorse, and continued fear over past actions. Second, it often results in mending relationships that were once broken by active alcoholism and drug addiction. In many cases, these mended relationships are ones critically important to the alcoholic's and addict's sense of community and self-esteem. Third, making amends permits the addicted person to see his/her past alcoholic and addicted behaviors clearly and for what they were by reducing the need for continued use of repressive defenses such as denial, minimization, and rationalization. In addition to the amends steps, persons in the AA fellowship program are urged to continue to take their personal inventories on a daily basis and when wrong to promptly admit it and take the necessary actions to correct the situation. This approach encourages the addicted person to own his/her actions and to take responsibility. Openness to self-criticism on a daily basis also reduces the addict's need to continue to use repressive defenses with regard to his/her behavior.

In a very real sense, the Buddhist concept of mindfulness characterizes the necessary passage of addicted people from states of blind acting out, lack of insight, and poor self-knowledge to the states of heightened awareness and joyful consciousness that are considered the hallmarks of ideal recoveries. Buddhists and others committed to spiritual growth and development utilize the tools of meditation, prayer, and other rituals to achieve mindfulness. In the fellowship of AA and in some formal 12-Step treatment programs, these tools encouraged as well.

PERSONAL RESPONSIBILITY,
POWERLESSNESS, AND HELPLESSNESS

It is sometimes argued that encouraging people to view their addictions as diseases takes away their sense of personal responsibility. From this point of view, alcoholics and addicts will simply continue to drink and use drugs while claiming that they have a disease and cannot help themselves. Twelve-Step theory neither endorses shirking of personal responsibility for one's addiction nor sees such shirking of responsibility as a necessary outcome of the teaching of disease models of addiction. The usual position taken on this matter by 12-Step theorists and clinicians is that because of genetic and other biological etiological factors, addicted people are not responsible for having developed an addictive disease, but they most certainly are responsible for dealing with the illness once they know they have it. Indeed, rather than encouraging addicted people to disclaim responsibility, 12-Step theory advocates a thoroughgoing sense of responsibility, not only for addictive behaviors but for all aspects of one's conduct in the world. In 12-Step approaches, people are held responsible generally for their actions and are not permitted to "cop out" by blaming their illness or, for that matter, anything else. Part of the misperception here stems from confusion of the concepts of powerlessness and helplessness. In 12-Step theory, addicted people are indeed encouraged to view themselves as powerless over their drug of choice, but they are not encouraged to perceive themselves as powerless in general. Because addicted people are powerless over a chemical does not mean that they are helpless. If one is an addicted person, many actions can be taken to help oneself. The addicted person may not be able to choose when to stop using cocaine in the middle of a cocaine run, but he/she is certainly able to choose to attend a treatment program or a Cocaine Anonymous group when not in the middle of a run. Addicted people can choose to become actively involved in their therapy groups if in treatment, or actively involved in their 12-Step fellowship groups if in one of these programs. Once clean and sober, addicted people can exercise choices about all aspects of their life, including jobs, relationships, marriages, parenting, investing, and so forth. In early stages of recovery, however, such choices are better made in consultation with professionals and, when appropriate, with sponsors in fellowship programs. As recovery progresses, the ideal outcome is a self-governing person with the ability to make choices that are in his/her best interests.

MENTAL ILLNESS AND 12-STEP THEORY

There is no conflict between psychiatric and 12-Step theories with regard to so-called dual diagnoses. It is well recognized and accepted by the majority of 12-Step theorists that some alcoholics and addicts may suffer from certain mental and emotional illnesses. These illnesses must be diagnosed and treated accordingly. In many cases, treatment will of necessity include use of antipsychotic and/or antidepressant medications. Twelve-Step theorists, however, do object to the overprescribing of psychoactive medications that can accompany poorly informed psychiatric treatment of alcoholics and addicts in early stages of recovery. As research has shown (e.g., Brown et al., 1991; Brown & Schuckit, 1988), most of the psychiatric symptoms seen in the first days and weeks of primary treatment are the outcome of alcohol and other drug use and do not constitute the bases for formal diagnoses of primary psychiatric disorders. Symptoms of depression and anxiety commonly seen in many alcoholics in the beginning of treatment usually resolve without psychoactive medication within 3 weeks of primary treatment in a supportive and caring environment.

On the other hand, 12-Step theorists stress the need for routine psychological assessments, psychiatric screenings, and intensive work-ups in individual cases when symptoms do not resolve and primary psychiatric disorders are suspected. Failure to treat an accompanying depressive disorder in an alcoholic is as serious a blunder as treating with antidepressant medications in the absence of a primary affective disorder.

In the past, 12-Step theorists were often in conflict with poorly informed and improperly trained psychiatrists who perceived alcoholism and drug addiction as symptoms of underlying psychiatric illness and who often produced secondary addictions by treating alcoholics inappropriately with benzodiazepines and other antianxiety agents with addiction potential. These conflicts, however, have been reduced considerably as more and better training in the addictions has been made available to psychiatrists and other medical personnel and as accurate information about addictive disease has become more widely available.

PRIORITY SETTING AND TIME BINDING

Most 12-Step theorists agree that the therapeutic change process should be an orderly one and should consist of clear priority setting activities. Newcomers to AA, for example, are often advised to deal with "first things first." This phrase is usually taken to mean that in the early stages of recovery, attempts to deal with issues other than those directly involved with drinking or drug use should be delayed until a stable base of sobriety has been achieved. It is not that 12-Step theorists and clinicians believe that other issues are unimportant and should be avoided permanently. It is more a question of *when* certain things get addressed and not a question of whether to address them at all. In the absence of sobriety, the problems of the vast majority of chemically dependent people do not improve

despite attempts at problem solving. As we have already noted, drinking
and drug use have important multiple impacts upon individuals, including
negative effects on the brain and cognitive processes involved with reasoning, judgment, problem solving, and decision making. As these cognitive deficits have been shown to improve as sobriety lengthens, it makes
very good sense to delay addressing complex problems for a time. Of
course, with regard to some problems, delay may not be possible and
issues other than drinking and drug use must be dealt with from the outset
of treatment. A primary affective disorder, for example, must be dealt with
early in recovery. Family issues also must be dealt with early in recovery.
However, in treating families, the same concern with priority setting
applies. Clinicians working from a 12-Step perspective generally endorse
more structured family therapy approaches with more modest initial
recovery goals and objectives in the beginning of treatment.

Throughout recovery, then, the phrase "First things first" serves as a
reminder that problem solving should proceed in an orderly fashion
moving from primary concerns to more secondary matters as treatment
proceeds. In a sense, this approach to problem solving encourages the
person to go at his/her problems in manageable units rather than flying
off in all directions at once. The phrase "Easy does it" is intended to
accomplish the same goal by slowing down the tempo of problem-solving
attempts and, hence, restricting the numbers of personal problems that
can be addressed at any one time. "Easy does it" also cautions the
alcoholic and addict to avoid a high-intensity, emotionally charged approach in which problems must be solved and solved now. Because most
problems in the real world often require considerable amounts of time to
solve and usually involve frustration and delay of gratification, problem-
solving styles characterized by impatience, impulsiveness, and inability to
delay gratification are not optimal for addicted people and are probably
associated with relapse.

Perhaps one of the more ingenious ideas to come out of 12-Step
theory is the simple but important concept of *time binding*. Newcomers
to AA and 12-Step-oriented treatment programs are constantly urged to
take life "24 hours at a time" because alcoholics and addicts seem to have
more difficulty than others in maintaining a here-and-now perspective.
Many chemically dependent people make themselves miserable by living
in the past or projecting into the future. A focus on the past can keep the
alcoholic stuck in the painful stuff of regret, guilt, and remorse over actions
and events that occurred while drinking. On the other hand, an obsessive
preoccupation with the future stirs anxiety, fear, and dread over events
that may or may not take place. By placing one's consciousness in the
reality of each day as it unfolds, addicted people can learn to avoid the

painful emotional triggers that are often associated with relapse. In effect, addicted people need to learn how to learn from their histories and not wallow in events they can no longer do anything about. And they need to learn how to plan for the future without projecting themselves into a future that may or may not unfold. In both cases, they need to learn to live in the reality of the here and now. Time binding is an important theoretical idea in helping them to do so.

CHANGE, ACCEPTANCE, AND GRATITUDE

The serenity prayer so popular in the fellowship of AA asks God to grant "the serenity to accept the things I cannot change, the courage to change the things I can, and the wisdom to know the difference." Curiously, most of the discussion in AA, however, seems to center around the need for acceptance and seldom on the courage to change. Perhaps this is because alcoholics and addicts perceive themselves and each other as having had major difficulties with acceptance in the past and now need to concentrate on that aspect of their development. In 12-Step theory, however, change is viewed as at least as important as acceptance for a stable, enduring, and fulfilling recovery. In many cases, alcoholics or addicts may make themselves miserable by persisting in attempts to accept some situations or problems that are, in fact, not in their best interests or even completely unacceptable. Difficult and destructive marriages and other intimate relationships that should be changed but are "accepted" are prime examples of situations that alcoholics and addicts in recovery often seem to be willing to put up with rather than address directly. Demeaning, unfulfilling, and boring jobs performed under the direction of impossible bosses in sick organizations are another situation in which recovering alcoholics and addicts find themselves stuck and miserable. Unfortunately, many alcoholics and addicts will choose relapse as a way of getting out of these difficult situations. By getting thrown out for being intoxicated, they allow alcohol and other drugs to make the decisions for them. Clearly, much more work needs to be done in 12-Step-oriented contexts on how addicted people can develop the attitudes and skills necessary for bringing about necessary and beneficial changes in their lives.

In general, however, change is an important ingredient of 12-Step theory and clinical practice. Treatment from this perspective is all about change—change in cognitions about self and others, change in the way problems are construed and solved, change in the way emotions are experienced and dealt with, and change in troublesome, difficult situations that reduce the quality of life in recovery or even increase the likelihood of relapse. If a person completes primary treatment and has changed nothing other than some verbal behavior concerning his/her intentions with regard to drinking or drug use, a continued stable and enduring recovery is not likely.

But despite all that has been said about the importance of change, acceptance is also critical. While actively drinking and using drugs, addicted people as a rule did not learn how to accept things very well. Disappointments were drowned in alcohol. Loss of a promotion or a job meant time to get drunk or high. Illness, death of a loved one, divorce, financial losses, or other major life reversals were not accepted but used as excuses for becoming intoxicated. Even the petty irritations of everyday life led to drinking and/or drug use. Hence, while 12-Step theory does stress the importance of changing those things that can and must be changed, it also emphasizes the need for addicted people to learn the skills and attitudes that comprise acceptance. As the saying in AA goes, sometimes alcoholics need to learn how to "sit still and hurt." That is, sit still and hurt without drinking or resorting to drug use.

Perhaps the single most crucial attitude that addicted people can learn is an "attitude of gratitude." The pessimism, cynicism, and chronic dissatisfaction that characterize active alcoholics and drug addicts and appear to drive the continuance of their addictions must yield to a degree of optimism, trust, and sense of fulfillment. By helping recovering alcoholics and addicts to see and appreciate the value of what they do have rather than complaining bitterly about what they do not have, 12-Step-oriented clinicians can encourage the development of cognitive structures in their patients that support decisions to remain abstinent and seek fulfillment in activities that do not involve the use of alcohol and drugs.

REFERENCES

Alcoholics Anonymous. (1976). *Alcoholics Anonymous.* New York: Alcoholics Anonymous World Services.

Brown, S. A., Irwin, M., & Schuckit, M. A. (1991). Changes in anxiety among abstinent male alcoholics. *Journal of Studies on Alcohol, 52,* 55–61.

Brown, S. A., & Schuckit, M. A. (1988). Changes in depression among abstinent alcoholics. *Journal of Studies on Alcohol, 49,* 412–417.

Cloninger, C. R. (1983). Genetic and environmental factors in the development of alcoholism. *Journal of Psychiatric Treatment and Evaluation, 5,* 487–496.

Dackis, C. A., & Gold, M. S. (1985). Bromocriptine as a treatment of cocaine abuse. *Lancet, 1,* 1151–1152.

Goldstein, D. B. (1983). *Pharmacology of alcohol.* New York: Oxford University Press.

Helzer, J. E., Robins, L. N., Taylor, J. R., Carey, K., Miller, R. H., Combs-Orme, T., & Farmer, A. (1985). The extent of long-term moderate drinking among alcoholics discharged from medical and psychiatric treatment facilities. *New England Journal of Medicine, 312,* 1678–1682.

Hunt, W. A. (1985). *Alcohol and biological membranes.* New York: Guilford Press.

Peele, S. (1985, January–February). Change without pain. *American Health,* pp. 36–39.

Peele, S. (1983, April). Through a glass darkly: Can some alcoholics learn to drink in moderation? *Psychology Today,* pp. 38–42.

Peele, S. (1988). Can alcoholism and other drug addiction problems be treated away or is the current treatment binge doing more harm than good? *Journal of Psychoactive Drugs, 20,* 375–383.

Peele, S. (1989). *Diseasing of America—Addiction treatment out of control.* Lexington, MA: Lexington Books.

Peele, S. (1990). Why and by whom the American alcoholism treatment industry is under siege. *Journal of Psychoactive Drugs, 22,* 1–13.

Pendery, M. L., Maltzman, I. M., & West, L. J. (1982). Controlled drinking by alcoholics? New findings and a reevaluation of a major affirmative study. *Science, 217,* 169–175.

Rychtarik, R. G., Foy, D. W., Scott, T., Lokey, L., & Prue, D. M. (1987). Five-to-six-year follow-up of broad-spectrum behavioral treatment for alcoholism: Effects of training controlled drinking skills. *Journal of Consulting and Clinical Psychology, 55,* 106–108.

Searles, J. S. (1993). Science and fascism: Confronting unpopular ideas. *Addictive Behaviors, 18,* 5–8.

Tabakoff, B., Hoffman, P. L., Lee, J. M., Saito, T., Willard, B., & Deleon-Jones, F. (1988). Differences in platelet enzyme activity between alcoholics and non-alcoholics. *New England Journal of Medicine, 313,* 134–139.

Tarter, R. E., Alterman, A. I., & Edwards, K. L. (1987). Neurobehavioral theory of alcoholism etiology. In C. Chaudron & D. Wilkinson (Eds.), *Theories of alcoholism* (pp. 73–102). Toronto: Addiction Research Foundation.

Tarter, R. E., & Edwards, K. L. (1986). Antecedents to alcoholism: Implications for prevention and treatment. *Behavior Therapy, 17,* 346–361.

Tarter, R. E., & Van Thiel, D. H. (Eds.). (1985). *Alcohol and the brain: Chronic effects.* New York: Plenum Press.

Tillich, P. (1952). *The courage to be.* New Haven, CT: Yale University Press.

Wallace, J. (1985). Predicting the onset of compulsive drinking in alcoholics: A biopsychosocial model. *Alcohol: An International Biomedical Journal, 2,* 589–595.

Wallace, J. (1987). Children of alcoholics: A population at risk. *Alcoholism Treatment Quarterly, 43,* 13–30.

Wallace, J. (1989a). Ideology, belief, and behavior: Alcoholics Anonymous as a social movement. In *Writings: The alcoholism papers of John Wallace* (pp. 335–352). Newport, RI: Edgehill.

Wallace, J. (1989b). The relevance to clinical care of recent research in neurobiology. In *Writings: The alcoholism papers of John Wallace* (pp. 85–207). Newport, RI: Edgehill.

Wallace, J. (1989c). A biopsychosocial model of alcoholism. *Social Casework: The Journal of Contemporary Social Work, 325–332.*

Wallace, J. (1990). Controlled drinking, treatment effectiveness, and the disease model of addiction: A commentary on the ideological wishes of Stanton Peele. *Journal of Psychoactive Drugs, 22,* 261–280.

Wallace, J. (1993). Fascism and the eye of the beholder: A reply to J. S. Searles on the controlled intoxication issue. *Addictive Behaviors, 18,* 239–251.

Wilson, B. (1953). *Twelve steps and twelve traditions.* New York: Alcoholics Anonymous World Services.

Wilber, K. (1993). *Grace and grit: Spirituality and healing in the life and death of Treya Killam Wilber.* Boston: Shambhala.

CHAPTER 2

Facilitating 12-Step Recovery from Substance Abuse and Addiction

JOSEPH NOWINSKI

This chapter presents a model for facilitating early recovery from alcohol or drug abuse or addiction. It is designed for use by practitioners who do not necessarily have a great deal of prior knowledge of 12-Step fellowships such as Alcoholics Anonymous (AA) or Narcotics Anonymous (NA) but who wish to actively facilitate their patients' use of such programs as a means of not drinking or using drugs. Patients need not be dependent on either alcohol or drugs in order to benefit from the model presented here. Rather, they need merely meet the primary criterion for being a member of AA (or NA), namely, a desire to stop drinking (or using drugs). (Alcoholics Anonymous, 1952, p. 139). However, the reader should be aware that these fellowships have as their overall goal abstinence from (as opposed to controlled use of) alcohol or drugs. By definition these fellowships were founded and exist for the benefit of those who have failed to control their use of alcohol and/or drugs. (Alcoholics Anonymous, 1976, pp. 21, 24, 30–31).

GOALS

Twelve-Step facilitation (TSF; Nowinski & Baker, 1992; Nowinski, Baker, & Carroll, 1992) is directed at what could be termed the "early" stage of recovery from alcohol or drug dependence. By early recovery we generally mean that process in which an individual moves from problem or compulsive use of alcohol or drugs toward abstinence. This process is typically marked by ambivalent motivation as well as any number of "slips" (actual use) and urges to use alcohol or drugs. TSF is intended to be a time-limited (12-to-15-session) intervention. It is a relatively structured intervention that focuses on a core of four objectives. Also included are a brief conjoint program for patients who are in a relationship and an elective program consisting of recovery-related topics that may be covered depending on the individual patient's progress in the core program. Sessions, with the exception of the initial (assessment) session, typically last 1 hour and follow a predetermined format. The model utilizes a range of interventions including education, confrontation, assigned readings, journaling, and behavioral assignments.

Early recovery can be broken down very broadly into two phases: acceptance and surrender. Acceptance refers to the process in which the individual overcomes "denial" or the belief that he/she can either control drinking or drug use or achieve sustained abstinence through sheer willpower. Another way to think of acceptance is that it represents an insight on the part of the patient that he/she has lost control. In the context of TSF, acceptance is marked by realization on the part of the patient that his/her life is becoming progressively more unmanageable as a result of alcohol or drug use and that willpower alone has not been a sufficient force to lead to lasting sobriety and a manageable life. Therefore, the only viable alternative to continued chaos and personal failure is to place one's faith in a "higher power" and to accept the need for abstinence.

AA and NA are programs of action, however, as much as they are programs of insight or spirituality. Surrender follows acceptance and represents the individual's commitment to making whatever changes in lifestyle are necessary in order to sustain recovery. Surrender requires action, including frequent attendance at AA and/or NA, being active in meetings, reading AA/NA literature, getting a sponsor, making AA/NA friends, and giving up people, places, and things that might represent a threat to recovery. In TSF the action and commitment that are the hallmarks of surrender are guided to some extent by the facilitator but also by those individuals the patient encounters and begins to form relationships with within 12-Step fellowships. To use AA jargon, if acceptance means "talking the talk," surrender means "walking the walk."

Involvement in 12-Step fellowships will inevitably expose both the patient and the therapist to a number of key (and possibly foreign) concepts, such as the spiritual concept of a "higher power" (Alcoholics Anonymous, 1976, p. 50), the advocacy of fellowship over professionalism (Alcoholics Anonymous, 1952, p. 166), and the concepts of group conscience and spiritual awakening (Alcoholics Anonymous, 1952, pp. 106, 132). Because these concepts are so central to 12-Step fellowships and their philosophy of recovery, the practitioner must not only be familiar with them but also prepared to discuss these concepts and their implications for action.

PRINCIPLES

It should be evident by now that TSF as a model of intervention seeks to be both philosophically and pragmatically compatible with the 12 steps of AA. Accordingly, TSF is based on certain principles, which follow from the 12 traditions of AA and which should be understood if the intervention is to achieve this desired compatibility. Potential facilitators might do well to reflect on these principles and to "work through" their reactions to them (if any) prior to embarking on an intervention.

Locus of Change

Perhaps more so than other therapies, TSF regards the agent of change with respect to patients' behavior as lying less in the therapist than in the fellowships of AA and NA. Therein lies the main reason why we prefer the word "facilitation" to "therapy" or "treatment." The facilitator is obviously a highly skilled professional who must possess not only good psychotherapy skills but also a working knowledge of 12-Step fellowships. The facilitator must also be able to resist *becoming* a patient's recovery program, as opposed to AA and/or NA becoming that program. In order to do this the facilitator must develop considerable skill in knowing when to provide advice and support personally and when to encourage the patient to seek these things through fellowship. As skilled as the facilitator may be, he/she must accept the idea that recovery is not dependent primarily on skills acquired through therapy but on active fellowship with other recovering persons. Such a therapeutic stance places the responsibility for recovery squarely on the shoulders of the patient and defines the facilitator–patient role as one of collaboration.

Motivation

AA has from its inception characterized itself as "based on attraction rather than promotion" (Alcoholics Anonymous, 1952, p. 180). This means that AA should never seek to attract members through advertising or promotion of any kind. Rather, AA's growth principle was based on the notions of identification and attraction. It was assumed that if an alcoholic attended meetings, listened to the stories of others, and identified with them, sooner or later he/she might be motivated to try the program laid out in the 12 steps. Although alcohol treatment, and even AA attendance, is frequently mandated today, in reality this approach is not consistent with the spirit of fellowship.

The philosophy of attraction implies that 12-Step fellowships may not in fact be the ticket to recovery for everyone. This philosophy also has definite implications for the 12-Step facilitator, who does best to take a low-key approach and emphasize basic ideas such as "giving it a try" and "keeping an open mind" when trying to motivate patients to become active in AA or NA. The effectiveness of coercive approaches to get patients to attend meetings and give up alcohol or drugs has not been thoroughly tested. Although some have argued cogently that most people who seek help are pressured to do so in some way or another (Anderson, 1981), it remains my conviction that involvement in AA or NA is more effectively accomplished through a shaping approach emphasizing positive reinforcement and progressive approximations than by coercion (e.g., threats of punishment), and that in any case a "shaping" approach is more consistent with the traditions of AA.

Spirituality

One aspect of 12-Step recovery that clearly separates it from other models of intervention is its active promotion of spirituality. The guiding books of AA—*Alcoholics Anonymous* (1976) and *Twelve Steps and Twelve Traditions* (1952)—are replete with references to the importance of spirituality to recovery. Here are some examples:

> We have learned that whatever the human frailties of various faiths, those faiths have given purpose and direction to millions. People of faith have a logical idea of what life is all about. Actually, we used to have no reasonable conception whatever. (Alcoholics Anonymous, 1976, p. 49)

> On one proposition, however, these men and women [alcoholics] are strikingly agreed. Every one of them has gained access to, and believes in, a Power greater than himself. (Alcoholics Anonymous, 1976, p. 50)

> ... as a result of practicing all the Steps, we have each found something called a spiritual awakening. (Alcoholics Anonymous, 1976, p. 106).

When conducting TSF the clinician should be prepared to discuss the issue of spirituality. At several different points in treatment (Nowinski &

Baker, 1992, pp. 73–81; Nowinski et al., 1992, pp. 2, 4, 47–48) the facilitator is asked to engage the patient in a specific discussion of his/her spiritual beliefs. Guidelines are provided for these discussions, which generally focus around the issues of willpower, powerlessness, and faith.

Pragmatism

Interestingly, although many people think of AA as a deeply spiritual program, pragmatism appears to be as much a part of AA tradition as is spirituality. One official AA publication, *Living Sober* (Alcoholics Anonymous, 1975), is subtitled *Some Methods AA Members Have Used for Not Drinking*. It contains a wealth of practical advice for avoiding taking "the first drink." Consider the following sampling from its table of contents:

Using the 24-hour plan
Changing old routines
Making use of "telephone therapy"
Getting plenty of rest
Fending off loneliness
Letting go of old ideas

In TSF the facilitator attempts to educate the patient with respect to some practical methods for staying sober. The facilitator consistently admonishes the patient to focus on "one day at a time" (another very pragmatic approach) and encourages the patient to solicit and follow practical advice from fellow AA members on how to deal with difficult situations, craving, and so on. Of course, the most basic practical advice given to all alcoholics and addicts is simple: Do not drink (or use) and go to meetings. Finally, each facilitation session ends with the facilitator assigning one or more *recovery tasks,* which are specific suggestions for reading and action. In this way the facilitation program mirrors the pragmatism of AA itself.

Constructive Confrontation

In setting a tone for intervention, the 12-Step facilitator takes an approach that could be described as collaborative. He/she attempts consistently to engage the patient in a constructive collaboration. Confrontation is common but does not take the form of threat. For example, the 12-Step facilitator will never terminate treatment simply because a patient drinks between sessions (or even shows up intoxicated).[1] On the other hand, the facilitator will consistently confront the patient about drinking and its connection to denial, acceptance, or surrender. The facilitator, committed to the idea that "90 meetings in 90 days" is the best strategy for the person in early recovery, will continue to ask for and encourage frequent attendance at meetings. The facilitator will "interpret" denial and talk frankly about "slips." However, the facilitator also accepts addiction as a "cunning and clever" illness and relapse (at least temporarily) as the rule rather than the exception. Again, the 12-Step facilitator seeks to be a shaper of behavior (sobriety) more than a mere monitor of it.

Focus

The focus of TSF is on helping the patient *begin* the process of recovery. Although collateral issues may be (and frequently are) raised by patients in the course of treatment, facilitators are advised to avoid "drift" (i.e., a loss of focus on drinking or drug use and on becoming active in AA or NA, in favor of some other issue). Facilitators make every effort to validate patients' legitimate concerns, for example, about work, marriage, or family issues. They also are alert for patients' use of collateral issues as a means of avoiding either the subject of alcohol or drug use or the facilitator's expectations of them. Although concurrent therapies may be necessary at times (e.g., for the acutely depressed patient), in general the TSF model advocates prioritizing problems, with early recovery at the top of the list.

OBJECTIVES

The primary goals of early recovery, namely, acceptance and surrender, are achieved not only through dialogue with the facilitator but also through action on the part of the patient. Toward this end, TSF seeks to achieve a number of specific objectives which can be broken down broadly into two categories: active involvement and identification.

Active Involvement

To be sure, active involvement in 12-Step fellowships such as AA and NA means going to meetings. Merely attending meetings, on the other hand, does not qualify as active involvement. Very often practitioners who are unfamiliar with the 12-Step model end their intervention on this level. "I told my patient to go to AA," the clinician might say, "but it didn't help him." Or: "I suggested AA to my patient, but she told me that she didn't like the meetings."

Much as any psychotherapy involves helping patients work through resistances (to insight, for example), facilitating active involvement means helping the patient to examine and work through resistances to active involvement in AA and/or NA. Working within a 12-Step framework one is apt to encounter the word "denial" instead of "resistance," though the two are in fact conceptually similar in many ways.

Getting active does begin with going to meetings. For the individual who is just beginning to give up alcohol or drugs (even after a prior period of sobriety), 12-Step fellowships have traditionally advocated attending 90 meetings in 90 days (i.e., a meeting a day [or more] as a minimum). The exact origins of this common wisdom are vague, as are the origins of much of the "culture" of AA. However, the advice squares well with research on relapse (Marlatt & Gordon, 1985), which shows consistently, across addictions, that the majority of relapses occur within 90 days of initial sobriety.

AA and NA meetings vary with respect to membership, tone, and agenda. Because AA is intentionally decentralized (Alcoholics Anonymous, 1952, pp. 160, 172), no two meetings will be alike. The facilitator must understand not only that there are discernible regional differences in overall tone, say, between New England and California, but that there is a growing trend toward homogeneity in certain meetings. It is common, for example, to find men's, women's, Latino, and gay AA and NA meetings. In larger communities one can typically locate meetings for professionals, clergy, and so on. Not all these meetings will be officially registered with AA's central office.

Though AA as an organization purposefully exerts no effort to ensure that meetings are organized or run a certain way, there are discernible types of meetings. These include "speaker meetings," where an individual tells his/her story (uninterrupted) of addiction and recovery, generally following the format of "how it was, what happened, and how it is now." Naturally the focus here is on how active involvement in a 12-Step fellowship led to recovery.

Another type of meeting is the "open discussion" meeting. Here a designated member or members raises an issue (resentment, loneliness, spirituality) to which members respond in turn, sharing their thoughts or experiences relative to the subject.

A third meeting is the "step meeting." Usually a group will focus on one of the twelve steps for a month at a time. At the beginning of the meeting the step is read aloud. Members then respond to the step, explaining how they are "working" it in their daily lives. Some step meetings go through the entire 12 steps in this way; other groups may limit themselves to certain steps only—say, 1, 2, and 3—and cycle through them several times a year.

Some AA and NA meetings are "open", meaning that one need not have a problem with alcohol or drugs to attend, whereas others are "closed" to persons who admit to alcoholism or addiction. And although there is no centralized monitoring of meetings, there are certain ethics that are traditionally observed. These include using first names only, never interrupting or questioning a person who is speaking, and welcoming newcomers. It is important for the facilitator to point out that one does not have to say that one is an alcoholic or addict in order to be welcomed at a 12-Step meeting. One only has to have the requisite "desire to stop drinking (or using)."

In facilitating early recovery the facilitator should monitor not only *how many* meetings a patient attends but also *what kinds* of meetings they attend. This can be done conveniently by asking patients to maintain a personal "recovery journal" in which they record meetings attended, what type they are, and their reactions to them. Exploring these entries at the outset of each session (review) can greatly enhance the overall facilitation effort.

Facilitators should make every effort to encourage patients to try out several different types of meetings, including open discussion, step, and speaker meetings. Attending one or two specialized meetings (e.g., a men's or women's meeting) is also recommended. After the patient has attended a number of different meetings several times each, he/she should be encouraged to begin thinking about making one of them his/her "home meeting." This means making a commitment to attending that meeting regularly and to accepting some responsibility at the meeting. This could be setting up (or folding up) chairs, making coffee, cleaning up, and so on. The secretary of the meeting is the individual who generally assigns such responsibilities, usually for a limited time.

Choosing a home meeting and accepting some responsibility for it moves the newly recovering patient to a deeper level of active involvement, which is one objective of the facilitation. Another level is achieved as the patient begins to get and use *telephone numbers*. Giving and getting phone numbers is another normal part of what could be called the 12-Step culture, and patients should be prepared for it. Of course, they may feel free to decline to give out their phone numbers, at least until they feel comfortable. Perhaps sooner than later, though, the therapist should encourage the patient to start getting phone numbers and using them. The primary purpose, of course, is to build a support network of people who are sympathetic to the goal of not drinking or using drugs, and who can be called in time of need. In this regard it is important to explain to patients who are not experiencing any urges to drink or use (and who may therefore be inclined to see no immediate need for such contacts) that it is important to establish a network of AA friends *before* one needs them.

On another level, getting and using phone numbers, like getting more active in meetings, serves to gradually reconstruct the patient's social circle. Over time it leads to less contact with drinking or using friends and more contact with new, sober friends. As research suggests that social support is a significant factor in recovery (Sobell, Cunningham, Sobell, & Toneatto, 1993), this process of progressively establishing a new social network can be thought of as a core objective of TSF.

The last objective with regard to facilitating active involvement in AA or NA concerns *sponsorship*. A sponsor—yet another integral part of the AA culture—is by tradition a sort of mentor: an individual who has traveled the road before you and who can serve as a guide. AA succinctly describes the role and significance of the sponsor in early recovery in this way: "Not every A.A. member has a sponsor. But thousands of us say we would not be alive were it not for the special friendship of one recovering alcoholic in the first months and years of our sobriety" (Alcoholics Anonymous, 1975, p. 26).

Sponsors typically establish a pattern of daily telephone (and sometimes face-to-face) contact with the newcomer. They may meet the newcomer at meetings and facilitate his/her meeting new people. The sponsor may suggest meetings that would be good ones for the newcomer to attend. Sponsors may also introduce newcomers to AA social events and may try to the best of their ability to answer questions about the steps or the fellowship. Because of the need to maintain clear boundaries, the facilitator (even if he/she were personally in recovery) cannot become a patient's sponsor. Nevertheless, the facilitator needs to take a proactive role in helping the patient to find at least a "temporary" sponsor very early in the recovery process.

Taken together, this set of objectives establishes a broad basis of social support for sobriety while simultaneously breaking the patient away from people, places, and things that have long been associated with alcohol or drug use. Along with identification it is a core aspect of 12-Step-oriented treatment. Obviously it goes well beyond the simple suggestion that a patient "try some AA meetings."

Identification

It is axiomatic within AA that the similarities among alcoholics, particularly with respect to not being able to control drinking, are much more important, at least to recovery, than their differences. Bill Wilson expressed it this way:

> We are average Americans.[2] 2. AA has grown considerably since these words were written. According to the AA General Services Office as of December 31, 1992, there were 87,300 AA groups spread out over 145 countries. Total membership at that time exceeded 2 million. All sections of this country and many of its occupations are represented, as well as many political, economic, social, and religious backgrounds. We are people who normally would not mix. But there exists among us a fellowship, a friendliness, and an understanding which is indescribably wonderful. (Alcoholics Anonymous, 1952, p. 17)

It is common for newcomers to AA and NA to experience discomfort. That is understandable. After all, addiction and alcoholism maintain a degree of social stigma. In addition, people who have little or no direct knowledge of 12-Step fellowships are apt to hold attitudes based on stereotypes, for example, that AA members are "holy rollers" obsessed with God, or that meetings are like religious services. On a deeper level they may resist identifying themselves with AA members out of shame.

The first thing the facilitator needs to do is normalize and empathize with the patient's initial reticence to identify. Reading the above quote can initiate a productive discussion of this issue, as can sharing the patient's entries in his/her recovery journal. The facilitator needs to remain alert for resistance to identification and to help the patient work it through. The first strategy for doing so is to ask the patient go to speaker and discussion meetings and to practice active listening. The facilitator routinely asks the patient whether there was a person, or a part of a story, that the patient related to (i.e., *identified with*). Building on this, the facilitator gradually shapes the patient's capacity for identification. Naturally this calls for no small amount of judgment and skill, for example, in knowing when to acknowledge that nonidentification is appropriate or identification too threatening to entertain.

Others methods for facilitating identification are the journal, already mentioned, plus reading AA material. Especially useful for purposes of promoting identification are the many personal stories of addiction and recovery that appear in *Alcoholics Anonymous* and *Narcotics Anonymous*. For patients with a great deal of social anxiety, attempting to identify through reading may be easier at first than identifying through listening.

However identification is achieved, it is a highly desirable outcome of TSF for it has the effect of *bonding* the patient to the fellowship. Often, in the very early stages of recovery, it is getting active that is most crucial. In order to sustain involvement and ensure sobriety over the long run, though, this bonding may be crucial. Furthermore, in general it is in the context of this bonding that many AA members begin to pursue more advanced work such as moral inventories (Steps 4 and 5) and to experience firsthand some of the spirituality that has long been associated with AA. In my experience with facilitating early recovery, it is rare for an individual to undergo a "spiritual awakening" without first bonding to the fellowship.

Taken together, active involvement and identification form a solid basis for recovery. The more effective the facilitator, in collaboration with the patient, is in establishing these dimensions of recovery, the more likely it is that the patient will sustain his/her sobriety.

ASSESSMENT

Facilitating recovery using a 12-Step model begins much as any good treatment for substance abuse should begin: with a thorough assessment. The specific approach to assessment employed in TSF has been described in detail elsewhere (Nowinski & Baker, 1992, pp. 35–53; Nowinski, Baker, & Carroll, 1992, pp. 21–33) and for reasons of space are described only briefly here.

Assessment is important for two reasons. The first and most obvious reason is that we want to determine whether the prospective patient is indeed addicted to alcohol or drugs. In reality, however, even problem drinkers can benefit from AA or NA and from TSF, as long as they are (or can be) motivated to stop drinking or using.

A second and perhaps less obvious objective underlying assessment has to do with the issue of motivation. Part of the purpose of taking a thorough alcohol and drug history, as well as a careful inventory of consequences, is to establish a collaborative therapeutic relationship with the patient and, ideally, to reach a *consensus* regarding diagnosis and treatment. This may require the facilitator to refer frequently in subsequent sessions to data collected during the assessment. Therefore, it is important that the clinician keep good records of information gathered. Toward this same end I recommend that the patient be given a copy of the assessment and be asked to review it as one of his/her first *recovery tasks* between sessions.

An alcohol–drug history is graphical representation of chronologic changes in the type and amount of mood-altering substances used by the patient, along with correlated events and effects. This is best done using a chart such as that shown in Table 2.1. In this hypothetical example, the patient reported his first use of alcohol at age 11. At that time he sipped from his father's beer, primarily on weekends. Drinking made him feel happy and sometimes sick. He reported that his mother and father fought often at about the same time. By age 13 his use of alcohol had increased to two or three beers, two or three times a week. This made him feel "cool." About this same time, his father left the home.

By the time he was 14 our hypothetical patient was drinking beer and smoking marijuana three to four times a week. He reports that this made him feel "mellow," which suggests that he is now using substances to control his mood. He also reports getting into trouble at school and having much conflict at home, presumably with his mother, at this point in time.

Although Table 2.1 is necessarily brief for purposes of illustration, the clinician should take care to fill it in as completely as possible, adding as much detail as the patient will offer. Again, the objective is to engage the patient in a collaborative effort in this instance of autobiography. If this takes more than one session, so be it.

After the alcohol–drug history is completed, the patient should be given a copy and asked to look it over between sessions. At the next session the facilitator should review it again with the patient, filling in any details that the patient recalled as a result of this recovery task.

The second major part of the assessment is an inventory of consequences of alcohol and drug use. Again, both for purposes of clarity and to enhance motivation, this is best done as a chronology. The facilitator can introduce this part of the assessment with an opening statement similar to the following:

> "Let's take some time to examine some of the issues, conflicts, and problems that you've experienced over your life, and let's see if any of them are connected in any way to your use of alcohol or drugs."

Negative consequences of alcohol or drug use should be explored chronologically and also categorically. Be sure not to leave out (or allow the patient to avoid) examining each of the following areas.

Physical Consequences

Included here (especially for older patients) are the physical consequences of long-term substance abuse, including hypertension, gastrointestinal problems, sleep disorders, weight loss, alcohol- or drug-related injuries and accidents, emergency room visits, blackouts, heart problems, liver disease, and kidney disease. Keep in mind that it is estimated that

TABLE 2.1. Alcohol–Drug History

Substance/ age	Type/ amount	Frequency	Effects	Significant events
Alcohol/11	Beer/sips from Dad's	Weekends	Happy/sick	Mom and Dad fighting
Alcohol/13	Beer/2–3	2–3 times/wk	"Cool"	Dad left
Alcohol, marijuana/14	Beer/2–3 1–2 joints	3–4 times/wk 3–4 times/wk	"Mellow"	Doing poorly in school/fighting at home

approximately 50% of all general hospital beds in the United States are occupied with patients whose medical illnesses are alcohol or drug related (National Institute on Alcohol Abuse and Alcoholism, 1990).

Legal Consequences

Alcohol and drug use often lead to legal troubles such as DWI (driving while intoxicated) arrests, arrests for possession or sale of illegal substances, arrests for disorderly conduct, and so forth. They also include alcohol- or drug-related illegal activities (e.g., sale, theft, and prostitution) for which the patient was neither arrested nor convicted.

Social Consequences

Social consequences of alcohol or drug use include relationship, family, or job conflicts. Substance abusers often alienate their partners, perform progressively more poorly at work, and are dysfunctional as parents. They may lose marriages, jobs, and friends. It is important to do a thorough inventory of such losses, in chronologic order, and to connect them to the patient's alcohol–drug history as appropriate.

Psychological Consequences

Habitual use of alcohol and drugs, even in the absence of clear dependency, typically leads to negative psychological consequences such as anxiety and depression. Other consequences include poor anger control, sleep and eating disorders, irritability, amotivational syndrome, and confused thinking. As habitual use gives way to dependency, and as negative consequences accrue, suicidal thinking and suicide attempts are not uncommon.

Sexual Consequences

Not only is alcohol and other substance abuse associated with sexual dysfunction in both males and females (Powell, 1984), but alcohol and drug use and dependency are often correlated with sexual victimization and exploitation. The facilitator should explore the patient's sexual history to determine whether sexual dysfunction, victimization, or exploitation is present, and if so whether it is correlated with substance abuse. Frank discussion of sexuality is often omitted from assessment even though it is often a potential motivator for recovery. Guidelines for conducting substance abuse-related sexual histories have been published elsewhere (Nowinski & Baker, 1992).

Financial Consequences

It is a good idea to have the patient estimate how much money he/she has spent on alcohol or drugs in the 2 years prior to the assessment. Included are the cost of the substances themselves and the costs of any consequences. The latter include the costs of traffic tickets, legal defense or representation, and lost income. For example, a cocaine addict may have spent $50,000 on cocaine over 2 years and also have lost a job worth $40,000 per year, had to hire one lawyer to represent him in court and another to represent him in divorce action, and had a bank foreclose on his house. These financial consequences are all justifiably included as costs of addiction.

Once the alcohol–drug history and the inventory of consequences have been completed, the assessment itself ends with the facilitator sharing a diagnosis and treatment plan. Obviously this should come as no surprise to the patient if the assessment process has truly been a collaborative venture. Still, the patient and clinician may disagree, especially if the clinician thinks the patient is addicted but the patient does not. What is important for the clinician to note is that it is not essential for the patient to acknowledge alcoholism or addiction in order to proceed with TSF. Remember, the sole criterion for making use of AA is a *desire to stop drinking*. Addiction is not a prerequisite.

TREATMENT

It is hoped that a successful assessment not only has confirmed a clinical diagnosis for the clinician but has also led the patient to discover within him/herself a desire to stop drinking or using drugs. This motivation will enhance treatment, especially if it means that the patient is willing to follow the facilitator's advice. One word of caution, however: Some patients may indeed express a desire to stop drinking yet lack a willingness to take the action that recovery requires. This is where being able to work effectively with the patient on the first three steps of AA becomes crucial to treatment outcome. Within AA and other 12-Step fellowships this transition—from passive acknowledgment of a problem to active participation in a fellowship—is known as "working the steps." This is the crux of what could be called early recovery. Two issues that this work centers around are *acceptance* and *surrender.*

Acceptance

The first Step of AA and NA as it appears in their respective "big books" reads as follows:

> We admitted we were powerless over alcohol—that our lives had become unmanageable. (Alcoholics Anonymous, 1976, p. 59)

> We admitted we were powerless over our addiction—that our lives had become unmanageable. (Narcotics Anonymous, 1982, p. 8)

Although many individuals take issue with the word "powerless," regarding it as counterproductive, it is important for clinicians who wish to facilitate 12-Step recovery to understand how that concept is used within the fellowships of AA and NA, which has to do with *acceptance of the limitations of willpower.* The fellowship of AA was built on the realization that in order to stay sober, the alcoholic first had to "quit playing God" (Alcoholics Anonymous, 1976, p. 62) and accept with humility the notion that "any life run on self-will can hardly be a success" (Alcoholics Anonymous, 1976, p. 60). Alcoholics were, after all, individuals who were intensely self-centered (Alcoholics Anonymous, 1976, p. 62) and lacking in humility, who were bound and determined to control their drinking through willpower alone and unwilling to accept the need for fellowship and support. They were, in a word, poor "therapy candidates" as much as they were poor candidates for sobriety.

The essence of the first Step, then, is that it represents a statement of humility. It reflects an acceptance of personal limitation—that life has become *unmanageable* and that willpower alone has not been enough to change that. Philosophically, the first Step (and AA itself) has been characterized as a challenge to the radical individualism that has been a central theme in American culture (Room, 1993).

In discussing Step 1 with patients it is extremely useful to have the alcohol–drug history and the chronology of consequences at hand. The focus of this dialogue should be on the *progressive pattern of unmanageability in the patient's life and the limitations of personal willpower.* If the history and chronology do not make a case for total loss of control, they should at least show a pattern of growing unmanageability that can be pointed out, repeatedly if necessary, to the patient. The patient can also be asked to describe some of the methods he/she has used in the past in order to limit or stop his/her use of alcohol and drugs. In this regard the facilitator would do well to share the following excerpt with the patient:

> Here are some of the methods we have tried: Drinking beer only, limiting the number of drinks, never drinking alone, never drinking in the morning, drinking only at home, never having it in the house, never drinking during business hours, drinking only at parties, switching fromscotch to brandy, drinking only natural wines, agreeing to resign if ever drunk on the job, swearing off forever (with or without a solemn oath), taking more physical exercise, reading inspirational books, going to health farms and sanitariums, accepting voluntary commitment to asylums—we could increase the list ad infinitum. (Alcoholics Anonymous, 1976, p. 31)

In the face of evidence of growing unmanageability and failure to control use, the patient who continues to resist suggestions that he/she needs to give up alcohol or drugs altogether, needs help doing so, and might give AA or NA a try, could be said to be in denial.

The discussion of Step 1, then, should proceed toward acceptance of the need for abstinence in a series of steps, as follows:

1. The patient acknowledges that he/she has a "problem" with alcohol or drugs—that life has become, or is becoming, unmanageable.
2. The patient acknowledges that individual efforts to limit or stop drinking or using have failed.
3. The patient acknowledges the need to give up alcohol and/or drugs and accepts with humility his/her inability to do so thus far.

As simple and straightforward as this acceptance sounds, clinicians find that it usually is more of a process than an event. For many individuals with alcohol or drug problems acceptance is a realization that is achieved gradually. It is also one that is frequently accompanied by emotional reactions (to acceptance of personal limitation and the loss of alcohol or drug as a "friend" and coping mechanism) with which the facilitator must be able to empathize. As a rule, acceptance without emotion is suspect. More typically, patients will be angry or depressed as they move through the stages of acceptance. The clinician does well to raise this issue of emotional responses to limitation and loss and explore it with the patient.

Surrender

Surrender follows acceptance and represents the patient's decision to humbly seek help and abandon personal willpower as a means of controlling or stopping use of alcohol or drugs. Like acceptance, surrender is more typically a process than an event, and one that evokes intense emotion. It is reflected in Steps 2 and 3 of Alcoholics Anonymous:

> We came to believe that a Power greater than ourselves could restore us to sanity.
>
> We made a decision to turn our will and our lives over to the care of God *as we understood Him.* (Alcoholics Anonymous, 1976, p. 59)

The italics at the end of the third Step appear in the original text and are emphasized in order to point out that the AA view of God or a Higher Power is a pluralistic one. There is no religious dogma within AA; on the other hand, there is a strong tradition of what could be called spirituality or faith, defined as follows: "Faith is a dynamic process of construal and commitment in which persons find and give meaning to their lives through trust in and loyalty to shared centers of value, images and realities of power, and core stories" (Fowler, 1993, p. 167).

If Step 1 involves accepting the problem (alcoholism or addiction), Steps 2 and 3 can be thought of as accepting the solution. In AA jargon this means "turning it over": moving away from self-centeredness and an excessive belief in the power of individual willpower toward a willingness to reach out for and accept the strength of fellowship. This is more than an abstract notion—it will be directly reflected in patients' *hope for recovery,* in their *willingness to become active in the fellowship,* and in their *openness to advice.* When the patient surrenders in this way, he/she begins to understand that powerlessness does not imply helplessness in the face of addiction.

AA and NA are fellowships that were established by and for the "hopeless," in other words, by and for people whose personal struggles with addiction led to personal defeat and desperation. Individuals whose problems with alcohol and drugs are less severe than that may have a harder time identifying with some of the shared images, values, and stories that form the spiritual foundation of these fellowships. Nevertheless, as long as life has become increasingly unmanageable as a result of drinking or drug use, the individual may become motivated to give up the addiction.

The clinician needs to engage the patient in a specific and ongoing dialogue about willpower, faith, and surrender. It is suggested that at least one entire session be devoted to reading Steps 2 and 3 and discussing the patient's reactions to them. Questions such as the following can be used as a guideline for this discussion:

- As a youth, who were your heroes, and who are they now?
- What are your most cherished values? In other words, what personal qualities in others do you admire most?
- How do you feel about people who ask others for help when they feel stuck, and why?
- Are you open to the idea that people struggling with similar problems can help each other more than each of those people can help him/herself?
- Whose advice are you most likely to follow?
- Do you ever pray? When and why?
- Are you open to the idea that there are some personal problems that a person can solve only by reaching out for help and support from others?
- Do you believe that others could help you stay clean or sober?
- What is your idea of God?
- Who in the world do you trust the most, and why?
- Are you willing to do what someone else who has overcome alcoholism or drug addiction tells you to do? When would you, and when wouldn't you, follow that person's advice?
- How do you feel about using the support of people in AA or NA to help you stay clean and sober?

Again, this sort of dialogue is more than an intellectual adventure. It is central to introducing the patient to the spiritual foundation of 12-Step fellowships. Therapists may not be comfortable engaging patients in this sort of dialogue. Others may wish to ponder such questions themselves before entering into this kind of dialogue. In the end, however, it is important to venture down this road, because it represents a highly effective route to working through patients' resistances to becoming active in AA or NA and making full use of their social and spiritual resources. In fact, merely accusing resistant addicts and alcoholics of being in denial is much like (and no more effective than) accusing resistant psychotherapy patients of being resistive. Rather than persisting in such a deadlock it is generally much more productive to name the resistance (or denial) and then explore its dynamics. In this case issues related to letting go of the illusion of personal omnipotence and overcoming distrust often are central dynamics underlying resistance.

Getting Active

The third and final part of early treatment centers around facilitating the patient's active participation in AA and/or NA. "Getting active," to use 12-Step jargon again, means "working the steps." AA puts it this way: "Just stopping drinking is not enough. Just not drinking is a negative, sterile thing. That is clearly demonstrated by our experience. To stay stopped, we've found we need to put in place of the drinking a positive program of action" (Alcoholics Anonymous, 1975).

A popular meditation book expresses similar sentiments in this way: "Work and prayer are the two forces which are gradually making a better world. We must work for the betterment of ourselves and other people. Faith without works is dead" (Anonymous, 1975, p. 83).

The meaning here is clear: Recovery requires faith, but it also requires action. Steps 1 and 2 in particular can be thought of as necessary but not sufficient conditions for staying clean or sober. To facilitate recovery, the clinician must be prepared to continually work with the patient toward the goals of active involvement described earlier, namely, going to meetings frequently and listening well, getting phone numbers and building a support network, seeking a home group and taking on a responsibility, seeking out a sponsor (or at least a temporary sponsor), and reading AA/NA material to understand the program.

Two useful vehicles for pursuing these goals are the *recovery journal* (described earlier) and the use of *recovery tasks*. The latter are not unlike "homework" that is often employed in cognitive-behavioral therapies, which, like TSF, also involve patient–therapist collaboration and active work on the part of the patient. It is recommended that the clinician end each session with a series of specific recovery tasks and begin each session with a review of the patient's "recovery week," including progress made on recovery tasks.

Recovery tasks and the subsequent review should cover each of the following areas:

Readings from AA and/or NA literature.
Suggestions about specific meetings to attend.
Progress made on the use of telephone therapy, selecting a home group, taking on responsibility, and getting a sponsor.

Clinicians may wish to employ techniques such as role playing in order to facilitate goals (e.g., using the telephone and speaking up at meetings) that are difficult for patients with high social anxiety. They must also be prepared to shape behavior through positive reinforcement of patients' efforts. It is not uncommon, for example, for patients to make several false starts when first trying to go to meetings. They may even get as far as the door, only to turn around and go home. Or, they may come late and leave early. Or, they may attend one meeting after they promised to attend three.

Obviously, to be able to shape behavior the facilitator must first know about it. A blaming or unreceptive attitude on the part of the facilitator is likely to cloud communication, when what is needed is openness. Patients should be made to feel safe disclosing what they actually did between sessions. This is not inconsistent with their also knowing what the clinician would *like* them to have done. Rather than scolding or punishing, a better approach is to reinforce positive efforts and identify the causes of any resistance. If the cause is something like social anxiety, techniques such as role playing may help. If the cause is linked to resistance to ideas such as powerlessness or turning it over, as described earlier, a different discussion may be in order.

Readings

Here are some suggestions for readings that might be assigned relative to the subjects of acceptance, surrender, and getting active:

Acceptance
Twelve Steps and Twelve Traditions: pp. 21–24
Alcoholics Anonymous: "The Doctor's Opinion," "Bill's Story,"
    "More about Alcoholism"
Narcotics Anonymous: "Who Is an Addict," "Why Are We Here,"
    "How It Works"
Living Sober: pp. 7–10

Surrender
Alcoholics Anonymous: "There Is a Solution," "More about Alco-
    holism," "How It Works"
Narcotics Anonymous: pp. 22–26
Twelve Steps and Twelve Traditions: pp. 25–41
Living Sober: pp. 77–87

Getting Active
Alcoholics Anonymous: Personal Stories (to be selected by facilitator)
Living Sober: Chapters 3, 6, 8, 10, 11, 13, 14, 15, 18, 22, 26, 27, 29

The facilitator should be familiar with any readings assigned and be prepared to discuss them during the review period at the outset of each session. Consideration should be given to the patient's reading level and available time when making reading assignments. For patients who cannot read (or who read only Spanish), suitable translations and audiotapes are available through Alcoholics Anonymous World Services (P.O. Box 1980, New York, NY 10163-1980).

Readings should not be limited to those mentioned here. Rather, these are offered as appropriate suggestions. With experience, the facilitator will develop personal preferences as well as a sense for "what fits who" with respect to readings.

Meetings

In order to make meaningful recommendations about which meetings to suggest to a patient, the facilitator must obtain current official AA and NA meeting schedules. These are available through regional AA or NA offices. Local numbers for AA and NA are listed in the white pages of many telephone books. They may also be obtained at AA and NA meetings. Clinicians wishing to conduct TSF owe it to themselves and their patients to attend open AA and NA meetings occasionally, to maintain current meeting schedules, and to develop their own small network of AA and NA "friends" who may be useful resources for getting shy newcomers to meetings, meeting them there, and so on. Many recovering persons express a great deal of gratitude to those first "friendly faces" encountered at meetings. The facilitator should not assume this responsibility personally; thus, he/she is wise to seek out a network of recovering men and women who are at a point in their own recovery where they are ready to do this sort of "twelfth-step" work. In this regard, the nonrecovering therapist should not feel guilty for calling on such help, as it is an integral part of the AA culture.

CONJOINT PROGRAM

It is not uncommon for interventions based on a 12-Step model to include a family and/or marital component. Doing so merely recognizes the reality that substance abuse affects not only the abuser but also his/her significant others. TSF incorporates a brief conjoint program into its model. The TSF conjoint program is consistent with the philosophy of Al-Anon, which is a 12-Step program for significant others (Al-Anon Family Group Headquarters, 1985).

The objectives of the TSF conjoint program, which generally spans no more than two or three sessions, are to provide a spouse or significant other with an overview of the facilitation program that the patient is undergoing, to do an initial assessment of possible partner substance abuse, and to introduce the significant other to Al-Anon and two of its key concepts: enabling and detaching.

TSF recognizes that the relationships, both marital and family, of alcoholics and addicts have often been rendered deeply dysfunctional as a result of the addiction. It recognizes that marital and/or family therapy is often appropriate. At the same time, TSF is based on the idea that *early* recovery is best served by focusing on acceptance, surrender, and getting active. In a similar vein, TSF seeks to help significant others get a *start* on recovering from the effects of addiction and believes that programs such as Al-Anon offer the best resources for that start. Accordingly, before a patient who is just beginning recovery, along with his/her partner or family, is referred for marital or family therapy, TSF attempts to engage the family in fellowships that can offer sympathy, support, and advice.

Partner Substance Abuse

The issue of partner substance abuse cannot be ignored by the practitioner working with persons in early recovery, for the obvious reason that it represents a threat to the early recovery of the primary patient. On the other hand, TSF does not insist on total abstinence from partners who are merely social drinkers. However, basic questions such as those listed below should be asked in order to determine whether a partner is best referred for treatment as well:

- Do you drink or use drugs at all? If so, what do you drink (use) and how often?
- Have you ever felt (or has anyone else ever suggested) that you have a problem with alcohol or drugs?
- Have you ever suffered any consequences of any kind related to alcohol or drug use?
- Has drinking or drug use ever interfered with your day-to-day life or made it "unmanageable" in any way?

Based on a simple and brief inquiry such as this, along with any information that the clinician has gathered from the patient, a decision can be made about whether it should be suggested to a partner that he/she seek further help. At the same time the facilitator will know whether partner substance abuse could be a complicating factor.

Introducing Al-Anon and/or Nar-Anon

Al-Anon and Nar-Anon are fellowships that parallel AA and NA but that exist for the benefit of those who are in relationships with alcoholics or addicts. As do AA and NA, both Al-Anon and Nar-Anon begin with statements of "powerlessness." In this case, however, it is the behavior of the alcoholic or addict over which the individual is powerless. Coming to terms with this personal limitation (Step 1 of Al-Anon) is a process that parallels the alcoholic's or addict's coming to terms with his/her powerlessness over alcohol or drugs. Many of the same psychodynamics (e.g., denial) must be acknowledged and worked through. Similarly, the decision to reach out to others (Al-Anon) for support and guidance has its parallels in Steps 2 and 3 of AA.

Learning to stop doing things that either purposefully or inadvertently allow the alcoholic or addict to continue drinking or using (*enabling*) and to let go of any illusion of being able to control the alcoholic or addict (*detaching*) is central to Al-Anon and Nar-Anon. It is only through learning detachment, it is believed, that partners and family members can begin to recover their own mental health. Al-Anon and Nar-Anon provide both the social and spiritual support for this process. Al-Anon expresses the overall goal this way: " 'Detach!' we are told in Al-Anon. This does not mean detaching ourselves, and our love and compassion, from the alcoholic. Detachment, in the Al-Anon sense, means to realize we are individuals. We are not bound morally to shoulder the alcoholic's responsibilities" (Al-Anon Family Group Headquarters, 1986, p. 54).

After giving partners an overview of the facilitation program and inquiring into their own use of alcohol or drugs, the facilitator devotes the bulk of the conjoint program to discussing the issues of enabling and detaching and encouraging the partner to get active in Al-Anon or Nar-Anon. In this way the conjoint program, however brief, parallels the facilitation program itself. Enabling is defined as any behavior that has the effect of allowing the alcoholic or addict to face the reality that drinking or drug use is making his/her life unmanageable. Examples are given, such as the following:

- Making excuses to cover up for the patient when he/she would otherwise get into trouble as a consequence of alcohol or drug use.
- Providing money or other support for acquiring alcohol or drugs.
- Justifying inappropriate or illegal behavior while under the influence of alcohol or drugs.

The significant other is asked to give specific examples of how he/she has enabled the patient to continue to drink or use. The motivations behind these actions are also explored. Typically it is concern for the well-being of the patient or fear of the consequences (e.g., to the family) of alcoholism or addiction that motivates enabling. Less often, it is a desire to avoid facing one's own alcohol or drug problem.

Detaching can be thought of as a process of learning not to enable, but it also can be conceptualized more positively (i.e., as learning what to do *instead of* enabling). The facilitator engages the partner in some discussion of this, using examples of enabling as a springboard. For example, instead of calling in "sick" for the alcoholic who in fact is hung over (enabling), the partner could sympathize with the dilemma but refuse to make the call (detaching).

Learning to detach takes courage. It can be supported by the therapist, to be sure, but it is in the fellowships of Al-Anon and Nar-Anon that partners will find the greatest amount of support and comfort for their task. Toward this end the facilitator should suggest several specific Al-Anon or Nar-Anon meetings that the partner could attend and follow up on these suggestions at the outset of subsequent sessions.

TERMINATION

If TSF has been successful, termination essentially consists of "turning over" the patient to the care of a 12-Step fellowship. The more successfully the patient and therapist have collaborated toward this end, the more likely it is that the patient will continue his/her progress toward lasting sobriety. This prediction is based on AA member surveys, which show that the best predictor of future sobriety is current active participation in AA (Alcoholics Anonymous General Services Office, 1990).

Because the overarching goal of TSF is involvement in AA and/or NA, termination should in part consist of an honest appraisal of how much progress has been made toward that end. Questions such as the following are in order:

- How many meetings per week, on average, do you now attend? What kinds of meetings are they?
- Do you have a home meeting?
- On average, how many AA/NA friends do you call by phone each week? How many AA/NA people call you?
- Have you taken on any responsibility at a meeting (making coffee, setting up, etc.)?

Besides monitoring activity per se, the facilitator does well to see whether the patient at termination has absorbed key concepts and whether his/her attitudes about addiction and recovery have changed at all as a result of the facilitation program. Questions such as the following are suggested for obtaining this information:

- Do you think that alcohol or drug use has made your life unmanageable?
- Do you believe now that alcoholics and addicts can "control" their drinking or drugging just by their own willpower (without asking for help from others)?
- What is your understanding of the following concepts: denial, enabling, higher power?
- What role, if any, has AA played so far in your effort to stay clean and sober?
- What are your plans relative to AA (or NA) now that this program (TSF) is coming to an end?

Finally, the facilitator needs to take a moment (preferably prior to the actual termination session) to reflect on the issue of the relative responsibilities of patient and therapist in this model. In this regard the concept of detaching is as relevant to the facilitator as it is to any significant other in the patient's life. Clinical experience suggests that the best the facilitator can hope to do is to introduce key concepts in ways that the patient can understand them, actively encourage the patient to give 12-Step fellowship a try, confront the patient constructively with the role that alcohol or drugs has played in making the patient's life unmanageable, and answer questions about AA or NA to the best of his/her ability. How many sober days the patient has had, and how active he/she has become in AA or NA, is not within the control of the facilitator. In the final analysis the facilitator must be able to "turn over" the patient and his/her future to the care of whatever higher power the facilitator happens to believe in.

ADVANCED WORK

This chapter has focused on a structured, time-limited intervention for "early" recovery. It is unlikely that any more ground than what has been described here could reasonably be covered in brief therapy. Indeed, the goals of TSF are ambitious. I do not recommend attempting to do more advanced work with patients until they have a minimum of 6 months of uninterrupted sobriety and have satisfied all goals of this core program, namely, becoming active. Toward this end patients who wish to continue treatment or discuss more "advanced" issues should be asked first to consolidate their recovery at least to this minimal level. On a practical level this means calling for a hiatus in treatment.

TSF as originally developed also includes an "elective program" (Nowinski & Baker, 1992, pp. 95–154; Nowinski et al., 1992, pp. 59–96), which provides therapist guidelines for covering the following topics: genograms; enabling; people, places, and routines; emotions; moral inventories; and relationships. A discussion of this material is beyond the scope of this chapter; however, parts of the elective program may be considered for patients who have consolidated their early recovery and are ready to work, for example, on Steps 4 and 5 (the so-called moral inventory) of AA.

CASE STUDY

The following is offered as an illustration of how the model of addiction and the interventions described in this chapter may be applied.[3]

Bob and Kathy, married for 20 years, came to see me ostensibly for help with long-standing marital difficulties that had reached crisis proportions since their youngest child left home for college. Though it was initially obscured by discussions and arguments about money and sex, it became apparent after a while that Bob had a drinking problem that needed to be evaluated. He was asked to come in individually for two sessions to talk about this.

The assessment sessions revealed that Bob had several signs of alcohol dependency. He had a powerful tolerance, drank daily, and had experienced a number of drinking-related consequences, not the least of which was a seriously strained marriage. In addition, he was in trouble at work as a consequence of drinking, a problem he had kept secret from his wife.

Bob at first was reticent to change the focus of therapy from his troubled marriage to his drinking. He was assured that his concerns about the marriage were legitimate and would be dealt with, but first he needed to examine his drinking and either take action or risk losing his job and/or his marriage.

The story of Bob's private struggle for control over alcohol was a testament to stubborn determination as much as it was a classic story of the power of addiction. Having started out sipping beers stolen from the refrigerator as a youth barely 12 years old, Bob had been drinking for nearly 30 years. Things did not get "really bad," though, according to him, until after he was married and the children were born. Two things happened then. First, he felt obligated to stay in a job that paid well but which he had previously intended to leave. Second, his relationship with Kathy, in his words, became "diluted" as a consequence of the demands of family life, meaning that sex between them became a very occasional thing, and she paid less attention to him than she did when there was just the two of them.

It was around this time that Bob developed the habit of having "a cocktail or two" every night after work and before dinner. For a long time Kathy went along with this, though she did notice that a cocktail or two eventually became three, four, or more. She did not much care for alcohol herself and had little personal experience with it in her own family. Out of naivete she took Bob's ability to "drink others under the table"—in other words, his tolerance—to be a good thing. Ironically, she believed that this ability to "hold his liquor" was actually a sign that Bob could *not* become addicted.

As time went on, the process of addiction gradually set in. Instead of eating lunch with his colleagues in the company cafeteria, Bob started going out alone for lunch two or three times a week, to a local bar where he would grab a sandwich and a couple of cocktails. By the time he got home he was anxious to "relax"—his euphemism for having more cocktails. Kathy and the children soon found that anything that stood between Bob and his cocktails made him irritable. He did not want to be bothered with problems until he was "relaxed." Of course, by that time he was also intoxicated, emotionally unstable, and prone to losing his temper. In time the family learned to avoid him. Kathy took to solving most of the household problems by herself, or else let them go. The kids, meanwhile, led their own lives and had minimal communication with their father.

Though he was very hesitant to admit it for a long time, privately Bob had struggled long (and ultimately unsuccessfully) to control his drinking. He had not wanted to be like his own father: a "quiet drunk" who was less flamboyant than Bob in his drinking but who had "liked his liquor" no less, and who had also been a social isolate and a "nonfactor" (as Bob described both himself and his father) within the family.

The story of Bob's private efforts to control his drinking sounded like something right out of the *Big Book*: drinking only wine, drinking only beer (no cocktails) at lunch, drinking from a smaller glass, adding more ice cubes to his cocktails, and so on. While he was conscious on some level of gradually losing control, he continued to tell himself that he was really all right. It was not until his boss smelled liquor on his breath that the shell of self-deceit that Bob had built was finally and abruptly shattered. He was called onto the carpet and told that a second such incident would result in disciplinary action. It also affected, he felt sure, his subsequent performance evaluation, which was lukewarm to say the least.

By the time he and Kathy came for "marriage counseling" Bob had managed to fall 2 years behind on his tax returns and owed the government several thousand dollars. According to Kathy, the house they lived in was falling apart faster and faster on account of maintenance projects that Bob refused to hire someone to do but kept putting off doing himself. Their son, who had just turned 18, was failing half his courses in his freshman year at college; meanwhile their daughter "hated" Bob and alternately fought with and ridiculed him. On top of all this, Kathy had been sexually turned off to Bob for some time, which left him feeling frustrated and filled with self-pity.

The assessment process involved carefully chronicling first the progression of Bob's drinking, from cocktails on weekends to cocktails at lunch, how he had built a tolerance, and how drinking affected him (i.e., making him irritable and withdrawn). We then proceeded to talk at length about the methods that Bob had used to "control" his drinking, followed by all the ways in which his life had become increasingly unmanageable. At the end of this process Bob was willing to admit that he had a drinking problem and "probably" needed to stop drinking altogether. At that point, however, he was not willing to entertain the idea of using AA as a resource for helping him implement his desire to stop drinking. On the other hand, he was willing to defer marriage counseling while he met with me to work on his drinking problem.

In a subsequent sessions Bob reported that he was drinking less than before but had not gone more than 1 day without a drink. At that point I moved ahead to a discussion of Step 1, reading it aloud and then talking with Bob about it at length, making sure he covered the following points:

- What does this statement mean to you? What is your initial reaction to it . . .
  —*Emotionally*: How does it make you feel?
  —*Intellectually*: What thoughts do you have in response to it?
- How do you relate to the concept of *powerlessness*? What kinds of things can people be powerless over in their lives?
- Can you see how some people might be "powerless" over alcohol or drugs?
- Have you ever felt powerless over something in your life? What have you felt powerless over?
- At this point do you believe that you can still control your use of alcohol? What makes you believe this?
- In what ways has your life become more *unmanageable* over the past several years? Where are the areas of conflict? In what ways are things not going well for you?

The *recovery tasks* discussed at this time focused on getting Bob to begin reading some of the material in the *Big Book,* especially "Bill's Story" and "We Agnostics." This material was particularly relevant to Bob, who was personally alienated from organized religion and who regarded AA as a religion of sorts. In addition, Bob was a strong believer in self-determination, to the point where it was all but impossible for him to find the humility necessary to admit that he had been ultimately unsuccessful, on his own, in controlling his drinking.

Reluctantly, and only after a frank discussion of humility combined with an appeal to be more open-minded, Bob agreed to try out a few different AA meetings. His assignment was to listen to the stories being told and to focus on *identifying* with as many as possible. Meanwhile, he was advised to avoid focusing his attention on how he was different from other people at these meetings in outlook, background, or circumstances.

One frequent problem of alcoholics who resist giving AA a try is their internalized stigma about alcoholism. Bob was no exception to this. He held very negative stereotypes about alcoholics and fully expected to discover himself in the company of derelicts and criminals when he went to AA. Of course, he discovered just the opposite, which made it easier to encourage him to continue. In fact, he made a friend at one of the very first meetings he went to, and this person eventually became his first sponsor.

The next focus of treatment was denial. Bob had attempted to avoid coming to terms with his loss of control over drinking as fiercely as any alcoholic. His first line of defense had always been to get angry whenever the subject was brought up by his wife. After blowing up he would usually change the subject, either launching into an attack on Kathy or else complaining long and loudly about some other problem, such as finances, his in-laws, or their sex life. In response to the ever growing list of household chores that went undone he pleaded fatigue—after all, he said, he worked hard all week and needed the weekends to "unwind."

Not surprisingly, Bob's denial extended outwardly to his behavior, and even inwardly to his own thought processes. For example, he went out of his way to associate with men who drank as much or even more than he did and then comforted himself by drawing the comparison between his own use and theirs. Of course, he concluded that he was merely "average" (and therefore "normal") among his peers. At times when he felt guilty pouring that fifth or sixth martini, he would tell himself that he "deserved" it, for example, because of the stress of having to endure an unsatisfying job. He tried to write off his trouble at work to a combination of bad luck and a vindictive boss, and he attributed his increasing tendency toward sexual impotence to his wife's rejection of him and her "preoccupation" with the children.

As is often the case, once Bob was able to admit to someone else (i.e., me) the ways in which he'd denied his drinking problem, the more open he became to accepting it. At this point he was even willing to admit it to Kathy and did so in a conjoint session. He continued to express reservations about whether he was a "true alcoholic" as he put it, but he was willing to keep going to AA on the premise that he did have the requisite desire to stop drinking.

As brief as this case example is, I hope it gives the reader a flavor for TSF as a mode of intervention. With respect to process it incorporates elements of education, confrontation, interpretation, and suggestion. It is based on the 12-Step model of addiction and recovery, and it clearly relies on sophisticated clinical skills for its successful implementation.

NOTES

1. TSF has specific guidelines for therapists to follow in the event patients show up for meetings intoxicated, if they binge, or if their overall mental status deteriorates. The general guideline is that sessions are terminated if the patient is intoxicated although the therapist's first task is to ensure the patient's safety and make suggestions regarding contacting the AA Hotline, getting to a meeting, and so forth. TSF may be temporarily suspended if patients require detoxification.

2. AA has grown considerably since these words were written. According to the AA General Services Office as of December 31, 1992, there were 87,300 AA groups spread out over 145 countries. Total membership at that time exceeded 2 million.

3. This case example is adapted from Nowinski and Baker (1992) and is used with permission of the authors.

REFERENCES

Al-Anon Family Group Headquarters. (1986). *Al-Anon faces alcoholism* (2nd ed.). New York: Author

Al-Anon Family Group Headquarters. (1986). *One day at a time in Al-Anon*. New York: Author

Alcoholics Anonymous. (1952). *Twelve steps and twelve traditions*. New York: Alcoholics Anonymous World Services.

Alcoholics Anonymous. (1975). *Living sober: Some methods A.A. members have used for not drinking*. New York: Alcoholics Anonymous World Services.

Alcoholics Anonymous. (1976). *Alcoholics Anonymous: The story of how many thousands of men and women have recovered from alcoholism* (3rd ed.). New York: Alcoholics Anonymous World Services.

Alcoholics Anonymous General Services Office. *Comments on A.A.'s triennial surveys.* New York: Author.

Anderson, D. J. (1991). *Perspectives on treatment: The Minnesota experience.* Center City, MN: Hazelden.

Anonymous. (1975, December 29). *Twenty-four hours a day.* Center City, MN: Hazelden.

Fowler, J. W. (1993). Alcoholics Anonymous and faith development. In B. S. McCrady & W. R. Miller (Eds.), *Research on Alcoholics Anonymous: Opportunities and alternatives.* New Brunswick, NJ: Rutgers Center of Alcohol Studies.

Marlatt, G. A., & Gordon, J. R. (Eds.). (1985). *Relapse prevention: Maintenance strategies in the treatment of addictive behaviors.* New York: Guilford Press.

Narcotics Anonymous. (1982). *Narcotics Anonymous* (4th ed.). Van Nuys, CA: Narcotics Anonymous World Services.

National Institute on Alcohol Abuse and Alcoholism. (1990). *Alcohol and health.* Washington, DC: Author.

Nowinski, J., & Baker, S. (1992). *The twelve-step facilitation handbook: A systematic approach to early recovery from alcoholism and addiction.* New York: Lexington Books.

Nowinski, J., Baker, S., & Carroll, K. (1992). *Twelve-step facilitation therapy manual: A clinical research guide for therapists treating individuals with alcohol abuse and dependence* (DHHS Publication No. ADM 92-1893, Project MATCH Monograph Series, Vol. 1). Rockville, MD: National Institute on Alcohol Abuse and Alcoholism.

Powell, D. (Ed.). (1984). *Alcoholism and sexual dysfunction: Issues in clinical management.* New York: Haworth Press.

Room, R. (1993). Alcoholics Anonymous as a social movement. In B. S. McCrady & W. R. Miller (Eds.), *Research on Alcoholics Anonymous: Opportunities and alternatives.* New Brunswick, NJ: Rutgers Center of Alcohol Studies.

Sobell, L., Cunningham, J. A., Sobell, M., & Toneatto, T. (1993). A life-span perspective on natural recovery (self-change) from alcohol problems. In J. S. Baer, G. A. Marlatt, & R. J. McMahon (Eds.), *Addictive behaviors across the life span: Prevention, treatment, and policy issues.* Newbury Park, CA: Sage.

CHAPTER 3

Psychoanalytic Theories of Substance Abuse

JEREMY LEEDS
JON MORGENSTERN

PSYCHOANALYSIS AND PSYCHOANALYTIC PSYCHOTHERAPY

Although it is probably the best known system and theory of psychotherapy, psychoanalysis is difficult to define. Controversy and innovation have been the rule since the theory's inception and have continued unabated through the present. Pine (1990), in trying to summarize and integrate various strains of psychoanalytic theorizing, speaks of the "central place of conflict and of the multiple functions of behavior" (p. 5). Gabbard (1992) characterizes psychoanalytic psychiatry as a "*way of thinking* about both patient and clinician that includes unconscious conflict, deficits and distortions of intrapsychic structures, and internal object relations" (p. 991). Other authors focus on how diffuse the concept of psychoanalysis is. Eagle (1984) notes the ferment within psychoanalytic theory. He points to the wide range of criticisms and innovations, some of which call into question the basic Freudian tenets. He ends his work by calling for "recaptur[ing] the early psychoanalytic and even pre-psycho-analytic emphasis on the disclaimed versus claimed, the impersonal 'it' versus the personal 'I,' the dissociated versus the integrated . . . " (p. 212). Greenberg and Mitchell (1983) categorize the "current diversity of psychoanalytic schools of thought" in two basic groups: those like Freud, who build around a concept of drives and their vicissitudes, and those like

Sullivan and Fairbairn, who give primary importance to "relations with others" (p. 3).

In this chapter, we use the broadest of these definitions of psychoanalysis. We use "psychoanalysis and psychoanalytic psychotherapy" to mean a theory and practice with a focus on making the unconscious conscious; in which the range of unconscious material extends from internal drives through representations of relations with others. Our purpose is to describe how theorists and clinicians from various points on the psychoanalytic spectrum have understood substance abuse and its treatment.

Psychoanalytic theories are theories of *motivation*—of why, for example, a person initiates or maintains a dependence on a substance or substances. "Motivation" implies both needs a person has and an absence of awareness of these needs and of their significance. Such "needs" often conflict with each other, with social norms, and so on, and come into awareness and behavior first in the form of "symptoms."

Originally, for Freud, "symptom" was the form in which a repressed idea or memory comes to consciousness. It does so in an unrecognizable form, because it is distorted by psychological defense. Thus a symptom is a *compromise*. It is the product of *conflict* between the repressed idea and the defense against it (Laplanche & Pontalis, 1973, p. 76).

Whether or not one maintains the original Freudian conception of drive and defense, the concept of symptom—the outward expression of an internal conflict, or of the conflict between an internal need and some external limitation—is one of the enduring ideas of psychoanalysis. Bringing to consciousness the underlying conflict that has resulted in symptoms is a goal of psychoanalytic therapy. It is usually assumed that "making the unconscious conscious" is a major contributor to the alleviation of the symptom, though the distance between insight and cure is often a wide and troubling one.

Substance abuse is generally understood within this psychoanalytic concept of symptom. However the underlying conflicts are conceptualized, it is generally assumed in psychoanalytic theory that substance abuse is a response to such conflict. A history of psychoanalytic concepts of substance abuse is therefore by and large a history of the kind of symptom psychoanalysts have conceptualized substance abuse as being.

It is a seemingly logical next step, after identifying what substance abuse is symptomatic of, to say that understanding the "underlying cause" of the symptom is the key to its removal. Perhaps logical but not necessary or, in fact, always valid. Often, psychoanalytic *understanding* has been confused with psychoanalytic *cure,* to the detriment of both. Whether psychoanalytic understandings of substance abuse are veridical is one major question; whether and how they are helpful in treatment are conceptually separate ones.

HISTORY AND CONCEPTS

As the range of ideas and techniques in psychoanalysis as a whole is wide, with a long and involved history, so it has been for psychoanalytic treatment of substance abuse. In part, the evolution of the theory of substance abuse treatment mirrors changes in psychoanalysis as a whole. Blatt, McDonald, Sugarman, and Wilber (1984), in an important paper on psychodynamic theories of opiate addiction, note that early psychoanalysts failed to distinguish between types of addiction, viewing all addiction as "oral phenomena" with similar unconscious meanings (p. 161). This was at a time when the field as a whole was concerned with "id" issues: the study of the internally based drives and how they played out in the patient's world.

Beginning with Rado (1926), analysts looked to formulate different typologies of addiction, based on the substance used and the internal state of the user. These early typologies were developed through the prism of the then current psychoanalytic focus on drives and defensive structure— what was known as ego psychology, as psychoanalytic interest evolved toward how people developed their own adaptations to the world. As we will see, other and often more recent psychoanalytic conceptions have mirrored the shift in the theory to the concern, noted by Greenberg and Mitchell (1983) above, with relations with other people, often under the broad rubric of object relations.

In the Blatt et al. (1984) schema, psychoanalytic theories of motivation for opiate addiction fall into three categories. The first is the "establishment of a need-gratifying, symbiotic state"; the second, "a defense against critical, harsh and dysphoric self-judgment (e.g., guilt and shame)"; and the third, "defense against potential psychotic disintegration" (p. 163). The authors developed these categories by "integrating the traditional emphasis of drives and defensive functions with object relations theory" (p. 163).

CURRENT STATUS

In a recent article, we (Morgenstern & Leeds, 1993) survey and discuss the current status of psychoanalytic theories of substance abuse. Readers with an interest in pursuing the topic in greater depth are encouraged to refer to this article. Based on that discussion, we will summarize the range of current psychoanalytic thinking (necessarily leaving out important points from our larger discussion) and briefly discuss its strengths and limitations.

In contrast to a wide range of other disorders, psychoanalysis has made rather meager recent contributions to the understanding of substance abuse. There are many possible explanations for this. One is the perception that drug abuse either renders one unsuitable for psychoanalysis or is a sign of such disturbance and weakness in ego strength that one would be considered unsuitable in any case. Hence the widespread refusal to treat these patients and the tendency to refer them to 12-Step programs. Another is that a history of poor outcome in attempts at treatment (Brickman, 1988) left a widespread feeling that psychoanalysis was not a treatment of choice for these disorders. Nonetheless, several psychoanalytic thinkers have made important contributions to the understanding of substance abuse. Four current authors are of particular interest and significance: Leon Wurmser, Edward Khantzian, Henry Krystal, and Joyce McDougall.

All four thinkers view substance abuse as a particular instance of a more general kind of disorder or pathology which is familiar to students of psychoanalysis. As such, the four theorists span the range of current psychoanalytic theorizing in general: drive theory (Wurmser), object relations (Krystal), self psychology (Khantzian), and McDougall's theory of psychosomatic disturbance. We have organized the thinkers in a chart (Table 3.1), based on what each considers to be wrong with the substance abuser and what effect each thinks an abuser seeks from a drug.

While all thinkers are aware and make note of the physiological aspects of substance abuse and addiction, their main focus is on the psychological aspects of the process.

Wurmser

Wurmser sees himself in a traditional psychoanalytic drive-theory context. While he favors a "deeply grounded combination treatment," involving self-help groups, pharmacologic treatment, education, and family counseling (1985, p. 95), he reserves a primary place for traditional psychoanalysis in treatment of substance abuse disorders. It is his theory that substance abusers suffer from overly harsh and destructive superegos, which threaten to overwhelm the person with rage and fear. Substance abuse is an attempt to flee from such dangerous affects. These emotions are the result of traditional *conflicts* between psychic agencies, specifically, by the harshness of the superego.

TABLE 3.1. Contemporary Psychoanalytic Theories of Drug Dependence

Theorist	Prototypic pathology	Vulnerability	Wished-for effect
Wurmser	Neurotic conflict	Condemned self	Liberation
Khantzian	Self deficit	Damaged self	Repair/regulation
Krystal	Impaired object relations	Borderline self	Merger/ecstasy
McDougall	Psychosomatic disturbance	Externalizing self	Avoidance/escape

Note. From Morgenstern and Leeds (1993, p. 196). Copyright 1993 by the American Psychological Association. Reprinted by permission.

Wurmser thinks actual, overwhelming early trauma are the origins of this state of being (1984, p. 230). He speaks of "unusually severe *real* exposure to violence, sexual seduction, and brutal abandonment, and/or of *real* unreliability, mendacity, betrayal, and abandonment, and/or of *real* parental intrusiveness or secretiveness" (p. 253). Such events lead to hostility to authority, rebelliousness, and defiance. They also lead to a harshness of internal authority and doubts about one's basic worth. One of his patients speaks of "a shadowy feeling of massive guilt, almost of mythical proportions" (1985, p. 90).

Drugs serve at least temporarily to disable the threatening internal authority and to neutralize the feelings of doubt and anxiety that appear so overwhelming. However, in disabling the superego, drugs do not affect only the specific, unwanted feelings and thoughts; they severely limit other superego functions as well. These include internal stability of mood and affect, the "ego ideal," self-observation, understanding of the boundaries of outer reality, and self-care (1984, p. 232). This accounts for the way substance abusers present to the therapist. They are often grandiose, avoidant, and manipulative; they are unaware of the dangers of their behavior. All this fits within Wurmser's notion of the use of drugs as an "archaic, global" way to avoid the feelings and impulses of pain, anxiety, and shame that so threaten the substance abuser.

Given this understanding, Wurmser's main focus in psychoanalytic treatment is the analysis of the superego. He believes that a moralistic stand toward addicts' behavior is counterproductive in that the problem is not too little superego but too much. The therapist needs a "strong emotional presence" and "an attitude of warmth, kindness and flexibility" (1985, p. 94).

Khantzian

Khantzian has developed a widely known group psychotherapeutic treatment for substance abusers. His work is based on the conception that *deficits,* not conflicts, underlie the problems of substance abusers. That is, weaknesses and inadequacies in the "ego" or "self," rather than conflicts between psychic agencies, are at the root of the problem.

For Khantzian, holes in the organization of the self—how a person protects, regulates, cares for, and thinks of him/herself—lead a person to seek the particular effect of a drug that will counteract the deficit. Khantzian is the only one of the four here surveyed who gives this degree of importance to the specific "drug of choice" for the abuser. For example, opiate addicts seek the drug's antiaggressive effect:

> Our experience suggests that the problems with aggression in such individuals are in part a function of an excess reservoir of this intense affect—partly constitutional and partly environmental in origin—interacting with psychological (ego) structures which are underdeveloped or deficient and thus fail to contain such affect. (1980, p. 35)

> On close examination, we have been impressed repeatedly that the so-called "high" or euphoria produced by opiates is more correctly a relief of dysphoria associated with unmitigated aggression. (1980, p. 32)

Cocaine addicts on the other hand exhibit a different range of predisposing factors:

1. Pre-existent chronic depression (dysthymic disorder)
2. Cocaine abstinence depression
3. Hyperactive/restless/emotional lability syndrome or attention-deficit disorder
4. Cyclothymic or bipolar illness. (Khantzian & Khantzian, 1984, p. 758)

Although difficulties in affect regulation and tolerance are common in all, the specific affects and the level of disturbance vary widely in Khantzian's schema. He does not consider abusers to be necessarily as disturbed as Wurmser or indeed the next two theorists do.

Khantzian and his colleagues have developed a modified dynamic group therapy (MDGT) (Khantzian, Halliday, & McAuliffe, 1990) to address the characterological underpinnings of substance abuse. The four foci of the groups are "1) affect tolerance, 2) the building of self-esteem, 3) the discussion and improvement of interpersonal relationships, and 4) the development of appropriate self-care strategies among the substance abusers" (McLellan, Woody, Luborsky, & O'Brien, 1990, pp. ix–xii).

Krystal

Krystal offers two theories of why individuals abuse substances. It is not clear if and how the two relate, but each makes an important contribution. Both presuppose severe disturbance in early development.

One theory is based on an object relations understanding of pathology. The drug is experienced by the abuser symbolically as a primary maternal object. That is, the drug stands in for the functions usually attributed to an actual maternal figure. The addict relates to the drug based on the disturbed pattern of relationship to such maternal figures as he/she has experienced developmentally. As Krystal says, "the drug dependent patient craves to be united with his ideal object, but at the same time dreads it" (1977, p. 243). This is a variant of borderline pathology. Krystal, like several other analysts (Kernberg, 1975; Rinsley, 1988), conceptualizes substance abuse in this light. The abuser's relation to the drug of abuse is an acting out in adulthood of primitive, infantile fantasies. Thus, the usual intense, unstable personal relations, rageful behavior, problems with self-care, and compulsive substance abuse are all part of an ongoing destructive drama. Krystal (1978) sees this as the "basic dilemma" of the substance abuser.

The second theory Krystal employs centers on the abuser's disturbed affective functions. This theory is known as "alexithymia."

Krystal believes that addicts differ from others in that they do not recognize the cognitive aspects of feeling states. That is, instead of experiencing differentiated feelings as "sad," "angry," "happy," and so forth, alexithymics experience global physiological states and tensions. This makes it difficult to use emotions as guides to self-understanding and eliminates or to some extent cripples an important source of information and feedback. It means one cannot read the significance of specific arousal states; and arousal itself becomes a source of anxiety. Therefore, one attempts to eliminate it by sedation or discharge. Substance abuse is one method of such sedation or discharge.

Krystal believes that severe disturbance in object relations is at the base of substance abuse. This is in contrast to the "conflict" or "deficit" models above. He is also more pessimistic about the treatment of substance abusers, as one would be with any such severe borderline pathology.

He advocates treatment in a program setting, with several therapists, to dilute transference, which would otherwise become too intense and possibly unmanageable. Although, like Khantzian, he recommends a focus on self-care and the tolerance of affects, he sees this as a first step in treatment, which must be accompanied by an analysis of the ambivalence and aggression being acted out by the patient through substance abuse.

McDougall

McDougall sees substance abuse as one of a variety of addictive behaviors, including eating disorders, compulsive sexual behavior, and addictive relationships. She sees all these as psychosomatic disorders. They are ways of dealing with distress that involve externalizing and physicalizing what are initially psychic disturbances. Psychosomatic phenomena are "all cases of physical damage or ill health in which psychological factors play an important role. These include: accident-proneness or the lowering of the immunological shield when under stress so that one more readily falls victim to infectious disease, as well as the problems of addiction, which are a 'psychosomatic' attempt to deal with distressful conflict by temporarily blurring the awareness of their existence" (1989, p. 19). Psychosomatic phenomena are a "discharge in action" rather than thought. Instead of elaborating feeling states internally, a psychosomatic solution is an externalization of the experience. Although everyone uses such defenses on occasion, substance abusers and others with psychosomatic disorders do so habitually. One outcome is that those feelings and experiences that would be painful or dangerous if actually experienced and felt internally are instead seen as unremarkable.

The psychosomatic–addictive solution is a defensive maneuver against unconscious emotions and fears. McDougall sees these as of a basic, akin to psychotic, nature: "deep uncertainty about one's right to exist and one's right to a separate identity . . . fear of losing one's body limits, one's feeling of identity or the control over one's acts" (1982, p. 382). Addiction is a way to avoid the internal feeling of deadness and emptiness that threatens the substance abuser. The use of drugs is part of the "false self" the person creates to ward off these painful and dangerous feelings.

While McDougall is more optimistic than many other analysts about the possible success of treatment with these patients, the extensive defenses against internal life make it a difficult and lengthy process. She advocates that attention be paid to the development of an internal life and, at the same time, to the patient's level of suffering and fear that increasing internal awareness may evoke.

CRITIQUE OF THEORY

Blatt et al. (1984) point out several difficulties with psychoanalytic studies of addiction from a rigorous methodological standpoint: "1) conclusions drawn from either single case studies or clinical reports based on only a few addicts, 2) a frequent failure to distinguish among different types of addiction or the level of severity of the addiction, 3) attempts to understand predispositional factors from data gathered after the addiction has taken place, and 4) difficulties establishing adequate control or comparison groups" (p. 161). These criticisms are similar to those often directed against psychoanalysis as a whole. They are, however, more telling in the case of addictions for two reasons. First, there is little evidence that unmodified psychoanalytic treatment is effective when provided to substance abusers. This is widely acknowledged even within the psychoanalytic community (Brickman, 1988; Gerald, 1992).

Second, significant advances have been made in understanding addictive behaviors during the last 20 years. Even contemporary analytic theories have largely ignored this important knowledge base. As a result, analytic theories and treatment techniques are out of step with an increasingly well-validated paradigm that views addictive disorders with an integrative biopsychosocial perspective. In looking at the current status of psychoanalytic theories and treatment, we must first summarize the new paradigms and their divergence from analytic models.

The analytic theories we have surveyed by and large share a common set of assumptions about substance abuse. First, they conceive of substance use as a symptom of an underlying disorder. As indicated, they differ concerning the nature of that disorder. Second, they tend to view the current psychological problems of the substance abuser as having existed prior to and causing the substance abuse. Third, they tend to conceive of substance use disorders as homogeneous, descriptively as well as etiologically. Although little attention is paid to definitions, all theories imply that compulsive use is categorically present or absent and degrees or dimensions of severity are not important. Similarly, each theorist views his/her theory as explaining all cases of substance use disorder and does not suggest that there may be different forms or subtypes of the disorder with different etiologies and psychodynamics. This is less so with a theorist such as Khantzian, who posits different varieties of self medication; however, he still puts all problems within this self-medication, drug-of-choice context. Fourth, most theories would consider the presence of substance use disorder in a patient as generally indicative of severe underlying pathology. As a result, most tend to be relatively pessimistic regarding the outcome of analytic treatment.

These assumptions diverge significantly from emerging knowledge about addictive disorders derived from empirical studies. The divergence of the psychoanalytic paradigm from empirically derived theories can be described succinctly as centering around three issues: (1) the homogeneity versus heterogeneity of substance abusers, (2) the impact of prolonged use on the personality and symptom picture of the substance abuser, and (3) the degree to which the pathogenesis of substance abuse can adequately be explained solely by psychogenic factors. We briefly summarize these points of divergence.

Homogeneity versus Heterogeneity

Studies from diverse areas such as psychiatric epidemiology (Regier et al., 1990), genetic epidemiology (Cloninger, 1987), clinical psychopathology (Babor, 1992), and treatment outcome (Kadden, Cooney, Getter, & Litt, 1989) indicate that substance abusers are a heterogeneous group differing in patterns of onset, course, symptom picture, family history and comorbid psychopathology. Of particular relevance are findings from the Epidemiologic Catchment Area study (Robins & Regier, 1991) indicating that substance abuse co-occurs with a wide variety of other disorders including personality disorders, bipolar disorders, schizophrenia, and anxiety disorders as well as alone without evidence of other psychopathology. This and other evidence (Meyer, 1986; Nathan, 1988) has led experts to reject the position that any one set of characterological features predisposes or is always involved in the pathogenesis of an addictive problem. This has indeed been acknowledged by analysts such as Krystal (1984), but the consequent expected reformulation of analytic positions has not yet been made.

In addition, empirically based paradigms consider specific patterns of substance use important in understanding and treating substance use problems. These paradigms reject the notion that substance use problems are either categorically present or categorically absent. Instead they view substance use problems as existing on a continuum of severity and attempt to provide clear operational criteria to establish whether use is normative or pathological. Such distinctions are important in determining appropriate treatment selection and goals.

Psychoanalytic approaches have not conceptualized this dimension and instead have focused on characterological issues. A significant limitation of analytic approaches is their failure to differentiate between patterns and severity of substance use. As a result, the analytic approach reinforces the homogeneity position by lumping together individuals with varying levels of problem severity.

The Impact of Substance Use
on Presenting Psychopathology

Psychoanalysts have generally assumed that the presenting psychological problems of substance-abusing patients were stable manifestations of underlying character and etiologically significant. However, current empirically based paradigms examining data from a variety of sources suggest that presenting psychological problems of substance abusers may be transient and may be the consequence rather than the cause of substance abuse. In particular, many have argued that the pharmacologic effects (e.g., on mood and anxiety) of substances and the loss of important social reinforcers that occurs during prolonged use are often responsible for the significant level of psychopathology found in substance abusers presenting for treatment. When considering the issue of additional psychopathology, empirical paradigms would classify substance users into a minimum of three types: (1) those with no additional problems, (2) those whose psychological problems are secondary to substance use, and (3) those whose psychopathology predates their substance use. Implications for the treatment of these groups would differ. Those with secondary psychopathology may not require additional treatment because their symptoms may remit after a period of abstinence, whereas those with primary psychopathology would require additional treatment. This can be contrasted to the analytic position that all substance abusers suffer from primary characterological problems and all require extensive treatment to address these problems.

Zinberg (1970), from within the psychoanalytic camp, has addressed these concerns by stressing the importance of drug, set, and setting in the development of addictive disorders. "Drug" is the pharmacologic effect of the substance, "set" is the frame of mind of the user; and "setting" is the social and environmental context in which the user finds him/herself (p. 5). He presents a critique of psychoanalytic thinking conceptually similar to that presented here, stressing the inadvisability of reading backward from substance abuse to "underlying" characterological issues.

The Pathogenesis of Substance Use Disorders

There is increasing empirical support for the dependence syndrome concept as a model to describe pathogenic processes in substance use disorders (Ziedonis & Kosten, 1993; Morgenstern, Langenbucher, & Labouvie, 1994). Overall, current consensus holds that most addictive behaviors are multiply determined by cultural, psychological, behavioral, and biological forces. In addition, a variety of clinical and laboratory studies offers strong evidence that more severe substance use is driven by biobehavioral forces and that cultural and psychological factors are of secondary importance (Babor, 1992).

Figure 3.1 illustrates this notion in a somewhat simplified manner. On the left, the dependence syndrome model is used to portray a transition from socially sanctioned drug use to mild, moderate, and severe forms of dependence. On the right are the dominant underlying mechanisms that control use at the various stages of the transition. Normal use is largely controlled by cultural and social factors. For instance, social modeling influences beliefs concerning the positive effects of alcohol and drugs. However, certain select individuals develop personal idiosyncratic beliefs in the power of alcohol or drugs to provide escape from painful affects or to escape from social responsibilities. For these individuals, substance use becomes driven by a need to regulate internal states and consumption of drugs deviates from normal to pathological use. Either because of internal conflicts or deficits or because of severe and/or prolonged stressors, these individuals are particularly vulnerable to the immediate positively reinforcing quality of drugs (i.e., their ability to alter mood quickly and effectively). At this level of mild dependence, motives and structures described by analytic theories may be the dominant underlying mechanisms that determine use.

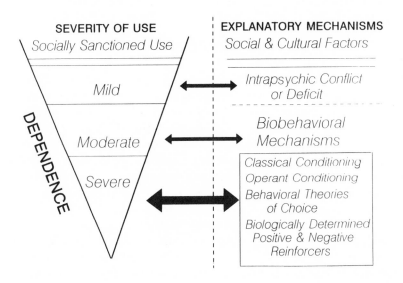

FIGURE 3.1. The relationship between dependence severity and pathogenesis.

However, if at this point drinking or drug use increases, an entirely different set of forces related to learning theory and biologically mediated reinforcement comes into play to determine use. Some of these biobehavioral mechanisms are listed in the figure. While it is beyond the scope of this chapter to describe these mechanisms, of particular importance is the notion that environmental stimuli—people, places, and things—become paired with biologically determined positive and negative reinforcers. With increasing use, concentrated cycles of reciprocal reinforcement occur and these stimuli function as powerful reinforcers which elicit overwhelming cravings. In addition, new studies indicate that alcohol and drugs act directly on pleasure and pain centers in the brain and thus are uniquely powerful reinforcers (Wise, 1988).

In sum, empirically based theories postulate that the biobehavioral mechanisms operative in moderate and severe dependence offer the most adequate explanation for the power, tenacity, and seemingly irrational character of drug addiction. In support of this position, they note that all widely used and effective treatments, whether drawn from behavioral or self-help traditions, use techniques designed to counter these biobehavioral mechanisms. Analysts have usually attributed the poor efficacy of insight-oriented techniques to the severe psychopathology of the addict. A more parsimonious explanation may be that insight does not work at moderate or severe levels of dependence because the dominant nature of the mechanisms driving addiction are not primarily psychological in nature.

CONCLUSION

What, then, is the future of psychoanalytic substance abuse treatment? Based on the above, it is not hard to see why there is currently a crisis of confidence from within psychoanalyis in the efficacy of psychoanalytic understanding and treatment of substance abuse. Brickman (1988), in a representative view, states that traditional psychoanalytic approaches to the treatment of addictions have been lacking in effectiveness. He questions the psychoanalytic presupposition that substance abuse patterns can be influenced by insight (p. 360). Several recent contributions to the literature advocate the use of 12-Step programs such as Alcoholics Anonymous as adjuncts to psychoanalytic psychotherapy (e.g., Brickman, 1988; Gerald, 1992). These approaches in essence divide the treatment of the abuser into two parts: The substance is addressed in 12-Step programs; character issues are addressed in psychoanalysis. Others would suggest that psychodynamic treatment not even begin until the resolution of the substance abuse problem and an extended period of abstinence (Kaufman,

1994). At the same time, there is an increasing interest in integrating various perspectives within the substance abuse field, and psychodynamic theorists and practitioners have been a part of this. One of the many examples is the Second Annette Overby Memorial Symposium, a meeting held in 1992, sponsored by the National Psychological Association for Psychoanalysis, entitled *Working with Alcoholics and Substance Abusers in Private Practice.*

It is clear that the field is in a period of flux, with the challenge of a new integration looming. Along with a growing contribution of research in understanding substance abuse patterns, psychoanalytic perspectives in understanding and treating addictive disorders have an important contribution to make. It seems clear that substance abusers are a heterogeneous group, and not all suffer from any one form of character pathology. Nevertheless, studies show that a significant portion do have character problems (Morgenstern, Langenbucher, Labouvie, & Miller, 1994). To date, there are no professional psychological treatments, with the exception of Khantzian's MDGT, that specifically target character problems within the context of substance abuse treatment. Whatever the empirical evidence shows about the overall psychoanalytic conceptions, it is imperative that clinicians make an attempt to understand the person who suffers, and not just "the substance abuser" in the abstract. This unified person, with thoughts, fears, needs, and anxieties that may or may not be related to substance abuse, is too often ignored in the design of treatments and the conceptualization of "who" a substance abuser is. Psychoanalytic theories will be crucial in addressing these concerns and in the creation of a new synthesis of empirical and clinical insight in the understanding and treatment of substance abuse.

REFERENCES

Babor, T. F. (1992). Nosological considerations in the diagnosis of substance use disorders. In M. Glantz & R. Pickens (Eds.), *Vulnerability to drug abuse.* Washington, DC: American Psychological Association Press.

Blatt, S., McDonald, C., Sugarman, A., & Wilber, C. (1984). Psychodynamic theories of opiate addiction: New directions for research. *Clinical Psychology Review, 4,* 1–34.

Brickman, B. (1988). Psychoanalysis and substance abuse: Toward a more effective approach. *Journal of the American Academy of Psychoanalysis, 16*(3), 359–379.

Cloninger, C. R. (1987). Neurogenetic adaptive mechanisms in alcoholism. *Science, 236,* 410–416.

Eagle, M. (1984). *Recent developments in psychoanalysis*. New York: McGraw-Hill.

Gabbard, G. O. (1992). Psychodynamic psychiatry in the "Decade of the Brain." *American Journal of Psychiatry, 149*(8), 991–997.

Gerald, M. (1992). Working with alcoholics and drug abusers in private practice: A psychoanalytic-chemical dependency model. *Psychology of Addictive Behaviors, 6*(1), 5–13.

Greenberg, J. R., & Mitchell, S. A. (1983). *Object relations in psychoanalytic theory*. Cambridge, MA: Harvard University Press.

Kadden, R. M., Cooney, N. L., Getter, H., & Litt, M. D. (1989). Matching alcoholics to coping skills or interactional therapies: Posttreatment results. *Journal of Consulting and Clinical Psychology, 57,* 698–704.

Kaufman, E. (1994). *Psychotherapy of addicted persons*. New York: Guilford Press.

Kernberg, O. (1975). *Borderline conditions and pathological narcissism*. New York: Jason Aronson.

Khantzian, E. J. (1980). An ego–self theory of substance dependence. In D. J. Lettieri, M. Sayers, & H. W. Pearson (Eds.), *Theories of addiction* (NIDA Research Monograph No. 30, DHHS Publication No. ADM 80–967). Washington, DC: U.S. Government Printing Office.

Khantzian, E. J., Halliday, K. S., & McAuliffe, W. E. (1990). *Addiction and the vulnerable self: Modified dynamic group therapy for substance abusers*. New York: Guilford Press.

Khantzian, E. J., & Khantzian, N. J. (1984). Cocaine addiction: Is there a psychological predisposition? *Psychiatric Annals, 14*(10), 753–759.

Krystal, H. (1977). Aspects of affect theory. *Bulletin of the Menninger Clinic, 41,* 1–26.

Krystal, H. (1978). Self-representation and the capacity for self-care. *Annual of Psychoanalysis, 6,* 209–246.

Krystal, H. (1984). Character disorders: Characterological specificity and the alcoholic. In E. M. Pattison & E. Kaufman (Eds.), *Encyclopedic handbook of alcoholism*. New York: Gardner Press.

Laplanche, J., & Pontalis, J. B. (1973). *The language of psychoanalysis*. New York: Norton.

McDougall, J. (1982). *Theaters of the mind: Illusion and truth on the psychoanalytic stage*. New York: Basic Books.

McDougall, J. (1989). *Theaters of the body*. New York: Norton.

McLellan, A. T., Woody, G. E., Luborsky, L., & O'Brien, C. P. (1990). Foreword. In E. J. Khantzian, K. S. Halliday, & W. E. McAuliffe, *Addiction and the vulnerable self: Modified dynamic group therapy for substance abusers*. New York: Guilford Press.

Meyer, R. (1986). How to understand the relationship between psychopathology and addictive disorders: Another example of the chicken and egg. In R. E. Meyer (Ed.), *Psychopathology and addictive disorders*. New York: Guilford Press.

Morgenstern, J., Langenbucher, J., & Labouvie, L. (1994). The generalizability of the dependence syndrome across substances: An examination of some properties of the proposed DSM-IV dependence criteria. *Addiction, 89,* 1105–1113.

Morgenstern, J., Langenbucher, J., Labouvie, L., & Miller, K. (1994, August). *The comorbidity of alcoholism and Axis II disorders in clinical population.* Paper presented at the annual meeting of the American Psychological Association, Los Angeles.

Morgenstern, J., & Leeds, J. (1993). Contemporary psychoanalytic theories of substance abuse: A disorder in search of a paradigm. *Psychotherapy, 30,* 194–206.

Nathan, P. (1988). The addictive personality is the behavior of the addict. *Journal of Consulting and Clinical Psychology, 56,* 183–188.

National Psychological Association for Psychoanalysis. (1992). *Working with alcoholics and substance abusers in private practice.* Second Annette Overby Memorial Symposium, New York, NY.

Pine, F. (1990). *Drive, ego, object and self.* New York: Basic Books.

Rado, S. (1926). The psychic effects of intoxicants: An attempt to evolve a psychoanalytical theory of morbid cravings. *Internal Journal of Psychoanalysis, 7,* 396–413.

Rinsley, D. B. (1988). The dipsas revisited: Comments on addiction and personality. *Journal of Substance Abuse Treatment, 5,* 1–7.

Robins, L. N., & Regier, D. A. (1991). *Psychiatric disorders in America.* New York: Free Press.

Wise, R. A. (1988). The neurobiology of craving: Implications for the understanding and treatment of addiction. *Journal of Abnormal Psychology, 97,* 118–132.

Wurmser, L. (1984). The role of superego conflicts in substance abuse and their treatment. *International Journal of Psychoanalytic Psychotherapy, 10,* 227–258.

Wurmser, L. (1985). Denial and split identity: Timely issues in the psychoanalytic psychotherapy of compulsive drug users. *Journal of Substance Abuse Treatment, 2,* 89–96.

Ziedonis, D., & Kosten, T. (1993). Behavioral pathology. In J. Langenbucher, B. McCrady, W. Frankenstein, & P. Nathan (Eds.), *Addictions research and treatment.* New York: Pergamon Press.

Zinberg, N. E. (1970). *Drug, set, and setting.* New Haven: Yale University Press.

CHAPTER 4

Exploration in the Service of Relapse Prevention: A Psychoanalytic Contribution to Substance Abuse Treatment

DANIEL S. KELLER

Advances in substance abuse treatment over the past two decades have been stimulated largely by developments from within the cognitive-behavioral, 12-Step/disease model, family therapy, and pharmacotherapeutic orientations. Increasingly, treatment as it is currently practiced relies on one or more of the therapeutic strategies deriving from these perspectives (Institute of Medicine, 1989). In particular, cognitive-behavioral approaches to addictions treatment (e.g., Marlatt Gordon, 1985; Monti, Abrams, Kadden, & Cooney, 1989) have begun to demonstrate both effectiveness (e.g., Carroll, Rounsaville, & Gawin, 1991) and increasing use across theoretical orientations (Morgenstern & McCrady, 1992).

During precisely this same period, a number of fairly well-developed psychoanalytic models on the nature of substance use disorders have emerged (e.g., Khantzian, 1980; Krystal, 1975; Krystal & Raskin, 1970; Wurmser, 1978). In addition, several psychodynamically-informed treatment approaches, which have been influenced to a greater or lesser degree by these models, have been generated (e.g., Galanter, 1993; Kaufman, 1994; Khantzian, Halliday, & McAuliffe, 1990). Yet by and large psychoanalytic ideas on substance abuse and its treatment have failed to find a place within the treatment techniques of most practitioners treating substance abusers (Leeds & Morgenstern, 1995, Chapter 3, this volume). This chapter examines the potential for a more robust psychoanalytic contribution to substance abuse treatment. To do so, I will (1) review current psychoanalytic psychotherapy indicating why it needs substantial modification in the treatment of substance use disorders; (2) provide a rationale for integrating aspects of psychoanalytic technique with cognitive-behavioral treatment for addictive disorders; and (3) illustrate how such an integrated psychoanalytic/cognitive-behavioral approach to substance abuse treatment, in which selected exploration of the substance abuser's attitudes, defenses, conflicts, and feelings as they are revealed within the moment-to-moment process of therapy, may be used to facilitate engagement in treatment and cognitive-behavioral relapse prevention.

One final word of introduction: Throughout the chapter psychodynamic therapy refers to the broad range of insight-oriented therapies based on psychoanalytic principles (e.g., Luborsky, 1984; Wallerstein, 1986) and not to orthodox or classical psychoanalysis per se (e.g., Greenson, 1967).

CONTEMPORARY PSYCHOANALYTIC PSYCHOTHERAPY

Psychoanalytic psychotherapy has undergone enormous development since Freud first invented it (e.g., Breuer & Freud, 1893–1895; Freud, 1894, 1896, 1905). Yet until relatively recently these developments, many of which are now decades old, have not been fully understood and appreciated by therapists of other orientations (see Safran & Siegel, 1990, for a notable exception). It has been my impression that many nonanalytically oriented therapists often believe that psychoanalytic psychotherapy focuses almost exclusively on "deep" unconscious conflicts rooted in the distant past and that such conflicts can be resolved only through "id interpretations," generally of an Oedipal cast. No doubt, at one time much analytic therapy was conducted along these lines as, for example, in Freud's (1905) "Dora" case. Yet the old caricature of a silent, depriving, incognito analyst whose utterances are limited to foisting interpretations, such as "You wanted to kill your father," on an otherwise reluctant or suggestible patient is certainly much less true today than a century ago and is more likely to be found in a cartoon in the *New Yorker* magazine than in the Park Avenue consulting room of a New York City analyst. For one thing, psychoanalysts have long recognized that for interpretations of repressed unconscious material to have any therapeutic effect, they must be preceded by an analysis of the elaborate layering of the patient's characteristic ego defenses and resistances (e.g., Fenichel, 1941; Freud, 1923; Greenson, 1967; Reich, 1933). Much of what constitutes contemporary psychoanalytic therapy is an analysis of such resistances (Schafer, 1976). Moreover, nowadays the analytically oriented clinician tends to focus on the here-and-now experience of the patient as revealed in the moment-to-moment process of their psychotherapeutic relationship (Gill, 1982; Schlesinger, 1981, 1982). Transference and resistance, for example, are regarded as having as much to do with the patient's present experience of him/herself, the therapist, and the therapeutic situation as they have to do with their infantile moorings. Furthermore, contemporary psychodynamic clinicians are far less likely to regard a patient's symptoms as the expression of a specific, circumscribed, drive–defense conflict the resolution of which is brought about by one fundamental penetrating insight into archaic experience but rather as the expression of well-integrated aspects of the patient's personality or character which ramify throughout the patient's contemporary life. As Wheelis (1973) put it: "The symptom does not afflict the patient, it *is* the patient" (p. 17). Thus, the locus of change in psychoanalytic therapy is the person, not symptoms. Much of the work of therapy investigates and attempts to alter the contemporary characteristic ways that the patient acts, feels, and relates to others.

An open-ended exploration and understanding of the meanings of these phenomena are the stuff of psychoanalytic psychotherapy, broadly speaking. Such exploration tends to reveal attitudes, postures, stances, feelings, ways of relating to others, and ways of thinking about things of which the patient has had perhaps only a dim intimation but about which he/she has been confused, puzzled, disturbed, or perplexed often over a period of many years. In the course of this exploration it is the therapist's task, in Shapiro's apt phrase, to "introduce the patient to himself" (1989, p. 10). In so doing, the patient may come to see that the very complaints that motivated him/her to seek treatment in the first place are brought about precisely through these characteristic yet obscure ways in which he/she thinks, feels, and relates. For example, a patient who wants a satisfying, intimate relationship but can never seem to find the right partner may come to discover a deep-seated fear of intimacy expressed perhaps only as an oddly peculiar uncomfortable feeling, vaguely experienced, followed by a curious loss of interest in the other when each new relationship "threatens" to become more intimate. Such an "insight" serves not merely as an end in itself but as yet another starting point for further exploration into yet other facets of the patient's experience. While the patient's fear of intimacy may have been forged initially in his earliest conflicts with parents—perhaps in how he learned to love—it is now likely that this and other unconscious conflicts have achieved a kind of autonomy, have become typical, characteristic modes of "being-in-the-world" (Binswanger, 1946). Insight into the *initial conflict* may be useful as a kind of basic formulation—a working hypothesis—but therapy must explore the myriad unknown ways in which this initial as well as other conflicts have been transmuted and now interpenetrate the patient's contemporary life.

In order for the patient's characteristic ways of thinking, feeling, and relating to emerge in therapy, the therapeutic situation is deliberately ambiguous. Apart from patients agreeing to communicate whatever occurs to them as best they can—the so-called basic rule of free association (Freud, 1900, p. 102)— there are no rules or directives for patients to follow. In contrast, the therapist reveals relatively little about him/herself. One of the results of such an ambiguous situation is that the patient's unconscious and preconscious fantasies as well as his defenses against them begin to emerge and, in particular, in relation to the therapist (i.e., the transference). Transference refers to the human inclination to distort one's experience of others based on fantasy rather than reality considerations and is potentially more likely under ambiguous circumstances. Transference distortions occur in all of us, as anyone who has gone on a job interview or out on a first date can attest. In therapy, transferences are at first more or less isolated reactions. As therapy develops, however, the patient's transference relationship to the therapist tends to blossom into what is known as a *transference neurosis* wherein the patient's prototypic pathology is "relived" or enacted. This provides the therapist the opportunity of working *in vivo* with the pathological aspects of the patient's personality. It is through the interpretation of the transference that the patient's pathological symptoms and character traits may be worked through and ultimately resolved. It is well beyond the scope of this chapter to discuss transference and its interpretation in any depth. The point I wish to make here is that the treatment situation is purposely designed to be ambiguous and nondirective so that these unconscious phenomena—especially the transference—may emerge.

Several important advances in psychoanalytic clinical theory which have evolved over the years deserve mention. These advances have had an enormous impact on contemporary technique and require a brief explication in order to understand many of the technical recommendations that follow in this chapter. First, in the early years in which psychoanalytic therapy was practiced, the central technical goal involved unearthing repressed wishes; that is, making the unconscious conscious. However, it was not long before analysts realized that in order for this to have a therapeutic effect, the patient's resistances—the dynamic, defensive forces that led to the repression in the first place—had to be analyzed first (Freud, 1912). This fact as well as other considerations actually led Freud (1923, 1926) to revamp his entire model of the mind ushering in the beginning of psychoanalytic ego-psychology. Thereafter, clinical work focused primarily on the patient's ego, not on the repressed unconscious (Fenichel, 1941; Greenson, 1967). In so doing, the therapist helps prepare the patient's ego to cope better with disturbing unconscious thoughts when they do emerge. In practice, this means that psychoanalytic therapists avoid attempting to "reach behind" the patient's resistances in order to "pull out" the unconscious material. Rather, resistances must be explored and worked through first. Greenson (1967), in his classic treatise on technique, summarized the technical rule that resulted from this change thusly: "Analyze resistance before content, ego before id, begin with the surface" (p. 137).

Second, when analysts began to focus on characterological patterns and traits (Reich, 1933), the therapist's attention expanded to include not only *what* the patient said (i.e., the content of the patient's communications to the therapist) but *how* the patient communicated; that is, the manner, form, and style in which the patient interacted with the therapist (i.e., the process of the patient's communications). A thought followed by a silence, a shifting emotional attitude, a stilted way of talking, a forced facial expression—all these and a multitude of other ways of behaving may indicate important resistances and require that the therapist remain attuned as much to how the patient thinks, feels, and relates as to what the patient thinks, feels, and relates. As we shall see later, these technical skills may be employed usefully in substance abuse treatment.

Despite the fact that no other therapy has yet evolved which permits so full an exploration of the total personality, there remain significant problems in recommending such unmodified psychoanalytic therapy as the *central* form of treatment for addictive disorders. First, on the basis of present knowledge, it seems reasonably clear that once the addictive disorder has achieved sufficient severity and chronicity, extrapersonality factors—behavioral, cognitive, environmental, and biological—are essentially responsible for maintaining the disorder (Marlatt & Gordon, 1985; Wikler, 1973). This is not to say that unconscious conflicts may not have initially contributed to the development of the disorder, nor is it to suggest that aspects of personality functioning do not play their part as well in sustaining an addiction. However, at least in the early to middle phases of treatment—when relapse is most likely to occur—these latter psychological factors are better considered as relatively *peripheral* as contrasted with the central task of achieving and maintaining abstinence. Therapy, to be effective, requires behavior change because the disorder is governed by behavioral laws.

Second, psychoanalytic conceptualizations of addiction (e.g., Khantzian et al., 1990; Krystal & Raskin, 1970; Wurmser, 1985) regard substance abuse as essentially rooted in some form of *underlying*, psychological disorder (see Leeds & Morgenstern, Chapter 3, this volume) despite the growing consensus among researchers and clinicians of the multiple biological, behavioral, and environmental factors involved in the etiology of addiction. To be sure, these analytic theorists have contributed immensely to elucidating important personality dynamics and deficits in substance abusers such as severe superego pathology, poor affect tolerance and expression, and the like. Yet again, while attention to such personality factors is important, these factors are, in my opinion, relatively peripheral as compared with the centrality of behavior change. Indeed, as I try to show in the next section, recent psychodynamically informed approaches to addictions treatment include cognitive-behavioral skills-building components.

Third, cognitive-behavioral treatments have emerged that directly address these behavioral, cognitive, and environmental factors associated with the maintenance of addictive processes (e.g., Marlatt & Gordon, 1985; Monti et al., 1989), and these therapies are beginning to demonstrate efficacy in controlled clinical trials (e.g., Carroll, Rounsaville, & Gawin, 1991; Institute of Medicine, 1989; Miller & Hester, 1986).

Fourth, as any clinician who works with substance abusers knows, the therapist must be active, directive, and prescriptive in working with such patients. However, dynamic therapy requires precisely the opposite. In order to foster exploration, in order to permit the patient's resistances to emerge, in order to nurture the transference, the therapist remains purposely nondirective and nonprescriptive. Yet to proceed this way with substance abusers before abstinence has been achieved and stabilized, the therapist risks entering into a collusion with the patient in which the patient's wish for a magic cure (i.e., that he/she needs to feel better before changing) is reinforced by the therapist's belief that insight into intrapsychic conflict must precede change in behavior.

RATIONALE FOR A COMBINED TREATMENT

Given this somewhat pessimistic preamble it might be asked: Is there any role at all for psychoanalytic ideas in the treatment of substance use disorders? It should be clear from the foregoing that some form of cognitive-behavioral therapy is indicated in the treatment of addictive disorders, particularly those of sufficient severity and chronicity. This is so because, as noted above, the primary factors maintaining the addiction tend to be behavioral, cognitive, and environmental. Nevertheless, in my opinion, cognitive-behavioral therapy for addictions may be enhanced by attention to defenses, resistances, and unconscious conflicts as expressed in the psychotherapeutic process and relationship, traditionally the central focus of psychoanalytic psychotherapy. There are several reasons for this. First, cognitive-behavioral therapy is undertaken within an interpersonal context, no less so than psychodynamic therapy. This interpersonal relationship acquires significant meaning for patients if one wishes to pay attention to it (Safran & Siegel, 1990; Wachtel, 1977). A focus on the nuances of the interpersonal process in therapy may well influence relapse prevention and outcome. Second, substance abusers exhibit a broad range of unconscious defense mechanisms, which often contribute significantly to exposures to risky situations and irrational thoughts and feelings which also predispose to relapse (e.g., Kaufman, 1994; Krystal, 1975; Wurmser, 1978). An understanding of defenses may also assist in surmounting various difficulties in acquiring and maintaining skills. Third, like other people, substance abusers experience unconscious conflicts that may also lead to relapse if left unattended (Kaufman, 1994). Fourth, the psychodynamic makeup of an individual will often exert a significant influence on how a structured task such as skills acquisition is approached and performed (Rapaport, Gill, & Schafer, 1968).

In recent years a combined psychodynamic/cognitive-behavioral approach to the treatment of general psychiatric disorders has found growing acceptance from within both psychodynamic (e.g., Wachtel, 1977) and cognitive-behavioral perspectives (e.g., Safran & Siegel, 1990). Moreover, initial integrative efforts have already begun to appear in the substance abuse field as well. In a recent book, Kaufman (1994) has delineated what he refers to as a pragmatic approach to the psychoanalytic treatment of addicted persons. In Kaufman's view, previous psychodynamic approaches to the therapy of alcoholics and addicts have met with little success because they have failed to sufficiently promote abstinence before engaging in psychodynamic exploration of the patient's conflicts. He describes a three-phase treatment in which the better part of the first two phases (i.e., the first 1 to 2 years of therapy) is spent attempting to secure and stabilize abstinence principally through rigorous application of cognitive-behavioral relapse prevention and 12-Step involvement. Psychodynamic therapy enters these phases only minimally, although a psychodynamic understanding of the patient is used to address patients with personality disorders and/or periodic intrapsychic conflicts that threaten sobriety. In the third phase, which Kaufman refers to as advanced recovery, therapy becomes more traditionally psychodynamic in the sense that the transference is permitted to develop more freely and is analyzed through an understanding of the transference–countertransference paradigms that emerge. Kaufman suggests that the typical conflictual themes that characterize this phase of treatment in addicts are mourning the loss of alcohol or other drugs as well as issues around intimacy and autonomy. These too are resolved within an understanding of the transference relationship.

Galanter (1993) has also recently described a treatment for substance abuse that combines both psychodynamic therapy and cognitive-behavioral methods, which he calls network therapy. Like Kaufman, Galanter believes that abstinence must be achieved and secured for therapy to be effective. Thus, the initial stages of his approach utilize cognitive-behavioral principles and techniques in order to achieve and maintain abstinence—but with a twist. The bulk of Galanter's cognitive-behavioral interventions are administered within the context of a network of supportive family members and friends who, along with the patient, meet regularly with the therapist. These network sessions, which augment the patient's concurrent individual treatment, focus on teaching the patient and his network the nature of craving as a classically conditioned response, identifying triggers and high-risk situations, and developing skills and strategies to prevent relapse. It is Galanter's contention that a patient's family and friends can be galvanized into a cohesive team in which network members actively partake in the patient's relapse prevention efforts, (e.g., in monitoring disulfiram [Antabuse] and executing avoidance strategies). In contrast to other forms of substance abuse treatment that involve family members (e.g., Stanton, Todd, & Associates, 1982), Galanter does *not* attempt to alter or restructure family systems, interpret "codependency," or in any way address network members' own psychopathology. Rather, when individual and/or group dynamics emerge, the therapist attempts to manage these as a good office manager might address staff difficulties.

Galanter (1993) does not expand at length on the nature of the patient's individual sessions because his volume is expressly concerned with the description of network therapy. However, in the early phase of treatment, psychodynamic conflicts or character traits are dealt with when they pose a threat to sobriety. For example, the network session of a patient who relapsed in the early phase of treatment focused on the cognitive and behavioral precipitants to the relapse and the development of more appropriate strategies. However, in the patient's next individual session attention was devoted to his marked impulsive character style, which had also played a role in his relapse (Galanter & Keller, 1994). According to

Galanter, once sobriety is stabilized, a more traditional psychodynamic treatment may unfold.

Although both Kaufman (1994) and Galanter (1993) have described innovative approaches in which the therapist utilizes techniques from both psychodynamic and cognitive-behavioral schools of thought, neither describes exactly how psychodynamic technique may be used to facilitate the cognitive-behavioral components of the treatment, though this is strongly implied in both. For instance, both recommend interpretation of unconscious conflict and character traits when these present a threat to abstinence. In the remainder of this chapter I attempt to illustrate more precisely how selected use of psychoanalytic technique may foster engagement in treatment and cognitive-behavioral relapse prevention.

INTEGRATED PSYCHOANALYTIC/
COGNITIVE–BEHAVIORAL THERAPY

An integrated model of psychodynamic and cognitive-behavioral therapy for substance abusers can be conceptualized as an admixture of supportive and expressive interventions (Schlesinger, 1969). In the early and middle phases of treatment, when the achievement and maintenance of abstinence are primary, the therapist will act in an essentially supportive, educative manner utilizing cognitive-behavioral techniques. However, when resistances, defenses, or unconscious conflicts pose a threat to treatment and/or sobriety, selective use of expressive–exploratory techniques are utilized. Conversely, in the advanced stage of treatment, when sobriety has been stabilized, a more expressive form of psychodynamic treatment may predominate in which unconscious conflicts are resolved within the traditional transference–countertransference matrix; however, selective reversion to supportive, cognitive-behavioral techniques is employed when abstinence is threatened.

In order to understand how cognitive-behavioral and psychodynamic components of this model interact, it may be helpful to briefly describe a purely didactic cognitive-behavioral approach to substance abuse treatment and then consider the central psychodynamic additions I am proposing here.

Cognitive-Behavioral Components

In general, the approach I am suggesting derives its cognitive-behavioral influence mainly from the relapse prevention model (RP) developed by Marlatt and Gordon (1985). Briefly, RP is essentially didactic and represents the supportive–educative emphasis of the integrated psychody-namic–cognitive-behavioral model. RP focuses on identification of a set of addiction-maintaining phenomena such as high-risk situations, condi-tioned cues for craving (triggers), and maladaptive thought processes operative within the patient's life, all of which increase the likelihood of relapse. In addition, RP addresses the substance abuser's general inclina-tion to unwittingly expose him/herself to such phenomena despite the effort to become sober (apparently irrelevant decisions). In this respect, as I try to show below, RP is quite compatible with psychodynamic clinical theory since such unwitting exposures are an illustration of unconscious motivation par excellence.

The RP approach is essentially psychoeducational in that it teaches patients to become aware of such addiction-related phenomena and assists them in developing coping skills and strategies that minimize the risk of exposure or the risk of using when exposure is unavoidable. In this respect the treatment is fairly straightforward, relying on common sense aug-mented by commitment to the change process. The goal is the achievement and maintenance of abstinence. Typical techniques might include avoid-ance of high-risk situations; understanding the nature of craving; strategies to endure craving, such as decision delay and self-monitoring; challenging maladaptive thoughts; drink refusal; and so forth (for a detailed discussion of these and related RP techniques for substance abuse treatment, see Marlatt & Gordon, 1985; Monti et al., 1989; Carroll, Rounsaville, & Keller, 1991; Kadden et al., 1992; and Morgan, Chapter 8, this volume).

Psychodynamic Components

In contrast to a purely didactic approach, the integrated psychodynamic–cognitive-behavioral model focuses selectively on the interpersonal proc-ess that develops between patient and therapist which may either facilitate or hinder skills acquisition and the attainment of abstinence. This inter-personal process can be viewed from a number of perspectives, but it may be most useful here to consider it from two interrelated vantage points: the working alliance and patient resistance. The working alliance (e.g., Greenson, 1967) refers to the ability of the patient to use his/her reason-able, observing ego to identify with the therapist's methods as they pursue mutually agreed on treatment goals. In contrast, resistance refers to the expression of defense within the treatment situation. As such, there may be times when the patient's resistances may temporarily impede his/her ability to maintain a good working alliance with the therapist. Such resistances may be blatant, such as noncompliance with treatment proce-dures, but more often are subtle or "quiet" such as a slight shift in the patient's attitude or nonverbal activity discordant with the patient's verbal communications (Schlesinger, 1982). At such times, the therapist in the integrated model would explore such resistances by interpreting defenses, unconscious conflicts, emotional or attitudinal shifts in the patient's demeanor, or the interpersonal process itself. The purpose of the exploration is to identify what is unconsciously bothering the patient at that moment in time so that a good working alliance may be reestablished and skills acquisition may proceed.

Clinical Illustrations

Let us now examine how psychodynamic exploration of the psychotherapeutic process can enhance RP efforts. I will focus on the assessment, early/middle, and advanced phases of treatment, respectively. Clinical examples are used to illustrate how selective exploration of ambivalence, resistances, defenses, painful affects, unconscious conflicts, and distorted cognitions may facilitate an otherwise cognitive-behavioral RP approach to treatment.

Assessment Phase: Addressing Ambivalence and Resistance

It is not uncommon for clinicians to think of the assessment or evaluation phase as somewhat distinct from treatment. In this view, assessment is a kind of information-gathering phase wherein the therapist amasses relevant data, arrives at a diagnosis, and recommends a treatment on which both patient and therapist agree. To be sure, we do gather a great deal of information during the assessment phase. For example, we would like to know the patient's substance abuse history in detail. We pay particular attention to when, how, and under what circumstances the patient's use began; how it made the patient feel; and how the patient's use has increased over time. We also want to know the patient's most recent use and whether he/she has developed tolerance or exhibits signs and symptoms of withdrawal. Moreover, we pay very special attention to previous attempts at abstinence and previous relapses. In addition to all this, we want to assess the problems the patient's substance abuse has caused in significant life areas (e.g., legal, financial, occupational, and with significant others such as family and friends). Finally, we want to make a careful assessment of the presence of concurrent psychiatric disorders. All this is important, indeed crucial, information for arriving at an accurate diagnosis and for tailoring an appropriately individualized treatment plan.

In the assessment phase, however, additional attention to the *way* the patient communicates offers another opportunity and one which, from the psychoanalytic viewpoint, may actually facilitate information-gathering activities. It is the opportunity for *engaging* the patient in the treatment process. Simply because a patient has presented in our consulting room does not mean that the patient feels that treatment is an undertaking upon which he/she wishes to embark. Indeed, quite a number of substance abusers present for treatment under a variety of conditions of duress, such as the importunings of a spouse, an employer, or the legal system. And even patients who present more or less willingly usually have some reservations. Our primary question must be: Does substance abuse treatment make sense to *the patient*? Not to his spouse, not to his employer, not to the courts, but to him?

The fact is that *ambivalence* typically characterizes the motivation of most patients (not just substance abusers) upon entering treatment. Sometimes the ambivalence is relatively mild and eliciting the array of negative consequences the substance use has engendered in the patient's life is enough to counteract the ambivalence, at least in the short run. At the other end of the spectrum, the patient may so disavow the need or desire for treatment that only external mandates ensure his/her participation. Usually, however, ambivalence is expressed more subtly. For example, the patient makes and keeps an initial appointment, but as we begin to query him his answers reveal hesitations of one sort or another. He "guesses" he has a problem despite a lifetime of unremitting drinking. Or, he may become more evasive or withholding about certain topics, thereby impeding our information gathering. The patient is physically present but not wholeheartedly psychologically present. Literally, he is in the office; figuratively, he has one foot in and one foot out the door.

The therapeutic task at this point is not to rid the patient of his ambivalence but to explore the curious obstacles he has put in his and our path. It may well be that the patient *does* feel the need for treatment but fears any number of implications it might entail.

For instance, a 34-year-old married alcoholic woman presents for an initial interview. Her mood is somewhat dysphoric and she states hesitantly that she "might" have a drinking problem, though her substance use history leaves little doubt that her problem is fairly severe. When I ask about her marriage, however, her dysphoria and hesitancy become intensified. Her answers are short, clipped, terse, and withholding. It is as if an invisible wall has gone up between us. I realize I have touched on a sore spot, but it is also clear that to proceed in this area *now* will likely only intensify her defensiveness. As we move on to other areas of her life, she begins to describe with much greater ease and animation a project she is involved with at work. I am struck by the difference in her overall psychological and emotional demeanor and say in a mildly upbeat way: "You know, as you talk about your project, you've really perked up." The patient reacts with a bit of a startle. She had not been aware of this significant shift in her mood until I had pointed it out to her. She continues to discuss her work a bit more and then falls silent. After a short period of quiet brooding, she openly begins to reevaluate her comparatively withholding attitude regarding her marriage. She then relates some serious difficulties in her marriage that are, not surprisingly, related to her drinking which she now states has "really gotten out of control lately."

Let us consider this clinical illustration further. First, by temporarily abandoning the pursuit of information and by focusing on the shifting emotional attitude of the patient, she is assisted in looking at herself in a way she was unwilling to do earlier. She is "introduced to herself," to quote Shapiro (1989) again. It is also important to note that the intervention was directed toward something positive—in this case the greater ease with which she began to communicate. Had I commented, for example, on her hesitancy to discuss her marriage she might have felt criticized. Or she might have grudgingly conceded the information I wanted. But it would not have been what *she* wanted to say at that point in time. It certainly would not have facilitated a good working alliance. Yet once she was able to acknowledge her concerns about her marriage, talking about her marital problems began to make sense to her and the previously held back information emerged easily. Second, this therapeutic fragment tells us much more than the extent of her marital problems or the extent of her drinking. It tells us that the patient is able to look at herself productively, that she has a good "observing ego," and that other similar interventions may also be indicated in working with this patient, particularly her resistances. Third, she becomes *engaged* in the therapeutic process. Whereas she starts out the interview stating that she "might" have a problem, she ends up with a new stance: namely, that she believes she does in fact have an alcohol problem and that it is related to a significant area of her life. She now has reasons for wanting to enter treatment.

Often therapists are tempted to avoid exploration of just these sorts of sore spots and just as often rationalize the avoidance as an attempt to build a positive rapport. Actually, such avoidance usually diminishes rapport in the long run. The patient will feel, in some corner of her mind, that she has "bested" or "hoodwinked" the therapist and how good can such a therapist be who can have the wool pulled over his/her eyes so easily? This is especially true for substance abusers.

To return to the clinical illustration: I do not suggest that this *particular* intervention would work with every patient. Patients vary in their degree of ambivalence and in their manner of expressing it. But I do think that the therapist's general attention to the process—in this case the patient's emotional attitude in relating her difficulties—can significantly enhance information-gathering efforts. In the above case, I think that the therapist's process comment made a decisive difference in the outcome of the session.

Early and Middle Phases of Treatment

In the early and middle phases of treatment the achievement and maintenance of abstinence are the central focus of therapy. Although there is debate within the literature regarding the feasibility of "controlled" drinking, as a practical matter, patients with moderate to severe substance abuse problems (i.e., most alcoholics, cocaine addicts, and heroin addicts) generally need to learn how to abstain and maintain their abstinence for treatment to succeed (Kaufman, 1994). This does not mean that the patient *must* be abstinent during all points of treatment. However, abstinence and its maintenance should be the central goals toward which both patient and therapist are striving. Generally, the early and middle phases occupy the first 6 to 9 months. It is here that RP techniques are most often utilized.

As delineated in cognitive-behavioral approaches (e.g., Carroll, Rounsaville, & Keller, 1991; Kadden et al., 1992; Marlatt & Gordon, 1985), treatment for substance abuse during these phases involves (1) identification of high-risk situations and classically conditioned cues (triggers) for craving and the development of strategies to limit exposure to them, (2) development of skills to successfully endure cravings and other painful affects, (3) learning how to challenge or better manage maladaptive thoughts about using, (4) learning how to avoid using when one is in an otherwise unavoidable high-risk situation, (5) generating a basic emergency plan for coping with high-risk situations in which other skills are not working, (6) learning to detect various ways in which one is "setting oneself up," and (7) generating pleasurable sober activities and relationships to offset feelings of emptiness and loss after removal of substance use from the patient's repertoire. During this phase, slips, lapses, and relapses are not uncommon and are regarded as opportunities to fine-tune one's future efforts to achieve abstinence.

How might the use of psychoanalytic technique facilitate this skills-building phase? I would like to focus on how knowledge of psychological defenses; attention to resistance and transference; and the use of free association, empathic listening, countertransference reactions, and inter-pretation might influence how one can promote abstinence and skills acquisition when working with (1) cravings, (2) apparently irrelevant decisions, (3) common maladaptive cognitions, (4) negative affects, and (5) intrapsychic conflict.

Working with Cravings. It has often been pointed out in the literature (e.g., Marlatt & Gordon, 1985; Wikler, 1973) that craving for substances is a classically conditioned response elicited by exposure to stimuli that have been repeatedly paired with substance use. Such stimuli are often *external*—such as bars, drug paraphernalia, substance-abusing friends and acquaintances, neighborhoods in which use occurred, and so forth—or *internal*—such as irrational thoughts or painful affect states which one has learned to temporarily abolish through substance use. In RP, the therapist teaches the patient the nature of the craving response by explain-ing Pavlov's learning paradigm and then helps the patient to develop strategies for limiting exposure to these conditioned cues as well as other ways to manage cravings once exposures have elicited the craving re-sponse.

Nevertheless, due to the nature of unconscious psychological defense mechanisms, not all craving is noticed or regarded as craving by the patient. For example, one chronically relapsing patient in group therapy for cocaine addiction, through the use of projection, would see signs of craving in other group members, though not in himself, generally in the week prior to *his* relapses.

Therapists who work with addicted people have long been aware of the use of the defense mechanism of denial in substance abusers. However, there has been an unfortunate tendency to mislabel other defensive processes as denial. One sometimes suspects that those who overuse the term "denial" are actually referring to a more general process, namely, resistance, which refers to the expression of all defenses within the treatment situation (Gill, 1982). Yet if we are going to help patients discover the many ways in which unconscious defenses operate so as to both express and disguise cravings, it is important to be as precise as possible. A good starting point is to study Anna Freud's (1936) classic articulation of this subject: *The Ego and the Mechanisms of Defense.* With respect to the use of defenses in substance abusers, Kaufman (1994) has provided an excellent discussion.

Although almost any defense mechanism may come into play, in my experience one of the most common defenses employed in the expression of craving is the defense of *displacement*. Displacement refers to an unconscious mental process through which feelings toward a person or object are transferred or shifted to some other person or object and experienced in relation to this new person or object (Fenichel, 1945). For example, transference is quintessentially a displacement (Greenson, 1967). With respect to craving, substance abusers frequently displace the urge to drink or use substances onto some other activity which may be extremely high risk but which they do not experience as risky at all. It is important to stress that the displacement takes place *unconsciously*. If, for example, a patient experiences a sudden urge to pay off the money he owes his dealer, it is not necessarily the case that he is aware of the desire to use drugs. If one told the patient at this point, "You really want to use drugs," it would likely increase his defensiveness, perhaps through the use of a variety of rationalizations.

Let us consider the operation of displacement in craving and the technique utilized to interpret it. A 33-year-old male alcoholic has been sober for approximately 2 months after beginning treatment in an outpatient chemical dependency rehabilitation program in which he has been receiving a combination of RP augmented by various 12-Step activities. During a group therapy session the patient, in the midst of relating to the group how well his recovery is going, casually adds that this upcoming weekend he is planning to go on the annual family fishing trip, which he eagerly looks forward to every year. He states this with a kind of avid enthusiasm and without the slightest trace of awareness that fishing trips are often high-risk situations because they are frequently accompanied by copious amounts of beer. Not too much time elapses before other group members inquire about the potential for beer to be present on the trip. The patient acknowledges that his uncle generally does bring four to six cases but states somewhat testily that he [the patient] is different now, he is in recovery, values his sobriety, and in any event is not going to drink. He adds that he "has" to go because it is also his uncle's birthday. The group becomes more confrontational (e.g., "You're in denial," "You're setting yourself up," "You're gonna drink, don't go"), which is followed by the patient, now somewhat angry, stating that his mind is made up, he is not going to drink, "I have to go!" After a brief silence, the patient looks up toward the therapist and asks what the latter thinks. The tone of the patient's voice sounds as if he expects the therapist to side with the group, but the therapist also senses a faint trace of honest curiosity in the way the patient asks the question. The therapist replies: "I think you want to go on this fishing trip *very* badly" and then adds somewhat ironically, "It sounds similar to a craving." The patient is slightly taken aback but then begins to mull over the therapist's comment. He has to admit that he had not thought about it that way but still believes he will not drink and reiterates his commitment to go on the trip. Nevertheless, his reiteration lacks the fire it had at the outset and seems somewhat empty, as if the patient were now only saving face. Two days later, at the next group therapy session, the patient informs the group that he has decided to forgo the fishing trip, adding that his recovery is more important.

I believe that this clinical vignette illustrates how the therapist's attention to the patient's displacement of craving from alcohol onto the fishing trip helps to facilitate the patient's RP efforts. It is important to note that the therapist does not say that the patient's desire to go on the trip masks his "real" desire to drink. Rather, the therapist states that the patient's desire to go contains an urgency that is similar to the urgency of a craving, something with which the patient is all too familiar and cannot reject out of hand. What makes the intervention effective is that it addresses what the patient is consciously experiencing (the urgency), not what is being hidden (the desire to drink), though it suggests a possible connection between this conscious experience and craving for alcohol in general. It is as if the patient must take this step first before he can even permit himself to entertain the possibility that he might actually want to drink on the fishing trip. The therapist addresses the defense rather than the motive underlying it.

It may be instructive to specify how a purely didactic RP approach might have differed from the one presented here. For instance, a didactically oriented RP therapist might have attempted to assist the patient in identifying the fishing trip as a high-risk situation in which cravings would emerge, in generating a list of pros and cons for going on the trip, and perhaps in utilizing the group to "brainstorm" or "problem-solve" a variety of alternative behaviors. From the psychodynamic point of view, however, such techniques are more likely to be effective when the patient is able to establish a good working alliance; that is, to identify with the therapist's methods and therapeutic goals. In this case, due to resistance, the patient was temporarily unable to identify with therapeutic behavior and goals he had largely embraced up to that point in the treatment. His resistance, as expressed in the displacement, had to be addressed first. He was then able to reestablish a good working alliance and was consequently able to "problem-solve."

Apparently Irrelevant Decisions. In working with substance abusers one is frequently impressed by the capacity of these patients to expose themselves to high-risk situations and conditioned cues with hardly the slightest awareness that they are headed for trouble. The patient who wanted to go on the fishing trip was certainly in that category. These sorts of setups are what Marlatt and Gordon (1985) have referred to as apparently irrelevant decisions. Essentially, the patient makes a decision or set of decisions that does not appear to be related to the desire to drink or use drugs but in fact brings the patient ever closer to risky environments in which cues for craving are likely to abound. It is as if these apparently irrelevant decisions are linked together in a chain, the last of which is the actual decision to use. However, it is often the case that the only decision the patient is aware of making is this final decision. In RP the therapist attempts to demonstrate that the final decision is only the last link in the chain of decisions, and skills are then taught to interrupt such decision chains earlier when cues, craving, and risky situations are more easily avoided.

From the psychoanalytic perspective one is impressed by the fact that such decisions, particularly the earlier ones, are experienced with varying degrees of unawareness. When one explores a chain of decisions, it is often difficult for the patient to remember very clearly what he/she was thinking and feeling at such decision points. From a psychodynamic perspective such vaguely articulated cognitive and affective states often indicate that unconscious factors are operative.

In fact, one is quite struck by the phrase itself—"apparently irrelevant decisions." It sounds so strangely psychoanalytic. After all, it was apparently irrelevant *thoughts* that Freud instructed his patients to report when he explained the basic rule of free association (Freud, 1900, p. 102). Let us consider how elicitation of the patient's associations may facilitate the articulation of a chain of apparently irrelevant decisions.

A 25-year-old single male cocaine abuser reports that he used cocaine during the interval between therapy sessions. Essentially, he had gotten off work and was driving home. Along the way he decided to take a different route and after awhile discovered that he was driving by a bar he used to frequent. He then decided to stop off, say hello, and have a soda. However, at the bar he told himself that as his problem was with cocaine, he could have a beer. After two beers he encountered a friend who "happened" to have a gram of cocaine—and the slip inevitably ensued. I would also like to note that the patient related these events in a bored, monotonous manner, which struck me as interesting.

In exploring the concept of apparently irrelevant decisions, the patient was able to see—somewhat intellectually—how his decisions to enter the bar and drink beer brought him closer to using cocaine. However, he reported that he was not aware of wanting to use cocaine until he ran into the friend. Moreover, he had greater difficulty connecting the events associated with the bar to taking a different route home. His experience of this action seemed limited to a sense of aimless drifting. I then asked whether he could recall what he was thinking or feeling around the time he decided to take the alternative route and he drew a blank. At this point I invited him just to let his thoughts flow and report what occurred to him. After a bit of silence, he reported that the word "relax" had popped into his mind, but it did not seem to have much significance. I then inquired, "What do you think of when you want to relax?" He paused for a moment, then broke out into a wide grin and said: "Gettin' high." Now the connection between the "apparently irrelevant" different route home and his ultimate decision to use had meaning. This also led him to recall that he had felt "uptight" at work that day and in fact had a fleeting thought about using, which he had brushed aside. When we explored what "uptight" meant (the patient tended to use this word somewhat indiscriminantly for many negative feelings), it turned out that he had felt bored. Thus, his uptight boredom led to a desire to "relax." Both the feeling and the cognition could now be used as red flags in the future.

Again let us attempt to distinguish the integrated approach from a purely didactic one. In the above case the didactic RP therapist might have attempted to educate the patient by explaining the concept of apparently irrelevant decisions and by illustrating how the patient's decisions appeared to be linked together. However, I doubt that such an approach alone would have produced in the patient the emotionally charged "aha" experience he had when we followed his associations. The concept now had experiential meaning and significance to him.

It has been my experience that apparently irrelevant decisions are often accompanied by just these sorts of obscure, fleeting, vaguely experienced words or feeling states that when fleshed out and explored help to reestablish the actual connections between the decisions. In this case, the word "relax" was a condensation of two thoughts into one, namely, "relax *and* get high." Obtaining the patient's associations was critical both in deciphering this condensed thought and in promoting RP skills.

Exploring Maladaptive Cognitions. It is quite common within the early and middle phases of treatment for patients to experience a variety of cognitions that may predispose to slips, lapses, or relapses. For instance, a patient may tell himself that "It would be all right to have just one drink," or that "It's okay to hang out in the bar; I just want to visit my friends," or "I'll keep some liquor in the house in case I have visitors." The tendency for patients to have these and a variety of similar thoughts is so common that Alcoholics Anonymous has developed the phrase "stinkin' thinkin'" to refer this class of cognitions, which captures their essence quite nicely.

From a psychodynamic perspective, these and other similar cognitions suggest that psychological defenses are at work. Many will recognize the defense of rationalization in the above examples. Cognitive-behavioral treatments recommend a variety of techniques to combat such rationalizations, such as challenging the thought or weighing the costs and benefits of drinking or using. It has been my experience, however, that such techniques work best the *poorer* the rationalization. For example, the thought that "I can have just one" is not as good a rationalization as "I'll keep some liquor around the house for guests." In the former, the intention to drink is explicit and can be challenged directly whereas in the latter the rationalization conceals the explicit intention to drink. While it is possible to challenge this latter thought, it may be met with a good deal of resistance. This is because effective rationalizations work precisely because they are *good* reasons. They are acceptable or "ego-syntonic" to the patient. In such cases, it may help to agree with the patient that there is some legitimacy in wanting to be a good host but point out that it becomes a problem in that it simultaneously permits alcohol to be available to him/her as well. Depending on the patient, one can even go a bit further and explain how rationalizations work and empathize with him/her as to how difficult it is to make such alterations in one's life, though it should also be stressed that such alterations are temporary and can be modified when sobriety is stabilized.

Not all maladaptive cognitions, however, are rationalizations. Another fairly commonly employed defense that produces maladaptive thoughts is the defense of reversal. In reversal, patients generally turn an unconscious feeling into its opposite before they can permit it to become conscious. In this respect, reversals are similar to reaction formations, although they differ in important respects (G. Mahl, personal communication, 1984). One often hears patients in early recovery wanting to "test" themselves by going to a bar. But what is it that these patients wish to test? Consciously, they may say they want to see whether they are strong enough to resume their normal activities without alcohol. However, in early recovery such tests are generally tests of weakness, not strength, and the therapist may wish to explore with the patient other indications of feeling weak. Or the therapist may by analogy suggest the idea of weakness. For example, I have told patients who wanted to test themselves that they remind me of someone who has just had major surgery and wants to work out.

Another illustration of reversal is often encountered in patients who want to "reward" themselves for their achievement of sobriety. One alcoholic patient, a sort of disheveled, sad sack of a man, during an assessment session described his longest period of sobriety, which had lasted a full year. When asked how he relapsed he said he had been feeling great about his success and had decided to "reward" himself. Unfortunately, but all too predictably, his "reward" led to heavy levels of drinking, loss of his job, and even homelessness. I responded to his statement that he had wanted to reward himself by suggesting, in a compassionate tone of voice, that his reward sounded more like a punishment. The patient, who had impressed me as both articulate and reflective, was startled, but the interpretation was on target and he began to view his behavior in this new light. Interestingly, over the course of treatment, in which the patient did quite well, the recognition that he punished himself by drinking helped him to avoid a number of slips.

Negative Affective States. Marlatt and Gordon (1985) have noted that empirical research supports the notion that negative emotional states frequently "trigger" relapses in substance abusers. Intolerance of negative affects and inability to verbalize them are at the heart of most contemporary psychoanalytic views on substance abuse (e.g., Khantzian, 1980; Krystal, 1975; Wurmser, 1978). There is some empirical evidence to support these psychoanalytic propositions. Keller and Wilson (1994) found that opiate and cocaine addicts were able to tolerate negative affects significantly less effectively than a group of matched normals. Taylor, Parker, and Bagby (1990) and Haviland, Shaw, MacMurray, and Cummings (1988) found significantly greater rates of alexithymia—the inability to verbally identify and differentiate affect states—in alcoholics. Recently, Keller, Carroll, Nich, and Rounsaville (1995) found high rates of alexithymia in a group of cocaine addicts.

Various means are available to the clinician in helping patients to tolerate negative affects more effectively. In some abusers, better articulation of affects tends by itself to promote affect tolerance. When affects are blended together or dedifferentiated they seem to be experienced as global, diffuse, overwhelming, and peremptory (Krystal, 1975). It is not that dissimilar from the way in which infants experience emotions. For example, when a baby feels frustration the emotion appears to radiate throughout its body from head to toe (Kernberg, 1975). The infant learns to manage and differentiate such emotions progressively better through its interactions with the primary caretaker and its own maturation (Greenspan, 1979; Stern, 1985). Ultimately, the toddler learns to label these emotions verbally. That is, the radiating effect of emotions in infancy appears to wane as the emotions become progressively more differentiated. Krystal and Raskin (1970) suggest that substance abusers may need a kind of remedial course in affect differentiation in therapy. They recommend a "pretreatment" phase prior to psychoanalytic psychotherapy in which the abuser is taught to identify and properly label affects.

Nevertheless, many affects that trouble addicts only become apparent during the course of treatment. If the therapist remains attuned to the patient's affective expression within the therapy hour, he/she may help the patient to articulate them. For example, let us return to the patient who took the alternate route home and ended up in a bar. As he recounted these events he sounded bored. This tone of voice in the therapy session impressed the therapist who pointed it out to the patient, and it turned out that indeed the patient had been feeling bored at work but had not articulated it. Identifying the feeling in the here and now greatly facilitates patients in being able to identify it later on their own.

Another way in which therapists can facilitate affect identification is through the use of their own countertransference reactions to the patient. In psychoanalysis, countertransference has traditionally referred to the therapist's *neurotic* emotional reactions to the patient (e.g., Freud, 1910; Gitelson, 1952; Reich, 1933). More recently, the concept has been broadened in which countertransference refers to the therapist's total emotional reaction (Kernberg, 1965; Racker, 1957). Patients stir up powerful feelings in therapists, and this is certainly the case with substance abusers (Kaufman, 1994). There are a number of typical such countertransferences and Weiss (1993) recently provided an excellent discussion. One of the most frequent is through the use of the defense known as projective identification (Ogden, 1979). In projective identification, the patient rids some unwanted part of him/herself such as a threatening affect, by inducing it in the therapist. It is as if the therapist becomes a "container" for feelings the patient has no other way of handling. The task for the therapist is to notice this in him/herself, analyze its meaning, and then take appropriate action.

For example, a 40-year-old heroin addict with bipolar disorder and a borderline characterological organization had been in substance abuse treatment on and off for many years. He generally never did well in treatment, often decompensated, and required multiple hospitalizations. The treatment staff in the clinic where he usually received his substance abuse treatment tended to regard him with disdain and derision. Upon his most recent presentation, however, he was assigned a therapist who treated him with interest, concern, and respect and after 18 months of hard work, he exhibited drastic and significant improvement. The therapy, unfortunately, was prematurely terminated when the therapist accepted another position elsewhere. Although the patient was assigned another therapist, he quickly deteriorated. One day he entered the clinic for an appointment with his new therapist and as he walked by the clinic secretary's desk he provocatively flipped up the bottom of his sportcoat which revealed a pistol in his back pocket. Security was summoned and, as it turned out, the gun was only a water pistol. Staff reactions, however, were intense, ranging from "We can't treat this guy" to "He's got to be discharged immediately" to recommendations for long-term psychiatric hospitalization. The fact that for much of the past 18 months the patient had been functioning extremely well and that he had just suffered a major loss appeared to evaporate into thin air. However, staff members eventually were able to recognize their own extreme responses as intense countertransference reactions induced by the patient's provocative behavior. The patient had acted out his feeling that without his first therapist he was worthless and untreatable. He, however, could not say this. He had to get the staff to say it for him. He was briefly hospitalized and returned to substance abuse therapy.

Use of Empathy and Interpretation of Conflict. Empathy is one of the key tools the clinician has at his/her disposal. It is through the act of empathic listening that the therapist gains access to the emotional life of the patient. Greenson (1960) has referred to empathy as a kind of "emotional knowing" (p. 418). One often has the impression that clinicians, especially beginners, think that empathy means listening supportively and sympathetically. These are indeed good therapist qualities, but they are not the same thing as empathy. Empathic listening is a specific attempt to understand the patient's emotional experience and convey this to the patient.

In psychodynamic terms, the act of empathic listening involves several steps (Greenson, 1960). First, the therapist temporarily suspends his/her observing functions in order to become a participant in the patient's emotional life, to see what it feels like to be the patient. The therapist makes a partial, temporary, "trial identification" (Fliess, 1942). Second, on the basis of this temporary identification, the therapist oscillates back into the role of observer and on a cognitive level attempts to articulate the meaning(s) of the emotion for the patient. Third, the therapist may communicate these "findings" to the patient in the form of a clarification or interpretation (Greenson, 1960).

It is important to note that the experience of oscillating back and forth between observer and participant is not based on a conscious attempt to follow this step-by-step breakdown of the empathic process. One does not say, "I am now going to empathize with the patient. First, I will adopt the role of participant. . . . " Rather, it seems to take place rather quickly, almost automatically, and only in retrospect does the empathic act appear to be sequenced.

Empathy may be used as (1) a gauge by which the therapist measures his emotional understanding of the patient, (2) a method for helping patients clarify and articulate their feelings more precisely and accurately, and (3) as a means for the patient to feel understood. It may also be used to facilitate the exploration of unconscious conflicts. Though RP for substance abuse focuses on behavior change that supports abstinence, it may be necessary from time to time to obtain insight into unconscious conflicts that might threaten the patient's abstinence if left unattended. Let me illustrate how empathic listening may be utilized toward this end.

A 22-year-old female college student with a history of alcohol and marijuana abuse has been sober approximately 6 months. Her recovery is generally stable although she has recently been musing over the possibility of controlled drinking in the future. The patient began drinking and using marijuana as a teenager in response to feelings of depression, but I subsequently learned that her use also coincided with an experimental homosexual relationship. The patient formerly thought of herself as heterosexual but shortly after beginning treatment had "come out" and now considers herself a lesbian. Despite the fact that she feels generally good about her choice, she has been grappling with a number of troubling implications of such a sexual orientation, not the least of which is telling her parents.

At the beginning of the therapy session in question she complains that she has been feeling sad for the past several months and does not know why. She is sober, her relationship with her girlfriend is in good shape, her grades have improved significantly; it just puzzles her that she should be feeling sad when "everything is going so well." She goes on to discuss a number of other things and midway through the session mentions that she has been teaching Sunday school at her church, which she has found to be enormously rewarding. I comment that this is certainly good news and add that I had not realized she had been teaching. I then asked her, essentially out of curiosity, how long she had been at it and she says "about two months." I then say, "You know that's interesting since it corresponds roughly to the time you've been feeling sad." The patient nods in agreement and then recalls that in fact she had first noticed feeling sad at the Sunday school. I am both struck and puzzled by this development. Why should she be saddened by this? I inquire as to her thoughts on the matter and as she begins to speak I find myself beginning to imagine being her in the Sunday school, looking out at a group of children. I see her now in a new light. In my office, I see her as a petite young woman just barely out of her teens. But in the Sunday school she is now a grown woman teaching little children and as I continue to imagine being her, looking out at the little children, I experience a kind of wistful sadness. I then imagine her thinking, "I love working with these children and I feel sad because as a lesbian I may not be able to have my own." At an appropriate moment, I tell her, "And you've been feeling sad with the children at Sunday school because it's sort of an unconscious reminder that it may be much more difficult to have your own children." The interpretation hit home. Whether she could become a mother as a lesbian had indeed been a troubling thought, one she had barely allowed herself to think. Nor had she connected it to the sadness she experienced in working with the children at Sunday school. We then raised the possibility that her thoughts about controlled drinking might also be related to these sad feelings, as painful feelings often trigger the desire to use. We were not able to reach a decisive conclusion, but the *patient* suggested intensifying her recovery program with extra group therapy and more Alcoholics Anonymous meetings.

In addition to explicating the empathic process, this clinical example illustrates several other points. First, the therapist helps the patient to articulate and establish meaning and significance for a previously inexplicable emotional experience. Second, the patient and therapist are able to connect these feelings with thoughts that might, if they are permitted to develop, lead to a slip or relapse. Third, the therapist does not explore in any great detail the unconscious determinants either now or in the past, of her conflicts regarding her sexual orientation. The exploration of the conflict takes place at the surface and its purpose is to promote relapse prevention.

Resistance and Transference. In psychoanalysis and psychoanalytic psychotherapy it is the analysis of resistance and transference that become the central focus of treatment. It may have struck the reader as somewhat peculiar that this chapter has thus far devoted relatively little attention to these variables. Actually, this is only apparently so at least with respect to resistance. In psychoanalytic clinical theory, resistance is defined as defense expressed within the treatment situation (Freud, 1912; Gill, 1982; Greenson, 1967). In an important sense, virtually everything we have thus far encountered regarding an exploration of the patient's cravings, apparently irrelevant decisions, distorted cognitions, affects, and conflicts are examples of working with resistances.

As noted earlier, far too often there is a tendency to think of resistance in its most egregious or blatant forms such as gross noncompliance. These "noisy" resistances do occur especially in the treatment of substance abusers. But as Schlesinger (1982) pointed out, it is far more often the case that we deal with "quieter" resistances, which demand attention to the therapeutic process. For example, a patient talks so fast he does not have time to hear himself think let alone mull over the implications of what he has said. Or, as in the case of the alcoholic woman we considered in the section on assessment, a patient's communications take on a relative withholding quality. The technique we have been describing for meeting these and other resistances deals with the resistance as it is presented and refrains from reaching behind the defense, as it were, in order to pull out the material it conceals.

From the standpoint of utilizing this sort of psychodynamic technique to promote relapse prevention through cognitive-behavioral skills acquisition, we pay *selective* attention to the patient's resistances. Thus, we want to examine those resistances that may lead to a slip or relapse. However, many resistances that might become the focus of therapy in standard psychodynamic treatment are passed over in this form of treatment. Indeed, some may be reinforced if they lead to relapse prevention and skills acquisition. For example, obsessional defenses that might be the principal source of resistance and central focus in the psychotherapy of certain patients often facilitate a substance abuser in creating distance from painful affects or in engaging in skills acquisition assignments. In the treatment described here I would support such defensive–resistive activity.

Transference, as defined earlier, refers to the patient's propensity to develop a fantasy-based relationship to the therapist. In standard psychoanalytic psychotherapy, the transference is allowed to flourish and the therapist's quiet, neutral, generally incognito manner creates a certain amount of ambiguity, which further augments the transference potential in the patient. In psychodynamically informed RP, however, we seek to *minimize* the transference potential in the patient. Treatment is essentially focused around reality factors and goals are well defined. That the therapist is more active, "real," and gives advice and support also tends to attenuate the transference. RP, as described here, also capitalizes on but leaves unanalyzed an important aspect of the positive transference: namely, the patient's capacity to form a moderately dependent relationship on a generally helpful therapist.

Nevertheless, this does not mean that transference reactions do not occur that require our attention. For instance, some substance abusers unconsciously attempt to cast the therapist into the role of a policeman, which, if successfully elicited, makes the patient feel justified in using. Some insight into how the patient does this may be helpful to avert a relapse. In addition, transference fantasies usually become intensified at termination and should always be explored as the termination phase is also a risky time for a substance abuser. The general principle here is the same as with other psychodynamic phenomena: We explore psychodynamically if the problem, feeling, conflict, or behavior increases the chances of relapse.

Advanced Phase of Treatment

Advanced recovery is a subject that occupies relatively less space in the literature than recovery in the early and middle phases of treatment. This is due in part to the recalcitrant fact that stable abstinence is so difficult to achieve (Institute of Medicine, 1989) relative to remission rates for other psychiatric disorders. Moreover, not all addicted individuals elect to continue psychotherapy once abstinence has been secured, often preferring to continue in 12-Step or other self-help treatment.

Nevertheless, some individuals do wish to continue in treatment and psychodynamic therapy may be of value (Kaufman, 1994). In the model of treatment delineated in this chapter as well as in other similar models (e.g., Kaufman, 1994), the advanced phase of treatment may become progressively more psychoanalytic in nature. In this respect, the therapist takes on a more neutral, exploratory role, which permits the patient's transference potential to emerge, the analysis of which may help to resolve a number of underlying conflicts. To a certain extent, some things the patient has learned in the earlier stages of treatment can actually facilitate this analysis. For example, I once treated a female alcoholic who, in resisting exploration of how she participated (unconsciously) in provoking arguments with her lover, eventually reminded herself, "If I could set myself up to drink, maybe I am setting up these arguments too." On the other hand, the essentially supportive, advice-giving, more "real" role that the therapist has adopted in the earlier treatment phases may hinder the patient from being able to tolerate the more depriving role the therapist assumes in psychodynamic treatment (Kaufman, 1994). In such cases, it may be necessary to refer the patient to a new therapist.

Owing to considerations of space, a full exposition of the advanced phase of psychoanalytic treatment with substance abusers is not possible. However, I would like to touch on three basic areas which generally become the focus of this latter phase: (1) exploration of critical affects, (2) the examination of unconscious conflicts, and (3) reconstructing and adjusting to a substance-free life.

As has been previously noted, substance abusers find managing and tolerating negative affects extremely difficult. In the advanced stage, further work in this area is possible. First, the abuser can be helped to express such emotions as guilt, shame, and rage. These are often extremely difficult to express in the transference as the patient, by this time, is often exceedingly grateful for the therapist's previous help (Kaufman, 1994). Often, it is more useful to explore such feelings through an examination of their expression to significant others in the patient's life. In this way, the transference can be interpreted within the "metaphor" of the significant other (Schlesinger, 1982). Assisting the patient to give expression to such affect also permits the therapist to help the patient learn to endure and tolerate the feelings without using (Khantzian et al., 1990). Gradually, greater self-regulation of emotional states may be achieved.

Kaufman (1994) has suggested that the central conflictual issues that characterize the advanced phase of treatment are intimacy and autonomy. Psychodynamically, substance abusers have developed an intense "object relationship" with their drug (Krystal, 1978). In a certain sense, this object relationship has served as a substitute for intimate relations with people. One frequently hears, for example, addicts describe their drug as "the best lover I've ever had," or some variation on this theme. For such people, intimacy with others carries the dual unconscious meaning of a kind of blissful merging and a simultaneous terrifying engulfment with the other (see Krystal, 1978; Leeds & Morgenstern, Chapter 3, this volume). What the addict needs, therefore, is to become capable of tolerating intimacy with people while simultaneously building a more autonomous sense of self, and it is through the analysis of the transference relationship to the therapist during the advanced stage of treatment that these conflicts may be more fully resolved.

Finally, the substance abuser must learn to adjust to a substance-free life. Cognitive-behavioral clinicians (e.g., Marlatt & Gordon, 1985) have suggested that such "lifestyle modification" can be accomplished by helping abusers substitute sober pleasurable activities for their substance-abusing ones. Often those activities abusers found pleasurable *prior* to the onset of their substance abuse are of great value. For example, one patient who had been an amateur artist but had given up the avocation during her many years of cocaine addiction was helped to resume this activity by encouraging her to paint cravings and other painful affects.

However, no matter how many sober pleasurable activities the therapist can promote in his/her patients, the fact is that for many patients life without alcohol or drugs is experienced as an arid, desiccated, empty existence. It is helpful to remember that the substance abuser is not merely someone with an alcohol or drug problem but a person who has *become* an alcoholic or addict. By the time he/she has reached the therapist's office, the "behavior" has become a way of life, has insinuated itself into areas the patient may not have even realized until sobriety has been achieved.

Giving up the substance use may be initially experienced as gratifying but later on experienced as giving up too much. A kind of mourning process must take place, not only over the loss of the substance but over of a way of life.

In addition, substance abusers must learn finally to renounce immediate blissful gratification and accept life's inevitable frustrations. Freud, in a much quoted passage, once remarked that the essential achievement of psychotherapy consisted of "transforming hysterical misery into common unhappiness" (Breuer & Freud, 1893–1895, p. 305). Yet it appears that "common unhappiness" is precisely what substance abusers find so intolerable. The normal aches and pains and frustrations of everyday life, which most of us accept as given, are for them deeply and profoundly disturbing. In this respect, a key aspect of the advanced phase of treatment is to nurture in the patient a kind of stoical acceptance that life's ordinary difficulties *are* tolerable and do not preclude the more enduring gratifications of love and work.

SUMMARY AND CONCLUSIONS

This chapter has focused on how psychodynamic therapy may contribute to cognitive-behavioral relapse prevention treatment of substance use disorders. It has emphasized that by focusing on the moment-to-moment process of psychotherapy, selected use of psychoanalytic technique may facilitate engagement in treatment, achieving abstinence, and preventing relapse. Several implications for the future development of substance abuse treatment are indicated. First, the treatment model suggested here is based on a cognitive-behavioral approach which has begun to demonstrate efficacy in controlled trials and the accrued clinical wisdom of psychodynamic technique whose efficacy is largely anecdotal. Such a model, therefore, needs to be tested under controlled conditions, particularly with reference to matching appropriate patients to this treatment type. Second, greater attention needs to be paid to the training of substance abuse therapists and, in particular, with reference to the process of psychotherapy, to the psychodynamics of the patient, and to the nuances of the interpersonal relationship that develops in treatment. Much of this can *only* be achieved through intensive personal supervision, which ought to be incorporated into existing training programs. Third, there is a paucity of articles in the clinical substance abuse literature that attempt to describe the therapeutic process through which techniques are actually administered. More are needed. This chapter has been an attempt to begin to address that need.

ACKNOWLEDGMENT

I wish to thank Drs. Jon Morgenstern, Edward Paul, Sally Satel, and Laurence Westreich for their many helpful comments and suggestions on an earlier version of the manuscript.

REFERENCES

Binswanger, L. (1946). The existential analysis school of thought. In R. May, E. Angel, & H. F. Ellenberger (Eds.), *Existence*. New York: Basic Books, 1958.

Breuer, J., & Freud, S. (1893–1895). Studies on hysteria. *Standard Edition, 2*, vii–309. London: Hogarth Press, 1955.

Carroll, K. M., Rounsaville, B. J., & Gawin, F. H. (1991). A comparative trial psychotherapies for ambulatory cocaine abusers: Relapse prevention and interpersonal psychotherapy. *American Journal of Drug and Alcohol Abuse, 17*, 229–247.

Carroll, K. M., Rounsaville, B. J., & Keller, D. S. (1991). Relapse prevention strategies in the treatment of cocaine abuse. *American Journal on Drug and Alcohol Abuse, 17*, 249–265.

Fenichel, O. (1941). *Problems of psychoanalytic technique*. Albany: NY: The Psychoanalytic Quarterly.

Fenichel, O. (1945). *The psychoanalytic theory of neurosis*. New York: Norton.

Fliess, R. (1942). The metapsychology of the analyst. *Psychoanalytic Quarterly, 11*, 211–227.

Freud, A. (1936). *The ego and the mechanisms of defense*. New York: International Universities Press, 1966.

Freud, S. (1894). The neuro-psychoses of defense. *Standard Edition, 3*, 43–68. London: Hogarth Press, 1953.

Freud, S. (1896). Further remarks on the neuro-psychoses of defense. *Standard Edition, 3*, 159–185. London: Hogarth Press, 1953.

Freud, S. (1900). The interpretation of dreams. *Standard Edition, 4 & 5*. London: Hogarth Press, 1953.

Freud, S. (1905). Fragment of an analysis of a case of hysteria. *Standard Edition, 7*, 3–122. London: Hogarth Press, 1953.

Freud, S. (1910). The future prospects of psycho-analytic therapy. *Standard Edition, 11*, 139–151. London: Hogarth Press, 1957.

Freud, S. (1912). The dynamics of transference. *Standard Edition, 12*, 97–108. London: Hogarth Press, 1958.

Freud, S. (1923). The ego and the id. *Standard Edition, 19*, 12–66. London: Hogarth Press, 1961.

Freud, S. (1926). Inhibitions, symptoms, and anxiety. *Standard Edition, 20*, 87–174. London: Hogarth Press, 1959.

Galanter, M. (1993). *Network therapy for alcohol and drug abuse*. New York: Basic Books.

Galanter, M., & Keller, D. S. (1994). *Network therapy for substance abuse: A therapist's manual.* Unpublished manuscript, New York University, New York, NY.

Gill, M. (1982). *Analysis of transference* (Vol. 1) (Psychological Issues, 353). New York: International Universities Press.

Gitelson, M. (1952). The emotional position of the analyst in the psycho-analytic situation. *International Journal of Psycho-Analysis, 33,* 1–10.

Greenson, R. R. (1960). Empathy and its vicissitudes. *International Journal of Psycho-Analysis, 41,* 418–424.

Greenson, R. R. (1967). *The technique and practice of psychoanalysis.* New York: International Universities Press.

Greenspan, S. I. (1979). *Intelligence and adaptation: An integration of psychoanalytic and Piagetian developmental psychology* (Psychological Issues, 47/48). New York: International Universities Press.

Haviland, M. G., Shaw, D. G., MacMurray, J. P., & Cummings, M. A. (1988). Validation of the Toronto Alexithymia Scale with substance abusers. *Psychotherapy and Psychosomatics, 50,* 81–87.

Institute of Medicine. (1989). *Prevention and treatment of alcohol problems. Opportunities for research: Report of a study.* Washington, DC: National Academy Press.

Kadden, R., Carroll, K. M., Donovan, D., Cooney, N., Monti, P., Abrams, D., Litt, M., & Hester, R. (1992). *Cognitive-behavioral coping skills therapy manual: A clinical research guide for therapists treating individuals with alcohol abuse and dependence* (NIAAA Project MATCH Monograph Series, Vol. 3, DHHS Publication No. ADM 92–1895). Rockville, MD: National Institute on Alcohol Abuse and Alcoholism.

Kaufman, E. (1994). *Psychotherapy of addicted persons.* New York: Guilford Press.

Keller, D. S., Carroll, K. M., Nich, C., & Rounsaville, B. J. (1995). Alexithymia in cocaine abusers: Response to psychotherapy and pharmacotherapy. *American Journal on Addictions, 4,* 234–244.

Keller, D. S., & Wilson, A. (1994). Affectivity in cocaine and opiate abusers. *Psychiatry, 57*(4), 333–347.

Kernberg, O. F. (1965). Notes on countertransference. *Journal of the American Psychoanalytic Association, 13,* 38–56.

Kernberg, O. F. (1975). *Borderline conditions and pathological narcissism.* New York: Jason Aronson.

Khantzian, E. J. (1980). An ego–self theory of substance dependence. In D. J. Lettieri, M. Sayers, & H. W. Wallace (Eds.), *Theories of addiction* (NIDA Research Monograph No. 30, DHHS Publication No. ADM 80–967). Washington, DC: U.S. Government Printing Office.

Khantzian, E. J., Halliday, K. S., & McAuliffe, W. E. (1990). *Addiction and the vulnerable self: Modified dynamic group therapy for substance abusers.* New York: Guilford Press.

Krystal, H. (1975). Affect tolerance. *Annual of Psychoanalysis, 3,* 179–219.

Krystal, H. (1978). Self-representation and the capacity for self-care. *Annual of Psychoanalysis, 6,* 209–246.

Krystal, H., & Raskin, H. A. (1970). *Drug dependence: Aspects of ego functioning.* Detroit: Wayne State University Press.

Luborsky, L. (1984). *Principles of psychoanalytic psychotherapy: A manual for supportive-expressive treatment.* New York: Basic Books.

Marlatt, G. A., & Gordon, J. R. (Eds.). (1985). *Relapse prevention: Maintenance strategies in the treatment of addictive behaviors.* New York: Guilford Press.

Miller, W. R., & Hester, R. K. (1986). The effectiveness of alcoholism treatment: What research reveals. In W. R. Miller & R. K. Hester (Eds.), *Treating addictive behaviors: Processes of change.* New York: Plenum Press.

Monti, P. M, Abrams, D. B., Kadden, R. M., & Cooney, N. L. (1989). *Treating alcohol dependence: A coping skills training guide.* New York: Guilford Press.

Morgenstern, J., & McCrady, B. S. (1992). Curative factors in alcohol and drug treatment: Behavioral and disease model perspectives. *British Journal of the Addictions, 87,* 901–912.

Ogden, T. H. (1979). On projective identification. *International Journal of Psycho-Analysis, 60*(3), 357–373.

Racker, H. (1957). The meanings and uses of countertransference. *Psychoanalytic Quarterly, 26,* 303–357.

Rapaport, D., Gill, M. M., Schafer, R. (1968). In R. Holt (Ed.), *Diagnostic psychological testing.* New York: International Universities Press.

Reich, W. (1933). *Character analysis.* New York: Orgone Press, 1945.

Safran, J. D., & Siegel, Z. V. (1990). *Interpersonal process in cognitive therapy.* New York: Basic Books.

Schafer, R. (1976). The idea of resistance. In *A new language for psychoanalysis.* New Haven, CT: Yale University Press.

Schlesinger, H. J. (1969). Diagnosis and prescription for psychotherapy. *Bulletin of the Menninger Clinic, 33,* 269–278.

Schlesinger, H. J. (1981). The process of empathic response. *Psychoanalytic Inquiry, 1*(3), 393–416.

Schlesinger, H. J. (1982). Resistance as process. In P. Wachtel (Ed.), *Resistance: Psychodynamic and behavioral approaches.* New York: Plenum Press.

Shapiro, D. (1989). *Psychotherapy of neurotic character.* New York: Basic Books.

Stanton, M. D., Todd, T. C., & Associates. (1982). *The family therapy of drug abuse and addiction.* New York: Guilford Press.

Stern, D. (1985). *The interpersonal world of the infant.* New York: Basic Books.

Taylor, G. J., Parker, J. D., & Bagby, R. M. (1990). A preliminary investigation of alexithymia in men with psychoactive substance dependence. *American Journal of Psychiatry, 147,* 1228–1230.

Wachtel, P. (1977). *Psychoanalysis and behavior therapy.* New York: Basic Books.

Wallerstein, R. S. (1986). *Forty-two lives in treatment: A study of psychoanalysis and psychotherapy.* New York: Guilford Press.

Weiss, R. (1993). Countertransference issues in treating the alcoholic patient:

Institutional and clinician reactions. In J. D. Levin & R. Weiss (Eds.), *The dynamics and treatment of alcoholism.* New York: Jason Aronson.

Wheelis, A. (1973). *How people change.* New York: Harper & Row.

Wikler, A. (1973). Dynamics of drug dependence. *Archives of General Psychiatry, 28,* 611–616.

Wurmser, L. (1978). *The hidden dimension.* New York: Jason Aronson.

Wurmser, L. (1985). Denial and split identity: Timely issues in the psychoanalytic psychotherapy of compulsive drug users. *Journal of Substance Abuse Treatment, 2,* 89–96.

CHAPTER 5

Theoretical Bases of Family Approaches to Substance Abuse Treatment

BARBARA S. McCRADY
ELIZABETH E. EPSTEIN

Mental health professionals have accorded the family a central role in the etiology, maintenance, and treatment of a variety of psychological and psychiatric disorders. Theoretical models of etiology have ranged from the notion of the schizophrenogenic mother (reviewed in Broderick & Schrader, 1981) to the heritability of depressive disorders (reviewed in Hammen, 1991). Maintenance models have conceived of individual symptoms as indicators of dysfunction in the family system (reviewed in Barton & Alexander, 1981) or focused on inept family management skills as important factors maintaining child behavioral problems (Patterson, 1986). Family-based treatments have evolved from a variety of theoretical models, ranging from treatments to teach spouses to model and reinforce appropriate eating behavior as part of treatment for obesity (Brownell, Heckerman, Westlake, Hayes, & Monti, 1978) to family educational models for schizophrenics (reviewed in Konstantareas, 1990) to family systems models for treatment of eating disorders (Dare, Eisler, Russell, & Szmukler, 1990). In short, although the U.S. government declared a "Year of the Family" and "family values" became an important topic of debate in the 1992 presidential campaign in the United States, the mental health field has made the second half of the 20th century the era of the family.

The family has been an integral part of the conceptualization of psychoactive substance use disorders since at least the 1930s, when social workers in state hospitals began to report the results of interviews and observations of the experiences of wives of alcoholics (Lewis, 1937). This chapter describes the historical roots of family approaches to conceptualizing the etiology, maintenance, and treatment of psychoactive substance use disorders, with a special emphasis on alcohol abuse and dependence. The chapter then presents key theoretical elements that serve as the basis for family-based treatment approaches, which will be described by McKay (Chapter 6, this volume).

HISTORICAL OVERVIEW

Psychodynamic Models

In the 1930s, many alcoholics received treatment in state mental hospitals. Social workers in those facilities began to interview the spouses (most often, wives) of the alcoholic patients and began to observe the significant distress that these women experienced. Lewis (1937), as the first to publish observations of this distress, and other authors continued to note that the women were anxious and depressed and reported experiencing a variety of psychosomatic symptoms. Theoretical models began to develop to attempt to explain these observations. The earliest model, the disturbed personality hypothesis, was derived from the psychodynamic models that predominated at the time and postulated that wives of alcoholics were disturbed women who resolved neurotic conflicts through their marriage to an alcoholic man. Although some authors postulated one primary underlying conflict (e.g., with aggression or dependence), Whalen (1953) hypothesized four different kinds of conflicts that could be resolved through marriage to an alcoholic and provided colorful names for each of these types of wives of alcoholics. She suggested conflicts with aggression ("Punitive Polly"), control ("Controlling Catherine"), masochism ("Suffering Susan"), and ambivalence ("Wavering Winifred").

A corollary to the disturbed personality hypothesis was the decompensation hypothesis. Central to psychodynamic models is the notion that neurotic conflicts serve as a defense against more basic or primitive conflicts. If defenses are removed, an individual would be expected to exhibit these more primitive conflicts and decompensate. Thus, it was hypothesized that if a married alcoholic successfully stopped drinking, his wife would decompensate and exhibit more severe psychopathology. MacDonald (1956) studied 18 women hospitalized in a state mental hospital, all of whom were married to alcoholics. He reported that 11 of these women had husbands who had decreased drinking recently, suggesting these observations as support for the decompensation hypothesis.

Sociological Stress Models

In the 1950s, alternative models began to develop. Jackson (1954) interviewed women who were attending Al-Anon meetings and developed a stress and coping model. She suggested that living with an alcoholic is stressful, and that most of the symptoms that wives of alcoholics experienced were common to any families living with long-term stressors, such as a chronically ill family member or a family member away in combat. She also suggested that families go through "stages" in coping with alcoholism, and that each stage is characterized by different psychological phenomena. Jackson suggested that family denial of the problem characterized the earliest stage of family coping, followed, in sequence, by attempts to control the problem, feeling hopeless and chaotic, attempting to maintain stable family functioning with the alcoholic present, attempting to escape from the problem through marital separation, organizing and maintaining the family without the alcoholic present, and a final adjustment phase if the alcoholic stopped drinking. Kogan and Jackson (1965) later tested Jackson's model of stress and coping by comparing the psychological characteristics of women whose husbands were actively drinking with women whose husbands had stopped drinking and with women whose husbands had never had drinking problems. They reported that women whose husbands were actively drinking were significantly more distressed than women in the comparison groups, who were indistinguishable from each other. Many years later, Moos, Finney, and Gamble (1982) reported results of a longitudinal study that followed alcoholics and their families for 2 years from the beginning of treatment and compared their functioning to sociodemographically matched community controls. The results of this prospective design supported Jackson's model—spouses whose alcoholic partners successfully resolved their drinking problems were indistinguishable on measures of psychological distress from spouses in the community control sample at follow-up.

Family Systems Models

By the 1970s, family systems models began to influence the alcohol field. In a series of studies, Steinglass and his colleagues observed the behavior of alcoholics hospitalized on an experimental unit, noting repetitive, patterned interactions between an alcoholic father and son, alcoholic brothers (Steinglass, Weiner, & Mendelson, 1971), and alcoholics and their husbands or wives (Steinglass, Davis, & Berenson, 1977) as well as significant differences in their patterns of interaction when sober and when intoxicated. These observations led to the hypothesis that alcohol performed certain positive functions in a family by stabilizing family roles, allowing for the expression of affect, allowing for greater intimacy among family members, or allowing for the exploration of topics that the family might avoid when sober. This set of positive functions was called the adaptive consequences of alcoholism (Davis, Berenson, Steinglass, & Davis, 1974). After these initial observational studies, Steinglass later studied alcoholic families in their homes as well as in the laboratory. He reported observable differences among families with an alcoholic family member who was drinking, sober, or in transition from one drinking status to another. Families with a sober alcoholic were most flexible in their functioning, having a balance between time together and time apart when at home (Steinglass, 1981) and showing more flexibility in solving structured tasks in the laboratory (Steinglass, 1979). Drinking families showed the most rigidity of family roles and interactions, while transitional families were intermediate in their functioning.

Wolin, Bennett, Noonan, and Teitelbaum (1980) provided a second family systems perspective on alcoholism, focusing primarily on the intergenerational transmission of alcoholism. Their work examined the family "rituals" that characterize all families—how families vacation, have dinner, celebrate holidays, and so on. They observed three types of ritual patterns in alcoholic families—intact rituals that were maintained despite drinking; subsumptive ritual patterns that were modified to incorporate the drinking, and disrupted rituals that were not maintained in the face of the drinking. They reported that those families whose rituals were maintained intact were least likely to have offspring who became alcoholic; those families whose rituals were most disrupted were most likely to have alcoholic offspring. A more detailed review of family ritual research is described later.

Family systems theory has contributed a number of constructs to the conceptualization of family functioning. Families are assumed to be governed by the law of *homeostasis*. All systems are assumed to operate to try to maintain balance, stability, and equilibrium. Factors that threaten to change the functioning of a family threaten that homeostasis, and the family system is assumed to function to try to avoid change. Thus, family systems models would assume, if an alcoholic family has functioned as a stable family unit with a drinking member, that introducing sobriety into the system would threaten homeostasis. A variety of aspects of the family's structure and functioning (*organization*) maintain homeostasis. Family members have defined *roles* that guide their actions. Roles may range from caretaker to bad child, but these roles are well defined and are assumed to be difficult to modify over time. Families also have unwritten family *rules* that govern the functioning of the family. These rules are not necessarily explicit or deliberate (e.g., the oldest child takes out the garbage) but are more likely to be implicit and unspoken (e.g., never talk about Mommy's drinking). Families also have a variety of *boundaries* that define relationships within the family and between the family and the rest of the world. Boundaries define alliances between family members, the degree to which information is available to different family members, the degree to which family members influence the decision making of the family, the degree to which outsiders are welcomed into the family, and the degree to which the family seeks interaction with outside persons and social institutions.

Behavioral Models

The fourth major group of family theoretical models that evolved was behavioral. Model development began with an observational study of the interactions between alcoholic men and their wives in a structured problem-solving task (Hersen, Miller, & Eisler, 1973). Careful coding of behavior during the interactions revealed that the wives looked at their husbands more when the husbands were discussing alcohol than when they were discussing a more neutral topic. Becker and Miller (1976) found that alcoholic husbands spoke more during alcohol-related conversations, while wives spoke more when discussing other topics. These researchers hypothesized that discussing alcohol was reinforced in the couple's interaction, either by increased attention from the spouse or by increased talking and dominance of the conversation by the alcoholic.

Later interactional research focused on the relationships between drinking and marital communication. Billings, Kessler, Gomberg, and Weiner (1979) made alcohol available to alcoholic couples and observed their interactions. Although half the couples did not drink at all, and most of those who did drank only one to two drinks, they found that alcoholics spoke more when drinking. Frankenstein, Hay, and Nathan (1985) administered a standard alcohol dose to all alcoholics in their marital communication study. They found that alcoholics spoke more when intoxicated than when sober, that couples emitted more positive verbal behaviors in drinking than in sober sessions, and that spouses were more positive verbally in the alcohol session. They also reported that alcoholics asked more questions when drinking, and that objective raters and the couples themselves rated the alcoholic as more dominant when drinking than when sober (Frankenstein, Nathan, Sullivan, Hay, & Cocco, 1985).

Jacob, Ritchey, Cvitkovic, and Blane (1981) initially reported findings contradictory to other interactional studies, finding that alcoholic couples became more negative when drinking, and that the wives of male alcoholics expressed more disagreements during drinking than during sober sessions. However, in later studies they identified two subtypes of alcoholics—steady, at-home drinkers and binge, out-of-home drinkers. Alcohol consumption was associated with positive familial consequences for the former group, but was associated with negative consequences for the latter group (Dunn, Jacob, Hummon, & Seilhamer, 1987; Jacob, Dunn, & Leonard, 1983).

Taken as a whole, these interactional studies suggest that interactions of alcoholic couples change when alcohol is present or discussed, and that these changes have a variety of positive features that may reinforce and maintain the drinking.

Family Disease Models

The family has been a focus of the disease model almost from the beginning of Alcoholics Anonymous. The primary publication of Alcoholics Anonymous, *Alcoholics Anonymous* (Alcoholics Anonymous, 1976) (often called the *Big Book*), includes a chapter with advice to family members in each edition. Al-Anon began in 1949 as an organization to assist the family and friends of alcoholics. The contemporary family focus of disease model approaches began with Cork's (1969) book on children of alcoholics, followed by Black's (1982) and Wegsheider's (1981) books about children in alcoholic families and the adult sequelae of their early experiences. Later authors began to focus on the partners of alcoholics and attempted to describe their problems (e.g., Beattie, 1987; Cermak, 1986). Although controlled research related to disease model conceptualizations is limited, these models have had a substantial impact on treatment and on popular thinking.

Contemporary disease model approaches describe alcoholism as a "family disease." Family members are seen as suffering from a disease, just as is the alcoholic. The "disease" of the family member is "codependence." Codependence has been described as a "recognizable pattern of personality traits, predictably found within most members of chemically dependent families" (Cermak, 1986, p. 1). Cermak proposed several specific symptoms of codependence: (1) investing self-esteem in controlling self and others in the face of serious adverse circumstances; (2)

assuming responsibility for meeting the needs of others before one's own; (3) experiencing anxiety and distortions of boundaries around issues of intimacy and separation; (4) being enmeshed in relationships with persons with personality disorders or alcohol or drug problems; and (5) having at least 3 from a list of 10 other signs and symptoms, that is, (a) using denial as a primary coping strategy, (b) having constricted emotions, (c) experiencing depression, (d) being hypervigilant, (e) displaying compulsive behavior, (f) experiencing anxiety, (g) being a substance abuser, (h) being a victim of physical or sexual abuse, (i) having stress-related illnesses, and (j) being in a relationship with a substance abuser for more than 2 years without seeking help.

Families members who are codependent are assumed to engage in a variety of behaviors that *enable* the substance abuser. Enabling refers to patterns of behavior that perpetuate the substance use, either by making it easier for the person to use or by providing positive responses to use and avoiding negative or limit-setting responses.

Current Status of Family Theory

Three models dominate contemporary family substance abuse treatment: family disease models, family systems models, and behavioral models. Most treatments provide some amalgam of these three models. For example, contemporary family disease models emphasize codependency, alcoholism as a disease, and family members' learning to focus on changing themselves—all concepts deriving from disease models. At the same time, many disease model treatment programs that include the family also emphasize communication, dysfunctional family roles, and family equilibrium—concepts derived from family systems theory.

Family systems models examine the functions the substance use serves for the family and attempt to change family roles, rules, and boundaries. At the same time, the treatment focuses on communication and problem solving and direct behavioral treatments to facilitate abstinence.

Behavioral family models examine family behaviors as antecedents to substance use and as reinforcing consequences and utilize treatments to modify antecedent and consequences of substance use. Behavioral therapists also examine repetitive relationship themes and communication and consider the functions that alcohol may play in maintaining stability of the relationship.

The next section describes how the historical trends in understanding substance use and family functioning and the terminology of behavioral, systemic, and disease model approaches are integrated into our model for conceptualizing the functioning of families with substance abuse.

KEY ELEMENTS IN THEORY

Etiology of Substance Abuse

The etiology of substance abuse is generally thought to be a complex, developmental phenomenon (Hill, 1994) with multiple determinants. Not only are there multiple environmental and biological pathways to substance abuse but there appears to be substantial variability in the expression of substance abuse and among substance abusers (Babor et al., 1992; Cloninger, Bohman, & Sigvardsson, 1981; Hesselbrock, 1986). Several models of alcoholism posit an ongoing interaction among environmental and genetic (including family of origin, extrafamily social network, and societal) factors in a developmental framework (Devor, 1994; Tarter, 1994). It is important to be cognizant of the complex nature of substance abuse and to be aware of its many faces in both the identified patient and his/her family members. A family therapist who adopts a simplistic model of substance abuse and does not consider empirical findings on variation in the presentation of substance use problems will lose a great deal of valuable information to help conceptualize the case and develop treatment strategies. The following section briefly reviews the literature on familial transmission of substance and related psychiatric disorders. Then, more proximate factors in etiology and maintenance of substance abuse are reviewed.

It is rarely the case that only one family member is substance dependent. Rather, family studies indicate that alcoholism has a high rate of familial transmission (Merikangas, Leckman, Prusoff, Pauls, & Weissman, 1985). Furthermore, alcoholism rates are elevated in family members of alcoholic probands (identified patients) but not of other substance abusers (Hill, 1994), indicating that "alcoholism (vs. abuse of other drugs) breeds true." However, other evidence (Cowley et al., 1992) suggests that offspring of alcoholics experience a heightened euphoriant effect from benzodiazepines.

Adoption and twin research suggests that transmission of substance abuse involves some genetic mediation (Cadoret, O'Gorman, Troughton, & Heywood, 1985; Kendler, Heath, Neale, Kessler, & Eaves, 1992; see also Hill, 1994). Further, rates of psychopathology are elevated in alcoholics (Hesselbrock, Meyer, & Keenen, 1985) and because these disorders are also transmitted in families, one can expect to see elevated rates of comorbid psychopathology in family members of substance abusers. Moos and his colleagues proposed a model of stress and coping, that posits that family members of alcoholics deal with a chronically stressful phenomenon and consequently are more likely to develop psychological or physical problems (Moos et al., 1982; Moos & Moos, 1984). Finally, assortative mating has been noted for substance abuse (Hall, Hesselbrock, & Stabenau, 1983a, 1983b). That is, many female substance abusers marry alcoholic or drug-abusing males; this pattern has implications both for the severity of pathology in the family and for increased risk of substance abuse by the children. Thus, family therapy with substance abusers is complicated by the probability that several family members may have current or past problems, including non-substance-related psychopathology, similar to those of the identified patient. Many spouses of alcoholics, whether substance abusing or not, have dealt with substance abuse problems in their parents or in other close relatives.

Research on the (postnatal) role of the family of origin of the drinker and spouse in the etiology of substance abuse problems has focused on family contact and interactions such as family rituals and behavior around drinking patterns. Bennett and Wolin (1990) have reported that transmission of alcoholism is more probable if there is continuing interaction between alcoholic parents and their adult offspring. Also, adult males are more likely to develop alcoholism if there is continuing contact between them and alcoholic parents of their spouses. Bennett, an anthropologist, attributes this transmission to an acceptance of alcohol as part of the "family culture" and an inculturation effect on the offspring. Wolin et al. (1980) also found that among 25 families with a history of alcoholism, those who kept family rituals such as dinnertime and celebration of holidays, even during heavy drinking periods, showed less alcoholism among the offspring. Furthermore, among 68 adult married couples from an alcoholic family of origin, deliberate and planned family rituals seemed to protect against transmission of alcoholism into their own families (Bennett, Wolin, Reiss, & Teitelbaum, 1987). Both of these studies have been quoted widely and treatment interventions have been based on these findings (Steinglass, Bennett, Wolin, & Reiss, 1987). One might ask whether the families most severely affected by alcohol were the ones with the most disrupted households and associated psychopathology, and whether the severity of the alcohol problem, not the "symptom" of disrupted family rituals, was responsible for increased transmission of alcoholism to the offspring. Bennett et al. (1987) checked for this possibility and found that the severity of alcoholism in the family of origin of the "transmitter" versus "nontransmitter" families was no different and concluded that transmission was not due to severity of the parental alcoholism. Steinglass et al. (1987) nevertheless note that the degree to which alcoholic families uphold and keep their family rituals is best used as a "marker," or a measure of family identity, regardless of whether it is "mechanistic" or not in transmission.

Family behavior around drinking patterns has also been implicated in transmission of alcoholism. Steinglass et al. (1987) report that the most important factor in cross-generation continuance of drinking is whether a family rejects or accepts intoxication during family rituals. Nontransmitter families did not tolerate the "intrusion of intoxicated behavior" (p. 321) during rituals, whereas transmitter families did not automatically and consistently reject the intoxicated family member from participating in the family ritual. That is, families that deliberately forbid intoxication and demanded sobriety as a prerequisite for participation were less likely to experience transmission of alcoholism to the offspring.

Maintenance of Substance Abuse

Just as etiology is multiply determined, so is maintenance. In this chapter we adopt a social learning framework that describes current factors maintaining drinking, regardless of etiologic underpinnings. Using this approach, we assume that genetic vulnerability, environmental influences, and other etiologic factors are not immutable. That is, we separate current antecedents from historic factors and believe that distal causes of the drinking do not prohibit an individual from changing problematic behavior. Perhaps, due to etiologic factors, attaining and maintaining sobriety are more difficult for some than for others; however, the following framework is generally applicable regardless of etiologic variables because it gives the drinker and his/her family a chance to analyze and change the immediate antecedents and consequences of drinking behavior.

The model emphasizes the drinker and spouse's roles (rather than other family members) as agents of change, because this paradigm has been studied and shown empirically to be useful in treating alcoholic couples (McCrady & Epstein, 1995; McCrady, Stout, Noel, Abrams, & Nelson, 1991). The model has been applied to alcohol problems but has not yet been studied in relation to other drugs. Presumably, families with other drug problems can be treated using a similar model. Several basic assumptions are put forth: (1) Reciprocal interactions between the drinker and his environment (in this model, primarily the spouse) determine repetitive, stressful intra- and interpersonal behavioral patterns; (2) external antecedents to drinking have a lawful relationship to subsequent alcohol consumption, through repeated associations with reinforcement or anticipation of reinforcement; (3) cognitive and affective events mediate the relationship between external antecedents and drinking; and (4) drinking is maintained by physiological, psychological, and/or interpersonal consequences (McCrady & Epstein, 1995). The model is further explicated here.

Several key concepts describe our model of maintenance of drinking. It is assumed that substance use occurs in response to *antecedent stimuli or cues.* These stimuli or cues precede the substance use, and their presence increases the probability that substance use will occur. External antecedents may include individual, dyadic, or other factors. They may be features of the physical environment (e.g., a bar or beer commercial), certain times of the day, or interpersonal events. Dyadic, or familial, antecedents might include arguments with one's spouse, particularly arguments resulting from the spouse's attempting to control the alcoholic's drinking. Dyadic antecedents are common in the alcoholic family, because such families often develop severe communication, sexual, and financial problems over time, all of which are reflected in an unhappy marriage and impaired ability to solve problems. Frequently, stress begets more stress, as the alcoholic responds to the spouse's intense anger, fanned over the years by accumulating alcohol-related incidents, by withdrawing and perhaps increasing alcohol intake as an "escape route."

Aspects of the environment become cues for substance use through repeated sequences of events that include the stimulus, substance use, the experience of *reinforcement* for use, and the lack of occurrence of *punishing stimuli.* Reinforcers are defined as stimuli that increase the probability that a behavior will occur, while punishers decrease the probability that the behavior will occur. It is important to note that reinforcers and punishers do not exist independent of behavior—they can be defined only in their effect on behavior. Thus, if a wife believes that wearing seductive clothing when her husband is sober will reinforce sobriety but her husband becomes anxious when he sees her scanty attire and then drinks, the seductive attire must be viewed as a punishment for sobriety rather than a reinforcer. Reinforcers and punishers together are termed "consequences" of substance use and are defined as stimuli that occur consequent to, or after, substance use. Positive reinforcers for drinking, at the individual level, may include, for instance, alleviation of withdrawal symptoms or temporary euphoria to replace a depressed mood. Drinkers list many short-term positive consequences of drinking, and these need to be addressed carefully—therapists cannot change an alcoholic's experience of organismic positive reinforcers but can challenge cognitive mediators of these reinforcers. For example, short-term effects of alcohol may be pleasing, but are they really as potent as expectancies would suggest? Are there any short-term negative effects that are equally or even more potent? Are the short-term positive effects worth longer-term, much more negative effects such as an unsuccessful marriage or serious health problems? Positive consequences of drinking should not be dismissed lightly in therapy. They need to be acknowledged and challenged, given up and mourned, and/or obtained via a route less hazardous than alcohol.

The spouse and other family members may also unwittingly supply positive consequences of drinking, for instance, by taking care of the intoxicated family member, pampering him/her when sick from drinking too much, or protecting the drinker from negative consequences at work (i.e., calling in sick for the drinker). For certain couples, alcohol may actually be associated with an increase in positive interactions. If an individual experiences a lightening of negative affect upon ingestion of alcohol, he/she may be more likely to be agreeable interpersonally, thus benefiting socially (or familially) from the drink.

The relationship between an antecedent stimulus and substance use is believed to be mediated by *organismic* events. These events are the constellation of experiences that occur "inside the skin" and include thoughts, feelings, and physiological reactions. Substance abusers may have a variety of positive expectancies about the reinforcing consequences of substance use and may use in response to negative affect or certain physiological cues such as decreasing blood alcohol level. Substance abusers may also have internal reactions to interpersonal situations such as an argument with a spouse, and they may drink in response to their affective reaction to the argument (e.g., anxiety or depression) or their cognitive interpretation of an interaction (e.g., "She is trying to control me . . . I'll show her she can't control me!").

A number of cognitive constructs are important to conceptualizing a couple's relationship from a behavioral perspective. Couples make certain *attributions* about the motivations underlying each other's behavior, assuming that they know the reasons for certain actions. They also have certain *expectancies* about each other's future behavior, based partly on past experience and partly on their distorted attributions about the partner's motivations. These cognitions are important to modify in therapy, as they may be significant sources of relationship conflict and thus generate cues for substance use.

The repertoire of behavioral *responses* available to the substance user and to the couple or family is important. Substance abusers may lack the requisite skills to deal with drinking antecedents such as social pressure to use substances, interpersonal conflicts, anxiety, or depression. Alcoholic couples often have a variety of *skills deficits* in that they may have difficulty coping with alcohol-related situations, expressing positive affect, disagreeing, making requests for change in the partner, listening to and understanding the partner's communication, providing positive support, or solving problems productively as a couple.

It is assumed that interactions within a relationship have a *reciprocity* (called *circular causality* in family systems models), in that the behavior can best be understood in its interactional context. Reciprocity refers to the pattern of behaviors that occur between two people, in which the behavior of one partner cues the behavior of the other partner, which in turn cues further behavior of the first partner. Each partner's behavior is best understood in its reciprocal relationship to the other person's behavior. Behavioral marital research has focused heavily on positive and negative reciprocity, finding that distressed couples in general have a higher rate of negative reciprocity (negative behavior begets negative behavior) while nondistressed couples have higher rates of positive reciprocity (positive behavior begets positive behavior).

The effect of alcohol on family and marital interaction is complex, and negative consequences are often quite prominent. Family members may avoid or criticize the drinker. In some cases, family members find it difficult to tolerate the drinking or the behavior of the intoxicated individual, and verbal or even physical assaults ensue. Typically, these negative consequences serve only to exacerbate the problem; the drinker may leave the house and drink elsewhere or may learn to drink secretly. In either case, a pattern of lying on the alcoholic's part and hypervigilance and mistrust by the spouse may result, severely damaging family functioning. Finally, because the alcoholic with a moderate to severe problem spends an inordinate amount of time seeking, consuming, or recovering from the effects of alcohol, he/she is typically unable to contribute fully to the daily functioning of the household. The nonalcoholic spouse and children must then take on more responsibilities around the house, leading to increased resentment and stress. All this may serve to deepen the unpleasantness in the home and cue the alcoholic to spend more time out of the home, drinking.

To summarize, problem drinking is maintained by many intersecting factors and involves the individual's intra- and interpersonal state, antecedent cues, and positive and negative consequences on the individual and family level. This complexity results in a spiral effect: Reciprocal interactions between drinkers and their social environment typically tend to worsen the drinking and drinking-related consequences over time, and dysfunctional patterns of individual and family patterns become overlearned and "automatic" through repetition. Families experiencing substance abuse may also be experiencing other individual and family problems.

Role of Research in Theory

Research has played a central role in the development of our behavioral–systems models for conceptualizing substance use and family functioning.

Jackson's early research challenged prevailing psychodynamic models, setting the stage for further stress and coping research and models that underpin contemporary theoretical models. The seminal observational research of Steinglass, Billings, Becker, Frankenstein, and Jacob provided major information on the importance of reinforcement and family organization. Clinical trials, which are not a focus of this chapter, have provided strong empirical support for the application of behavioral and integrated models for couples and family-involved treatment for alcohol and drug problems (e.g., Cadogen, 1973; Corder, Corder, & Laidlaw, 1972; McCrady et al., 1991; O'Farrell, Choquette, Cutter, Brown, & McCourt, 1993; Szapocznik et al., 1988; Thomas & Ager, 1993).

Before turning to a consideration of treatment implications of the model, some of the complicating factors, including other psychopathology and heterogeneity of substance-abusing families, are considered.

Relationship between Substance Abuse and Other Psychopathology

As mentioned above, research indicates that rates of psychopathology are elevated in substance-abusing populations. Estimates of lifetime drug use disorders comorbid with alcohol dependence are as high as 80% (Carroll, 1986; Ross, Glaser, & Germanson, 1988). Comorbid antisocial personality disorder rates among male alcoholics range from 23% (Morgenstern & Langenbucher, 1994) to 53% (Ross, Glaser, & Stiasny, 1988), depending on recruitment site (e.g., rates tend be higher in Veterans Administration populations) and diagnostic instrument used. For mood disorders, Ross, Glaser, and Stiasny (1988) cited rates of 23% and 60% for depressive disorders and anxiety disorders, respectively, in men and 35% and 67%, respectively, for women.

The relationship between substance abuse and psychopathology is complex. Simple models do exist; for instance, the classic disease model contends that psychopathology in both the identified patient and his/her family members is a result of chronic substance abuse and abates after the abuser is able to maintain sobriety. There is no empirical evidence to support this hypothesis, and, in fact, several studies indicate that a substantial proportion of psychopathology is primary (i.e., predates substance abuse) (Epstein, Ginsburg, Hesselbrock, & Schwarz, 1994). Khantzian (Khantzian & Khantzian, 1984) is a proponent of an alternative theory, that substance abusers use alcohol and drugs to self-medicate preexisting conditions. For instance, narcotics addicts, according to this view, are not seeking euphoria but are attempting to alleviate dysphoria associated with intense affect and drive states such as rage and depression. Further research is needed to evaluate this view and in general to untangle the relationship between substance use and psychopathology.

Family systems models view psychopathological symptoms as serving particular functions in the family interaction. In general, psychopathological symptoms are an integral part of and help maintain the "family identity." Because, according to family systems models, stability and predictability are important to maintain a homeostatic balance (Steinglass et al., 1987), behaviors and interactions, including psychopathology, become incorporated into the system. For instance, in a family in which the husband is alcoholic, a child who behaves badly at school can serve as a focus for the nonalcoholic spouse. In this way, rather than concentrating on her unhappiness and frustration with her husband and thus jeopardizing the stability of the marital relationship and viability of the family as a whole, the wife concerns herself with the poor behavior of the child. Thus, the psychopathology of the child serves as a distraction from the alcoholism in the family.

Regardless of the etiology of individual psychopathology in the family, one point is clear: It must be assessed in terms of severity, need for treatment, and impact on the family functioning and maintenance of substance abuse. For instance, if in the context of family therapy it becomes apparent that the alcoholic father is suffering symptoms of a major depression, strategies must be devised to address the depression. Does it persist for at least 2 weeks after the individual becomes sober? Is it so severe that it is interfering with the individual's ability to stop drinking? Is the individual a suicide risk? If the answer to any of these questions is yes, the therapist needs to consider a referral for a medication evaluation or for other treatment specific to the depression. Sometimes character disorder, either in the spouse or in the abuser, interferes with couple treatment. In our clinic, for example, a couple in which the alcoholic man was 15 years younger than his female partner presented for treatment. As treatment progressed the woman became more volatile and unpredictable emotionally. She either cried uncontrollably and begged for understanding or became irate and verbally abusive. At home, the man dealt with her violent mood swings by spending very little time with her while sober. In session, he had trouble tolerating the intensity of her attacks, and she had difficulty controlling them. It became apparent that the depth of the woman's psychopathology (i.e., borderline personality disorder) rendered marital therapy for the man's alcohol problem inappropriate. Each partner was referred for individual therapy.

Heterogeneity of Substance Abuse Problems in Families

Both behavioral and family systems models of family therapy assume heterogeneity among substance abuse problems and among families of substance abusers. Behavioral approaches typically begin with functional analysis—an individualized analysis of the substance abuse pattern, its particular antecedents (i.e., triggers or cues), the amount and type of substance consumed, and the particular pattern of reinforcing and punishing consequences that typically ensue in various circumstances. This method recognizes that each substance abuser has an idiosyncratic use of and array of associated problems with alcohol and/or drugs.

Two models of alcoholism and family factors explicitly address the notion of heterogeneity among families of substance abusers. Steinglass, Bennett, Wolin, and Reiss (1987) contend that though alcoholic families are characterized by life structured around alcohol as a "central organizing principle," there is substantial variability among facets of each family. Families vary along particular dimensions of family temperament and family identity and also according to the family's developmental stage (early, middle, or late phase). According to Steinglass et al. (1987), varying configurations of three family temperaments render uniqueness among alcoholic families: energy level (high vs. low), preferred interactional distance (less vs. more permeable), and behavioral range (flexible vs. inflexible). Family identity is defined as an underlying cognitive structure (i.e., a set of shared beliefs and rules). Steinglass et al. (1987) have stressed the heterogeneity among alcoholic families they have studied and treated, arguing against simplistic models of etiology and treatment of problems in the alcoholic family.

Jacob and Leonard (1988; Leonard, 1990), in an attempt to resolve discrepancies in the literature regarding the positive or negative effect alcohol had on marital interactions (Frankenstein, Hay, & Nathan, 1985; Jacob & Krahn, 1988), segregated a sample of 49 alcoholic couples into steady versus episodic/binge drinkers (there was no indication of how many steady versus other drinkers there were in the sample). Depending on the alcoholic's drinking pattern, alcohol had different effects on the marital interaction. Wives of episodic drinkers became less negative when their husbands drank, and wives of steady drinkers became more negative in the same context. Earlier, Jacob, Dunn, and Leonard (1983) found that steady drinkers' wives reported higher marital satisfaction and lower scores on the Minnesota Multiphasic Personality Inventory than did wives of episodic drinkers. Using sequential analysis of drinking and marital satisfaction in a relatively small sample, Dunn, Jacob, Hummon, and Seilhamer (1987) reported that the marital satisfaction of in-home steady drinkers' wives was increased after the husband's drinking, whereas for out-of-home steady drinkers' wives, the husband's drinking predicted decreases in marital satisfaction. Thus, preliminary evidence suggests that alcohol has varying impact depending on characteristics of particular families and drinkers.

Tasks Required for Treatment to Be Successful

The application of the above-described theoretical model to family-involved substance abuse treatment requires several elements. The first tasks revolve around engagement in the therapy. Ideally, several family members and the identified substance user would all be involved in the treatment. If only one family member is willing to become involved, however, the clinician can still incorporate family conceptions into the treatment.

The second major task of therapy is assessment. Assessment focuses on identification of antecedent stimuli for use, organismic mediating variables, and consequences of use. The relative role of individual, familial, and other interpersonal systems in maintaining the substance use must be assessed. Additionally, assessment of the problems and functioning of individuals within the family unit is appropriate to determine whether any family member is experiencing distress so severe that other treatment is warranted. Assessment also addresses the role of substance use in the family and the overall patterns of interaction in the family in terms of patterns of communication, problem solving, and behavioral control; roles and family rules; and family boundaries.

The third major task of therapy is the introduction of change procedures to affect the substance use. Most contemporary family models first focus on stabilizing abstinence or nonproblem use before addressing family functioning. A variety of behavioral techniques may be used to achieve this goal, and pharmacologic adjuncts may be considered as well.

The fourth major task is the modification of antecedents to substance use, reinforcing consequences of substance use, and the introduction of reinforcing consequences for abstinence or nonproblem use. This is the first phase of therapy to require significant behavior change from family members other than the substance user.

The fifth task is the modification of patterns of family interaction, communication and problem-solving skills, and consideration of family themes, rules, and roles that interfere with effective family functioning.

Although these phases of therapy are described as sequential, therapy often requires the clinician to be flexible in sequencing of therapy. For example, if physical abuse and threats are used a primary mode of behavioral control in a family, such a pattern would need to be addressed immediately to ensure the safety of family members.

Application of the Family Therapy Models of Alcoholism Treatment to Other Psychoactive Substances

Research on family models of treatment has focused on alcohol problems. Limited attention has been given to treatment of other drug use; most of this work has focused on family treatment of adolescent drug abuse. Adolescent drug use is currently treated in the context of a more general framework of adolescent problem behaviors, and family-based treatments typically address the entire set of problems (Liddle & Dakof, 1994). Prevailing family therapy techniques for substance-abusing adolescents include structural family therapy (Stanton, Todd, & Associates, 1982), strategic (Lewis, Piercy, Sprenkle, & Trepper, 1990), behavioral (Bry, 1988), multidimensional, and multisystemic (Henggeler & Borduin, 1990) approaches. Liddle and Dakof (1994) provide a review of the efficacy of family-based treatments for adolescent substance abusers. In general, they report that family treatment is effective in engaging and retaining substance-abusing adolescents and their families in treatment and in significantly reducing drug use.

Stanton et al.'s (1982) model of structural–strategic family therapy for drug addicts, is one of the only well-developed family approaches for adults. It has been used primarily for narcotics-dependent individuals but can be adapted for any type of drug addiction. This method is short term and goal directed and involves the addict's family of origin in the treatment. Focus is on the addict–parents triad, because the addict's dyadic or marital relationship is seen as a repetition of the nuclear family of origin. However, the drug use is also dealt with in the context of the "family of procreation" because the identified patient's drug taking is seen as a part of the current interactional behavior of the whole family. Goals for the treatment are prioritized in the following way: (1) abstinence from drugs, (2) productive use of time (i.e., employment or school), and (3) stable and autonomous living situation. In addition, home detoxification is encouraged. Stanton et al. (1982) have provided evidence for success using their structural–strategic approach. In a random assignment study, at 1-year follow-up individuals who underwent family therapy were using significantly less psychoactive substances (in every drug category except alcohol) than those who underwent nonfamily treatment. Nearly two thirds of the family-treated subjects were abstinent from drugs at follow-up. This study has been replicated in the Netherlands (Romijn, Platt, & Schippers, 1990;

Romijn, Platt, Schippers, & Schaap, 1992). Romijn et al. (1990) found that 18 months after treatment, 64 to 81% of the family-treated subjects were abstaining or rarely using illegal and legal opiates, nonopiates, and alcohol. Far fewer of the non-family-treated subjects were similarly abstinent at 18 months follow-up; however, the differences between the family-treated and control groups were not statistically significant. Other researchers (i.e., McLellan, Arndt, Metzger, Woody, & O'Brien, 1993) are beginning to incorporate generic forms of family therapy into psychosocial treatment packages as adjuncts to methadone maintenance programs with good success.

In terms of behavioral family therapy for adult substance abusers, now that the efficacy of such family treatments for alcohol problems is fairly well established, future research might test their applications to problems with other drug classes. There is no reason to assume that the behavioral marital therapy model, for instance, would need to be altered in a substantive way to be applied to other drugs such as marijuana or cocaine. Other behavioral treatments have been successfully used to treat these disorders (Grabowski, Rhoades, Elk, Schmitz, & Creson, 1993), and their continued application to other drug use disorders is encouraged (Onken, Blaine, & Boren, 1993). Of course, differences in the interventions would need to be tailored to the particular sequelae of various drugs, and variations in populations using certain drugs might present a problem. For instance, it would be more difficult to recruit a large sample of middle-class, married heroin addicts on which to test behavioral marital therapy for opiate use than it is to recruit such a sample for alcohol use. However, it would be possible to extend the model used currently with "purely alcoholic" couples to couples where the alcoholic is a polyabuser.

In summary, most family therapy work with substance abusers has been done with families of adolescent addicts who are also treated for more general patterns of deviant behavior. The limited work done thus far to develop and test various types of family therapy with adult substance abusers indicates that such treatment approaches have merit and should be further developed.

ADVANTAGES AND DISADVANTAGES
OF A FAMILY APPROACH

There are several advantages to a family-based approach to conceptualizing and treating substance use disorders. Most important is the strong empirical base for the theoretical models and for treatments derived from family models. Family models also direct the theoretician's attention to the environmental contexts in which alcohol and other drug use occur and direct the clinician to consider maintaining factors beyond the individual. Family involvement is associated with better compliance with treatment (e.g., Berger, 1981) and with better treatment outcome. By directing attention to the family, the clinician increases the probability that the identified client will comply with treatment and have a successful outcome. In addition, ample research supports the negative impact that substance use has on the functioning of the rest of the family, and involving the rest of the family in treatment may ease the distress of other family members as well. Family models provide a framework for conceptualizing the interrelationships between substance use and family functioning and can be used as a guide for treatment with any member of the family who is available for treatment.

One disadvantage of family models is their greater complexity. Theoreticians must account for multiple interactive relationships, and clinicians must be able to attend to the complexities inherent in dealing with several individuals and the interactions among them. Working with families requires specialized skills and training.

Family models also have some limits from a theoretical perspective. The models lack a conceptualization of the limits of family treatment. The models do not address the complexities introduced by families with multiple substance-abusing members, families with members with other kinds of psychopathology, or families characterized by an extremely high degree of disorganization or destructive interactions. The models also give no explicit attention to the relative importance of the needs of various family members. For example, although the presence of a supportive spouse might increase the probability of a successful treatment outcome, continuing in a relationship might have adverse consequences for the non-substance-abusing partner. Family models also have no explicit theory to facilitate decision making about the focus of intervention (i.e., individual, familial, or other social systems).

SUMMARY AND CONCLUSIONS

In summary, family models have evolved over the past 60 years into contemporary models that emphasize the multiple determinants of psychoactive substance use disorders, the multiple factors that maintain these disorders, and the complex interrelationships between the substance user and the familial and other interpersonal environments in which he/she exists. A rich body of empirical literature provides strong support for family-based models and for the effectiveness of treatments based on these models. Research knowledge is limited by its lack of attention to gender, cultural, racial, and sexual orientation issues among subjects, the lack of couple treatment research on drug users, and the lack of family treatment research on alcoholics. The practicing clinician will be confronted repeatedly with family issues among substance-abusing clients and concerned family members and should incorporate family models into everyday clinical practice.

ACKNOWLEDGMENT

Preparation of this chapter was supported in part by grants RO1 AA07070 and P50 AA08747 from the National Institute on Alcohol Abuse and Alcoholism.

REFERENCES

Alcoholics Anonymous. (1976). *Alcoholics Anonymous: The story of how many thousands of men and women have recovered from alcoholism* (3rd ed.). New York: Alcoholics Anonymous World Services.

Babor, T. F., Dolinsky, Z. S., Meyer, R. E., Hesselbrock, M., Hofmann, M., & Tennen, H. (1992). Types of alcoholics: Concurrent and predictive validity of some common classification schemes. *British Journal of the Addictions, 87,* 23–40.

Barton, C., & Alexander, J. F. (1981). Functional family therapy. In A. S. Gurman & D. P. Kniskern (Eds.), *Handbook of family therapy* (pp. 403–443). New York: Brunner/Mazel.

Beattie, M. (1987). *Co-dependent no more.* Minneapolis, MN: Hazelden.

Becker, J. V., & Miller, P. M. (1976). Verbal and nonverbal marital interaction patterns of alcoholics and nonalcoholics. *Journal of Studies on Alcohol, 37,* 1616–1624.

Bennett, L. A., & Wolin, S. J. (1990). Family culture and alcoholism transmission. In R. L. Collins, K. E. Leonard, & J. S. Searles (Eds.), *Alcohol and the family: Research and clinical perspectives* (pp. 194–219). New York: Guilford Press.

Bennett, L. A., Wolin, S. J., Reiss, D., & Teitelbaum, M. A. (1987). Couples at risk for transmission of alcoholism: Protective influences. *Family Process, 26,* 111–129.

Berger, A. (1981). Family involvement and alcoholics' completion of a multiphase treatment program. *Journal of Studies on Alcohol, 42,* 517–520.

Billings, A. G., Kessler, M., Gomberg, C. A., & Weiner, S. (1979). Marital conflict resolution of alcoholic and nonalcoholic couples during drinking and non-drinking sessions. *Journal of Studies on Alcohol, 40,* 183–195.

Black, C. (1982). *It will never happen to me!* Denver, CO: M.A.C.

Broderick, C. B., & Schrader, S. S. (1981). The history of professional marriage and family therapy. In A. S. Gurman & D. P. Kniskern (Eds.), *Handbook of family therapy* (pp. 5– 35). New York: Brunner/Mazel.

Brownell, K. D., Heckerman, C. L., Westlake, R. J., Hayes, S. C., & Monti, P. M. (1978). The effect of couples training and partner cooperativeness in the behavioral treatment of obesity. *Behaviour Research and Therapy, 16,* 323–333.

Bry, B. H. (1988). Family-based approaches to reducing adolescent substance use: Theories, techniques and findings. In E. R. Rahdert & J. Grabowski (Eds.), *Adolescent drug abuse: Analyses of treatment research* (NIDA Monograph 77, Publication No. ADM-88-1523 pp. 39–68). Rockville, MD: U.S. Department of Health and Human Services.

Cadogen, D. A. (1973). Marital group therapy in the treatment of alcoholism. *Quarterly Journal of Studies on Alcohol, 34,* 1187–1194.

Cadoret, R. J., O'Gorman, T. W., Troughton, E., & Heywood, E. (1985). Alcoholism and antisocial personality: Interrelationships, genetic and environmental factors. *Archives of General Psychiatry, 42,* 161–167.

Carroll, J. F. X. (1986). Treating multiple substance abuse clients. *Recent Developments in Alcoholism, 4,* 85–103.

Cermak, T. (1986). *Diagnosing and treating co-dependence.* Minneapolis, MN: Johnson Institute.

Cloninger, C. R., Bohman, M., & Sigvardsson, S. (1981). Inheritance of alcohol abuse. *Archives of General Psychiatry, 38,* 861–868.

Corder, B. F., Corder, R. F., & Laidlaw, N. L. (1972). An intensive treatment program for alcoholics and their wives. *Quarterly Journal of Studies on Alcohol, 33,* 1144–1146.

Cork, M. (1969). *The forgotten children.* Toronto: Addiction Research Foundation.

Cowley, D. S., Roy-Byrne, P. P., Godon, C., Greenblatt, D. J., Ries, R., Walker, R. D., Samson, H. H., & Hommer, D. W. (1992). Response to diazepam in sons of alcoholics. *Alcoholism: Clinical and Experimental Research, 16*(6), 1057–1063.

Dare, C., Eisler, I., Russell, G. F. M., & Szmukler, G. I. (1990). The clinical and theoretical impact of a controlled trial of family therapy in anorexia nervosa. *Journal of Marital and Family Therapy, 16,* 39–58.

Davis, D. I., Berenson, D., Steinglass, P., & Davis, S. (1974). The adaptive consequences of drinking. *Psychiatry, 37,* 209–215.

Devor, E. (1994). A developmental/genetic model of alcoholism: Implications for genetic research. *Journal of Consulting and Clinical Psychology, 62,* 1108–1115.

Dunn, N. J., Jacob, T., Hummon, N., & Seilhamer, R. A. (1987). Marital stability in alcoholic–spouse relationships as a function of drinking pattern and location. *Journal of Abnormal Psychology, 96,* 99–107.

Epstein, E. E., Ginsburg, B., Hesselbrock, V., & Schwarz, J. C. (1994). Alcohol and drug abusers subtyped by antisocial personality disorder and primary or secondary depressive disorder. *Annals of the New York Academy of Sciences, 708*, 187–201.

Frankenstein, W., Hay, W. M., & Nathan, P. E. (1985). Effects of intoxication on alcoholics' marital communication and problem solving. *Journal of Studies on Alcohol, 46*, 1–6.

Frankenstein, W., Nathan, P. E., Sullivan, R. F., Hay, W. M., & Cocco, K. (1985). Asymmetry of influence in alcoholics' marital communication: Alcohol's effects on interaction dominance. *Journal of Marital and Family Therapy, 11*, 399–411.

Grabowski, J., Rhoades, H., Elk, R., Schmitz, J., & Creson, D. (1993). Clinicwide and individualized behavioral interventions in drug dependence treatment. In L. S. Onken, J. D. Blaine, & J. J. Boren, (Eds.), *Behavioral treatments for drug abuse and dependence* (NIDA Research Monograph 137, DHHS Publication No. 93-3684, pp. 73–77). Rockville, MD: National Institute on Drug Abuse.

Hall, R. L., Hesselbrock, V. M., & Stabenau, J. R. (1983a). Familial distribution of alcohol use: I. Assortative mating of alcoholic probands. *Behavior Genetics, 13*(4), 373–382.

Hall, R. L., Hesselbrock, V. M., & Stabenau, J. R. (1983b). Familial distribution of alcohol use: II. Assortative mating in the parents of alcoholics. *Behavior Genetics, 13*(4), 361–372.

Hammen, C. L. (1991). Mood disorders (unipolar depression). In M. Hersen & S. M. Turner (Eds.), *Adult psychopathology and diagnosis* (2nd ed., pp. 170–207). New York: Wiley.

Henggeler, S. W., & Borduin, C. M. (1990). *Family therapy and beyond: A multisystemic approach to treating the behavior problems of children and adolescents*. Pacific Grove, CA: Brooks/Cole.

Hersen, M., Miller, P. M., & Eisler, R. M. (1973). Interactions between alcoholics and their wives. A descriptive analysis of verbal and nonverbal behavior. *Quarterly Journal of Studies on Alcohol, 34*, 516–520.

Hesselbrock, M. (1986). Alcoholic typologies: A review of empirical evaluations of common classification schemes. *Recent Developments in Alcoholism, 4*, 191–206.

Hesselbrock, M., Meyer, R., & Keener, J. J. (1985). Psychopathology in hospitalized alcoholics. *Archives of General Psychiatry, 42*, 1050–1055, 698–704.

Hill, S. (1994). Etiology. In J. Langenbucher, B. McCrady, W. Frankenstein, & P. Nathan (Eds.), *Annual review of addictions research and treatment* (pp. 127–148). New York: Pergamon Press.

Jackson, J. (1954). The adjustment of the family to the crisis of alcoholism. *Quarterly Journal of Studies on Alcohol, 15*, 562–586.

Jacob, T., Dunn, N. J., & Leonard, K. (1983). Patterns of alcohol abuse and family stability. *Alcoholism: Clinical and Experimental Research, 7*, 382–385.

Jacob, T., & Krahn, G. L. (1988). Marital interactions of alcoholic couples: Comparison with depressed and nondistressed couples. *Journal of Consulting and Clinical Psychology, 56*, 73–79.

Jacob, T., & Leonard, K. (1988). Alcoholic-spouse interaction as a function of alcoholism subtype and alcohol consumption interaction. *Journal of Abnormal Psychology, 97,* 231–237.

Jacob, T., Ritchey, D., Cvitkovic, J. F., & Blane, H. T. (1981). Communication styles of alcoholic and nonalcoholic families when drinking and not drinking. *Journal of Studies on Alcohol, 42,* 466–482.

Kendler, K. S., Heath, A. C., Neale, M. C., Kessler, R. C., & Eaves, L. C. (1992). A population-based twin study of alcoholic women. *Journal of the American Medical Association, 14,* 1877–1882.

Khantzian, E. J., & Khantzian, N. J. (1984). Cocaine addiction: Is there a psychological predisposition? *Psychiatric Annals, 14*(10), 753–759.

Kogan, K. L., & Jackson, J. (1965). Stress, personality and emotional disturbance in wives of alcoholics. *Quarterly Journal of Studies on Alcohol, 26,* 486–495.

Konstantareas, M. M. (1990). A psychoeducational model for working with families of autistic children. *Journal of Marital and Family Therapy, 16,* 59–70.

Leonard, K. E. (1990). Marital functioning among episodic and steady alcoholics. In R. L. Collins, K. E. Leonard, & J. S. Searles (Eds.), *Alcohol and the family: Research and clinical perspectives* (pp. 220–243). New York: Guilford Press.

Lewis, M. L. (1937). Alcoholism and family casework. *Social Casework, 35,* 8–14.

Lewis, R. A., Piercy, F. P., Sprenkle, D. H., & Trepper, T. S. (1990). The Purdue brief family therapy model for adolescent substance abusers. In T. Todd & M. Selekman (Eds.), *Family therapy with adolescent substance abusers.* New York: Allyn & Bacon.

Liddle, H. A., & Dakof, G. A. (in press). Family-based treatment for adolescent drug use: State of the science. In E. Rahdert (Ed.), *Adolescent drug abuse: Assessment and treatment* (NIDA Research Monograph Series). Rockville, MD: National Institute on Drug Abuse.

MacDonald, D. E. (1956). Mental disorders in wives of alcoholics. *Quarterly Journal of Studies on Alcohol, 17,* 282–287.

McCrady, B. S., & Epstein, E. E. (1995). Marital therapy in the treatment of alcohol problems. In N. S. Jacobson & A. S. Gurman (Eds.), *Clinical handbook of couple therapy* (pp. 369–393). New York: Guilford Press.

McCrady, B. S., Stout, R., Noel, N., Abrams, D., & Nelson, H. F. (1991). Effectiveness of three types of spouse-involved behavioral alcoholism treatment. *British Journal of Addiction, 86,* 1415–1424.

McLellan, A. T., Arndt, I. O., Metzger, D. S., Woody, G. E., & O'Brien, C. P. (1993). The effects of psychosocial services in substance abuse treatment. *Journal of the American Medical Association, 269*(15), 1953–1959.

Merikangas, K. R., Leckman, J. F., Prusoff, B. A., Pauls, D. L., & Weissman, M. M. (1985). Familial transmission of depression and alcoholism. *Archives of General Psychiatry, 42,* 367–372.

Moos, R. H., Finney, J. W., & Gamble, W. (1982). The process of recovery from alcoholism. II. Comparing spouses of alcoholic patients and matched community controls. *Journal of Studies on Alcohol, 43,* 888–909.

Moos, R. H., & Moos, B. S. (1984). The process of recovery from alcoholism. III. Comparing functioning of families of alcoholics and matched control families. *Journal of Studies on Alcohol, 45,* 111–118.

Morgenstern, J., & Langenbucher, J. (1994, August). *Comorbidity: Recent findings and their implications for understanding and treating addictive disorders.* Symposium for presentation to the annual meeting of the American Psychological Association, Los Angeles.

O'Farrell, T. J., Choquette, K. A., Cutter, H. S. G., Brown, E. D., & McCourt, W. F. (1993). Behavioral marital therapy with and without additional couples relapse prevention sessions for alcoholics and their wives. *Journal of Studies on Alcohol, 54,* 652–666.

Onken, L. S., Blaine, J. D., & Boren, J. J. (1993). *Behavioral treatments for drug abuse and dependence* (NIDA Research Monograph 137, NIH Publication No. 93-3684). Washington, DC: U.S. Government Printing Office.

Patterson, G. R. (1986). Performance models for antisocial boys. *American Psychologist, 41,* 432–444.

Romijn, C. M., Platt, J. J., & Schippers, G. M. (1990). Family therapy for Dutch drug abusers: Replication of an American study. *International Journal of the Addictions, 25*(10), 1127–1149.

Romijn, C. M., Platt, J. J., Schippers, G. M., & Schaap, C. P. (1992). Family therapy for Dutch drug users: The relationship between family functioning and success. *International Journal of the Addictions, 27*(1), 1–14.

Ross, H. E., Glaser, F. B. & Germanson, T. (1988). The prevalence of psychiatric disorders in patients with alcohol and other drug problems. *Archives of General Psychiatry, 45,* 1023–1031.

Ross, H. E., Glaser, F. B. & Stiasny, S. (1988a). Sex differences in the prevalence of psychiatric disorders in patients with alcohol and drug problems. *British Journal of Addiction, 83,* 1179–1192.

Stanton, M. D., Todd, T. C., & Associates. (1982). *The family therapy of drug abuse and addiction.* New York: Guilford Press.

Steinglass, P. (1979). The alcoholic family in the interaction laboratory. *Journal of Nervous and Mental Disease, 167,* 428–436.

Steinglass, P. (1981). The alcoholic family at home. Patterns of interaction in dry, wet, and transitional stages of alcoholism. *Archives of General Psychiatry, 38,* 578–584.

Steinglass, P., Bennett, L. A., Wolin, S. J., & Reiss, D. (1987). *The alcoholic family.* New York: Basic Books.

Steinglass, P., Davis, D. I., & Berenson, D. (1977). Observations of conjointly hospitalized "alcoholic couples" during sobriety and intoxication: Implications for theory and therapy. *Family Process, 16,* 1–16.

Steinglass, P., Weiner, S., & Mendelson, J. H. (1971). Interactional issues as determinants of alcoholism. *American Journal of Psychiatry, 128,* 275–280.

Szapocznik, J., Perez-Vidal, A., Brickman, A. L., Foote, F. H., Santisteban, D., Hervis, O., & Kurtines, W. M. (1988). Engaging adolescent drug abusers and their families in treatment: A strategic structural systems approach. *Journal of Consulting and Clinical Psychology, 56,* 552–557.

Tarter, R. E. (1994). Alcoholism: A developmental disorder. *Journal of Consulting and Clinical Psychology, 62,* 1096–1107.

Thomas, E. J., & Ager, R. D. (1993). Unilateral family therapy with spouses of uncooperative alcohol abusers. In T. J. O'Farrell (Ed.), *Treating alcohol problems: Marital and family interventions* (pp. 3–33). New York: Guilford Press.

Wegsheider, S. (1981). *Another chance: Hope and health for the alcoholic family.* Palo Alto, CA: Science & Behavior Books.

Whalen, T. (1953). Wives of alcoholics: Four types observed in a family service agency. *Quarterly Journal of Studies on Alcohol, 14,* 632–641.

Wolin, S. J., Bennett, L. A., Noonan, D. L., & Teitelbaum, M. A. (1980). Disrupted family rituals: A factor in the intergenerational transmission of alcoholism. *Journal of Studies on Alcohol, 41,* 199–214.

Yates, W. R., Petty, F., & Brown, K. (1988). Alcoholism in males with antisocial personality disorder. *International Journal of the Addictions, 23,* 999–1010.

CHAPTER 6

Family Therapy Techniques

JAMES R. McKAY

The central premise underlying family therapy approaches to addictions treatment is that it can be beneficial to involve significant others in the treatment process. There are two basic types of family-based interventions: couple therapy and family therapy. In couple therapy, participation is limited to the substance abuser and one other family member, who is often a spouse or romantic partner. In family therapy, other family members, such as children or grandparents, are also involved. Couple therapy tends to be used more often with adult substance abusers, whereas family therapy is more common with adolescents. In this chapter, several approaches to family therapy are presented and key clinical issues are identified. Therapeutic techniques common to all approaches and those that are unique to each approach are outlined. Case material is used to illustrate how clinical issues surface and can be addressed in family therapy sessions. Finally, future directions for family therapy and the limitations of the approach are discussed.

Family therapy techniques from four different orientations are presented: psychodynamic, behavioral, family systems, and family disease approaches. Although these four orientations share a number of techniques, each has a different primary focus. The psychodynamic approach places particular emphasis on unconscious interpersonal processes, such as the repression of wishes and other feelings and the ways family members work to either support or undermine each other's defensive structures. Behavior therapy places a greater emphasis on assessment, goal setting, and practicing new and more adaptive behaviors through in-session role playing and between-session "homework" assignments. Family systems therapy is designed to address problems with boundaries and role functioning within families that produce a "symptom," in this case substance abuse, in a family member. In the family disease approach, substance abuse is viewed as a disease that affects all family members. Treatment therefore focuses on issues such as enabling, codependency, detachment, and the use of 12-Step programs for other family members.

WHEN IS FAMILY THERAPY WARRANTED?

Family therapy is difficult. Rather than having one person to contend with, the family therapist must deal with two or more patients in the same room at the same time. The therapist has to process and attend to two or more sets of feelings and points of view. The therapist may also be faced with having to work hard to set limits within the session as tempers rise and arguments break out. Finally, the more people that are involved in the treatment, the more difficult it is to keep everyone engaged and coming to the sessions.

Despite the difficulties in conducting family therapy with substance abusers, it can be a very useful approach in some cases. Family therapy is recommended when current interpersonal conflicts or relationship problems are directly contributing to substance abuse. For example, a substance abuser may drink or take drugs after a bitter argument with a spouse or after feeling badly let down or disappointed by a parent (Maisto, O'Farrell, Connors, McKay, & Pelcovits, 1988; Marlatt & Gordon, 1985). Family therapy can also be important when family members are somehow enabling the identified substance abuser. Enabling occurs when family members inadvertently support an individual's use of alcohol or drugs by not speaking up about the seriousness of the problem or taking other steps to confront and deal with the problem (Brown, 1988). In some situations, family therapy can also be used by family members to organize an intervention designed to convince a resistant substance abuser to enter treatment (Johnson, 1986). Finally, family therapy can be used to help other family members who have been adversely affected by the behavior of the substance abuser.

TECHNIQUES AND GOALS COMMON
TO ALL FAMILY-BASED APPROACHES

Although the four approaches to family therapy for the addictions differ in many ways, they also share certain techniques and therapeutic goals.

These techniques and goals are important in all forms of family therapy because they concern forming and maintaining alliances with each family member and facilitating better communication and interpersonal functioning.

Joining

One of the first tasks for the family therapist is to make connections with each member of the couple or family. The goal of this process, which is known as joining, is for the therapist and family members to feel that they can work together on the problem (Kaufman & Pattison, 1981). The first part of this process involves careful listening on the part of the therapist. At the beginning of the first session, for example, the therapist might ask each family member to talk about his/her perceptions of what is wrong in the family and his/her feelings about it. Although each person will probably say something about the substance abuse problem in the family, the person may not agree on whether there are problems in other areas. For example, one study investigated differences between alcoholics and their spouses in their perceptions of the functioning of their families prior to entering treatment (McKay, Maisto, Beattie, Longabaugh, & Noel, 1993). There was relatively good agreement about how well the family functioned in some areas, such as problem solving, communication, and sharing of emotions. However, there was essentially no agreement on how well the family dealt with establishing and adhering to rules of conduct and the appropriateness of the level of involvement between family members (e.g., overly intrusive vs. underinvolved). By paying equal attention to each person, the therapist conveys that he/she is interested in what everyone has to say and expects that there may be differences in their perceptions of the family. This stance on the part of the therapist makes it less likely that some family members will feel ignored or devalued.

The second part of the joining process requires that the therapist be able to communicate to the family that he/she has (1) an understanding of each member's perceptions of the problem and (2) a clear idea about how to address the issues raised by each member. Often, families with substance abuse problems are demoralized and pessimistic when they seek help. The process of joining may therefore stretch out over several sessions, as family members gradually begin to have more hope that things might actually improve. However, it is particularly important for the therapist to make connections with family members as soon as possible, as families with substance abuse problems are already at heightened risk to drop out of treatment.

Establishing the Ground Rules

It is also important early on to establish the ground rules for the therapy. Issues such as the time and length of sessions, the expected duration of the treatment, procedures for changing or canceling sessions, and the cost of each session and how payments will be made should ideally be discussed in the first session. With substance-abusing patients, it is also crucial to discuss how urges to use and any episodes of substance use will be dealt with. Although the various therapeutic orientations have somewhat different approaches to addressing substance use during treatment, each orientation strongly advocates that substance abusers openly discuss both their urges to use and any episodes of actual use.

Conducting outpatient family therapy with an active substance abuser can be extremely difficult. Therefore, another issue that should be addressed early on is what the family members should do if the identified patient begins to use again or is not able to completely stop using at the beginning of treatment. For example, should they still come to a session if the substance abuser is nowhere to be found? Or, should they bring an intoxicated substance abuser to the session if he/she is willing to come? In cases in which the substance abuser continues to use heavily at the beginning of family treatment, it may be necessary for that person to enter a more restricted treatment setting for detoxification or rehabilitation before family therapy can commence. When the substance abuser comes to a family session under the influence, Kaufman (1985) recommends that the session be held. However, the therapist should leave it to the family members to deal with the substance abuser rather than taking control of the situation. Substance abusers will frequently fail to come to sessions if they have started using again. Family sessions can still be held to discuss ways to motivate the patient to return to therapy or to provide a place for family members to talk about themselves. However, the session should not be used to discuss other issues that concern the substance abuser and thus need to be brought up with that person present.

Eliciting Each Member's Experience

As the therapy progresses, it is important that the therapist continue to express a genuine interest in each family member's perceptions and feelings. This helps each member to feel engaged in the treatment process. Furthermore, by demonstrating an interest in each member and curiosity about his/her experience, the therapist provides a model to family members of how they should listen and respond appropriately to each other (Shapiro, 1982a).

Identifying Central Areas of Interpersonal Dysfunction

One of the primary tasks in all forms of family therapy is to identify central areas of interpersonal dysfunction. In families with substance abuse problems, for example, there is often difficulty with trust, boundaries, role functioning, communication, and setting appropriate limits on behavior (McCrady, 1986; Moos & Moos, 1984; Stanton, Todd, & Associates, 1982). These problems can sometimes act directly to trigger substance abuse, as when a vicious argument with a spouse prompts an alcoholic to go off on a binge. Even when interpersonal dysfunction does not lead immediately to episodes of substance abuse, it increases the likelihood that more drinking or drug use will occur over time (McKay, Longabaugh, Beattie, Maisto, & Noel, 1992, 1993a). Furthermore, other members of the family are adversely affected by difficulties in interpersonal functioning. It is therefore important to identify areas of interpersonal dysfunction early in either family or couple therapy.

Improving Communication of Thoughts and Feelings

Many families with substance abuse problems are characterized by major problems around the communication of thoughts and feelings (Billings, Kessler, Gomberg, & Weiner, 1979; Jacob, Richey, Cvitkovic, & Blane, 1981; McCrady, 1986; McKay, Murphy, Rivinus, & Maisto, 1991). These problems include difficulty recognizing feelings, fear about expressing anger or disappointment, lack of control over anger, lying to cover up unacceptable behaviors, and so forth. Problems with communication may play a role in the etiology of substance abuse, as individuals who have difficulty recognizing and expressing their feelings might be more prone to use drugs or alcohol either to defend against or allow the expression of their feelings. Often, the substance abuser has desperately been attempting to either hide substance use or convince the family that the problem is under control. Therefore, the central communications in the family are organized around the substance abuser's attempts to mislead, or in some cases deceive, other family members. By the time the couple or family comes to therapy, communication problems are likely to be profound. These issues should be identified and addressed in therapy.

Addressing Enabling

In families with addiction problems, there is a tendency for the non-substance-abusing members to want to make things easier for the substance abuser. Although this may seem paradoxical, given the pain and suffering addiction causes other family members, it is nonetheless a common occurrence (Brown, 1988). Examples of enabling include the spouse who calls in sick for an intoxicated or hungover mate, the parent who ignores obvious evidence of substance use in a teenager, and family members who do not challenge extremely unlikely excuses offered up by substance abusers to explain their behavior. Family therapy can be particularly effective in decreasing enabling, as other family members are involved in the therapeutic process.

SPECIALIZED TECHNIQUES AND GOALS

Although certain techniques and goals are common to all approaches to the family treatment of substance abuse, major differences also exist. In this section, specialized techniques and goals from psychodynamic, behavioral, family systems, and family disease approaches to family therapy are identified and discussed.

Psychodynamic Approach

In psychodynamic treatment, there is a strong emphasis on discovering and working with unconscious material. In family therapy, this is done by (1) uncovering unconscious interpersonal processes; (2) exposing and working through forbidden feelings, such as anger and disappointment; and (3) helping family members to understand how they support each other's defensive structure. Unconscious interpersonal processes are thought to affect family functioning in a number of ways. For example, the term "projective identification" is used to describe a process in which family members unintentionally elicit certain behaviors from other members (Zinner & Shapiro, 1972). A father with a drinking problem may express considerable remorse and cut way back or stop drinking entirely. However, at the same time he may deny or repress feelings of anger and resentment that others expect him to quit drinking or the feeling that he is entitled to drink despite his lack of control. These denied or repressed aspects of himself might then be projected out onto his son and might contribute to the son's defiant, "no one's going to tell me what to do," stance toward substance use. The father communicates this attitude to the son through subtle, indirect messages, which nonetheless can be quite powerful.

Psychodynamic therapists also pay close attention to wishes, beliefs, and feelings that go unexpressed in families because they are viewed as unacceptable. Sometimes family members will state that certain wishes or feelings are "bad," such as when a parent says, "quit acting like a baby," when an adolescent boy is upset over something. Often, however, the communication is not direct. Family members can express their displeasure by ignoring the individual or by becoming cool and aloof. Under these circumstances, the family member learns not to express such thoughts or feelings. Over time, he/she may even lose the capacity to recognize that these internal states are being experienced (Meeks, 1988; Modell, 1975; Stolorow & Brandchaft, 1987).

Another unconscious process that can cause problems in families or couples is the tendency of members to support each other's defensive structures (Stolorow & Brandchaft, 1987). For example, an adolescent might become sensitive to the fact that his father seems to withdraw and avoid him when he expresses painful affects, such as anger or sadness. According to psychodynamic theory, the father has difficulty tolerating these feelings in his son because he has difficulty tolerating them in himself. In other words, the father's defenses are oriented around avoiding painful feelings. In order to stay close to his father, the adolescent learns not to express these feelings. This process occurs at a preconscious or unconscious level; the message is conveyed even though family members rarely say something as direct as "If you want to be close to me, don't cry like that!"

In treating families or couples with addiction problems, psychodynamic family therapists listen carefully for evidence of unconscious processes in the family, such as unexpressed wishes and feelings and the support of other family member's defenses. Therapists will try to elicit these feelings by encouraging family members to give voice to what they are experiencing and then listening in a noncritical fashion. When family members are struggling to understand their own feelings, the therapist might offer an interpretation—a comment that captures the therapist's perceptions of repressed or denied thoughts and feelings, as well as the interpersonal dynamics within the family. In some families, for example, members may find it difficult to recognize and express the depth of their anger at or disappointment in the substance abuser. Interpretations can also be helpful in situations in which the family is perpetuating a maladaptive pattern of interacting but is largely unaware of it. In families with acting-out adolescents, for example, the therapist may observe and comment on a pervasive lack of curiosity on the part of the parents concerning their adolescent's thoughts, feelings, and behaviors (Shapiro, 1982a).

Learning how to formulate interpretations and when to deliver them is one of the most difficult tasks encountered by psychodynamic therapists. However, Luborsky (1984) has developed an approach to interpretation, called the core conflictual relationship theme (CCRT), that simplifies the learning process somewhat. Luborsky (1984) suggests that therapists offer interpretations that consist of a statement of the patient's (1) main wish, (2) expectation concerning the response of the other, and (3) response from the self. For example, a therapist treating a couple might say, "John, it seems to me that you wish that Sara would have faith and confidence in you, but you believe that she considers you a failure. You then deal with the feelings by saying to yourself, 'to hell with her,' and going out drinking." The goal of the CCRT method is for patients to understand how their wishes and expectations concerning interpersonal relationships are related to their behavior. This emphasis on interpersonal functioning makes the technique very appropriate for family or couple therapy. In conjoint therapy, the therapist can make interpretations on the basis of what goes on between family members in the session itself rather than relying on descriptions of relationship episodes outside of the therapy session, as must be done in individual therapy.

Behavioral Approach

The behavioral approach to couple and family therapy differs in a number of important ways from the psychodynamic approach. The therapist is more active and the sessions are more structured, greater use is made of assessments to guide the sessions and determine treatment goals, weekly homework assignments are typically given in each session, progress is often monitored through rating scales and checklists, and little attention is paid to unconscious processes. In the addictions, behavioral treatment has been used more often in couple therapy than in family therapy. This may be because the techniques of behavior therapy are easier to implement with two adults than with a room full of family members. In any case, behavioral marital therapy (BMT) has been compared with other treatments for alcoholism in a number of rigorous research studies and has done very well (Holder, Longabaugh, Miller, & Rubonis, 1991).

O'Farrell (1993) and McCrady (1982) have developed BMT protocols that share many techniques and goals. Both authors stress that couple treatment for alcoholism must address the drinking of the alcoholic member as well as the overall health of the relationship in order to be successful. O'Farrell (1993) recommends 10 to 15 couple sessions to produce and stabilize short-term changes both in the drinking behavior of the alcoholic and in associated marital discord. During this initial period, some of the interventions are focused specifically on eliminating or controlling drinking, whereas others are intended to improve the marital relationship. Interventions to control drinking include establishing drinking goals, structuring each member's role in the alcoholic's recovery process, establishing agreements concerning the use of disulfiram (Antabuse), employing techniques to reduce hazardous drinking, and identifying and decreasing family members' behaviors that trigger or enable drinking (McCrady, 1982; O'Farrell, 1993; O'Farrell & Cowles, 1989). Interventions to improve family relationships include increasing positive interchanges, such as pleasing behaviors and shared recreational and leisure activities, and resolving conflicts and problems through training in communication and problem-solving skills. After changes in drinking behavior have been maintained for 6 months or so, interventions are geared toward preventing relapse and addressing long-term marital and family issues (O'Farrell & Cowles, 1989).

The behavioral approach strongly emphasizes the importance of setting goals and practicing new ways of interacting during the treatment sessions and at home between sessions. Couples are often instructed to role-play new behaviors during a session, such as giving and receiving positive comments and planning shared leisure activities, before attempting them outside the session. When practicing these behaviors between sessions, couples are told to record information about the homework assignment (e.g., frequency of the new behavior, what each person did, and the outcome) so that the couple and the therapist can monitor progress.

In BMT, there is a strong emphasis on behavioral contracting. For example, a contract can be used to specify the spouse's and the alcoholic's roles in the recovery process (O'Farrell & Cowles, 1989). This type of contract spells out the drinking goal for the alcoholic (e.g., 6 months of abstinence), what the alcoholic commits to doing to achieve that goal (e.g., going to Alcoholics Anonymous three times per week), what the alcoholic will do if abstinence is not achieved (e.g., start taking Antabuse), what the spouse will do to facilitate recovery (e.g., not nag about prior drinking), and what the spouse will do if the alcoholic begins to drink again (e.g., refrain from arguing and leave the home until the drinking bout is over).

One example of a behavioral contract that is frequently used in BMT is an agreement between an alcoholic and spouse (or significant other) that the alcoholic will take Antabuse every day while the spouse observes (Azrin, 1976; O'Farrell, Cutter, & Floyd, 1985). Antabuse is a medication, intended to be taken daily, that will make someone who has taken it violently ill if he/she drinks that day. Antabuse therefore tends to discourage drinking as long as an individual takes it every day. In return for the alcoholic's willingness to take Antabuse, the spouse agrees to reward the alcoholic positively and not bring up past drinking episodes or voice concern about future drinking (O'Farrell & Cowles, 1989). Because the

Antabuse contract establishes a specific protocol for the taking of Antabuse, alcoholics and spouses are clear on what behaviors constitute a violation of the contract. For example, an alcoholic who says, "Oh, I forgot to tell you; I took my Antabuse while you were out of the room," will have violated the contract, as the spouse did not see him take the medication. The clear delineation of rules and procedures provided by the Antabuse contract increases the likelihood that the alcoholic will continue to take Antabuse.

Family Systems Approach

According to family systems theory, substance abuse in either adults or adolescents can develop during periods in which the family as a whole is having difficulty with an important developmental issue, such as separation, or when the family is experiencing a crisis, such as marital problems (Stanton et al., 1982). During these periods, substance abuse can serve to distract family members from their central problem. A typical example of this might be an adolescent who goes on a binge during a period in which his parents are considering divorce. Substance abuse can also serve to slow down or even stop a transition to a new developmental stage that is being resisted by the family. For example, it is normal for young adults in their early 20s to separate from their families of origin and move toward establishing families of procreation. However, this transition can be very anxiety provoking to some families as it threatens the equilibrium of the family. Alcohol and drug use interferes with important developmental tasks, such as establishing oneself in a trade or career and forming intimate relationships. This means that a young adult remains dependent on his/her parents. Therefore, the behavior of the substance abuser "helps to maintain the *homeostatic balance* of the family system" (Stanton et al., 1982, p. 2).

The family systems approach to treating substance abuse focuses on identifying and addressing underlying family issues or processes that have necessitated the development of a "symptom" (i.e., substance abuse). By shifting the attention of family members away from the behavior of the substance abuser and onto whatever central issue or crisis the family is experiencing, the therapist initiates a process that should make it possible for the substance abuser to give up his/her symptom. To determine the nature of the family's central problem, the therapist makes use of theoretical material about family processes and developmental stages, information provided by family members during therapy sessions, observations of interactions between family members during therapy sessions, and the family's response to clinical interventions.

In the family systems approach, therapists use a number of techniques to clarify the nature of the central issues in the family and prompt changes in patterns of interaction and other aspects of family functioning. These techniques include reframing, enactment, and boundary making. Substance abusers are often thought of or described in negative terms by other family members; he/she may be said to be selfish, thoughtless, irresponsible, and so forth. According to family systems theory, however, the behavior of the substance abuser is actually serving an important function for the family. Once the therapist understands the function of the substance abuse, he/she can "reframe" it by explaining how the behavior has come about and the function it serves in the family (Fishman, Stanton, & Rosman, 1982; Minuchin, 1974). According to Kaufman and Pattison (1981):

> A family with a drinking teen-ager may frame his behavior as simply bad or selfish. The therapist may reframe the behavior by pointing out that one motive is to gain the parents' attention as a couple and prevent an impending divorce. The therapist may then point out that as a consequence of concern about the adolescent's drinking, the parents are indeed working together. Reframing can be used to move the family from preoccupation with just the drinking behavior to a consideration of related motives and consequence. (pp. 958–959)

In family therapy sessions, family members often tend to talk about events from the prior week or the more distant past. Frequently, this involves individual family members talking to the therapist rather than to each other. Although this material can certainly be useful, the family systems approach stresses the importance of family members directly addressing each other about current problems or issues during the therapy session. This brings the family's dysfunctional patterns of interacting into the session, where interventions can be directed toward effecting change.

For example, an adolescent was brought into inpatient treatment because his parents were unable to control his substance abuse and aggressive behavior. When the adolescent would become angry or frustrated at the therapist or his parents during family therapy sessions, he would storm out of the room. At first, his parents would sit quietly in their chairs and take no action in the face of their son's rage. The therapist asked whether they had considered going after their son and insisting that he return to the session. The parents reported that it had not really occurred to them to do anything like that, and they could not imagine that it would do any good anyway. This situation was therefore an *enactment* of the kind of interactions that had occurred at home prior to the adolescent's hospitalization. With the encouragement and support of the therapist, the parents were together able to confront their son and demand that he return to the session. He resisted at first, making derogatory comments about his parents' passivity, but when they persisted, he came back with them to finish the session. In this family therapy session, the enactment of problematic family functioning during the session itself made it possible for the therapist and parents to work out a potentially more adaptive mode of functioning and determine whether it would be effective.

Another technique frequently used in the family systems approach concerns making adjustments to boundaries within the family. According to family systems theory, healthy family functioning requires that there be an appropriate degree of distance or separation between individuals within the family as well as between subsystems of the family (e.g., parents and children) (Minuchin, 1974). Furthermore, the roles and responsibilities of each family member should be clearly defined (Kaufman & Pattison, 1981). In families with substance abuse problems, however, there are frequently major difficulties around boundaries. When the substance abuser is an adolescent or young adult, family systems therapists often observe that there is a lack of closeness between the parents and overinvolvement between one parent (usually the mother) and the substance-abusing son or daughter (Fishman et al., 1982; Kaufman & Kaufmann, 1979). Therefore, the boundary around the parental subsystem is not as strong as it should be. When the substance abuser is an adult, the spouse and in some cases the children may begin to take on the roles or responsibilities of the substance abuser or become overinvolved in other ways leading to enmeshment. In these cases, boundaries between the substance abuser and other family members have become overly permeable.

Family systems therapists address boundary problems in a number of ways. First, family members are advised that they should speak directly to each other and not answer for other members (Kaufman & Pattison, 1981). If a family member persists in responding to comments or questions addressed to other members, the therapist will separate these individuals by moving them further apart in the room or, in some cases, actually sitting between them (Minuchin & Fishman, 1981). With adolescent drug abusers, the therapist may direct the adolescent to sit quietly while the parents work out a problem (Minuchin & Fishman, 1981). This reinforces the appropriate boundary between the parental subsystem and the adolescent. The therapist may also give the family tasks to do between sessions that reinforce boundaries, such as setting aside specific periods for the parents to have time alone together.

Family Disease Approach

According to the psychodynamic, behavioral, and family systems perspectives discussed above, processes in the family can contribute to the onset, course, and outcome of substance abuse in a family member. The family disease perspective also asserts that processes in the family contribute to addiction. However, according to this perspective, substance abuse is thought of as a disease that affects all (or nearly all) family members. To successfully address an addiction problem, all family members are thought to require 12-Step focused treatment interventions. For the substance abuser, this means Alcoholics Anonymous, Narcotics Anonymous, or Cocaine Anonymous. Spouses are urged to attend Al-Anon, a 12-Step self-help program for the adult significant others of substance abusers, whereas younger family members are sent to a 12-Step self-help program for young people, Alateen (12-Step theory and techniques are discussed in other chapters in this book). The family disease perspective also encourages family members to seek out family and/or individual therapy, provided it is compatible with the 12-Step approach to recovery.

Key clinical issues in the family disease approach to treatment are denial, enabling, codependency, and detachment. Denial refers to the tendency in other family members to not acknowledge or accept the severity of the substance abuser's problem (Brown, 1988; Steinglass, Bennett, Wolin, & Reiss, 1987). For example, a wife may realize that her husband drinks too much but will attempt to normalize the problem by saying, "But he still goes to work everyday," or, "He doesn't really drink any more than his friends." Similarly, the children of a substance abuser may attempt to minimize or deny that there is a problem in the family (see the family therapy case presented later). Enabling refers to the tendency of family members to do things that actually make it easier for the substance abuser to continue to use alcohol or drugs. Examples include making excuses for the substance abuser, avoiding confrontations about binges, bailing the substance abuser out of jail, and so forth. Enabling is therefore closely related to denial.

According to the family disease perspective, other family members frequently become codependent as the substance abuser's disease progresses. This means that they become preoccupied with the substance abuser and begin to organize their lives around that person. Eventually, codependent family members spend much of their time reacting to the behavior of the substance abuser (Brown, 1988), and they neglect other family members and their own interests, health, and well-being. Codependency is seen as an attempt on the part of the spouse or family member to gain some control over the unpredictable behavior of the substance abuser (Brown, 1988). For example, a codependent spouse might believe that if she is particularly vigilant, she will be able to keep her husband from drinking too much, or at least limit the extent of the damage when he goes on a binge.

In the family disease approach, the primary goals of treatment are to (1) help all family members to recognize that they have a disease, (2) help significant others detach to some degree from the substance abuser, and (3) get all family members involved with 12-Step programs. Detachment is seen as the process by which family members are able to live meaningful, enjoyable, and productive lives no matter what the substance abuser does. In other words, detachment is the key to overcoming codependency. Family members are taught that there is nothing they can do to help the substance abuser stop using other than to quit enabling. Instead, they are directed to concentrate on their own issues through individual or group therapy and regular attendance at the appropriate 12-Step program.

The family disease approach is therefore different from the other approaches to family therapy discussed here in that it stresses separate treatments for each family member. The problem is in the family, but the solution is for family members to work their own programs of recovery. Family or couple sessions may be used at the beginning of treatment to explain the disease concept to the family and outline the steps each member must take to initiate and maintain recovery. However, only a small number of such sessions are generally used with this approach.

KEY CLINICAL ISSUES IN FAMILY THERAPY

When attempting to work with substance abusers, clinicians are usually faced with a number of difficult issues and decisions. These include which intervention to use; how many sessions to recommend; how to address resistance, declining motivation, and relapses; detecting and treating additional psychopathology; and working with self-help programs. Most of these issues become even more complicated when family therapy is undertaken, due to the additional people who must be attended to during the course of the treatment.

Timing and Duration of Conjoint Interventions

Marital or couple therapies for substance abuse, such as BMT (McCrady, Dean, Dubreuil, & Swanson, 1985; O'Farrell, 1993), can be used during the primary rehabilitation phase of treatment, during aftercare, or during both phases. O'Farrell, for example, has developed a BMT protocol that involves group marital therapy during rehabilitation and individual couple relapse prevention marital therapy during aftercare (O'Farrell, 1993; O'Farrell, Choquette, Cutter, Brown, & McCourt, 1993). In most cases, marital therapy runs for 12 to 20 consecutive weekly sessions during the rehabilitation phase of treatment. In the study by O'Farrell et al. (1993), couples also received up to 15 aftercare sessions over a 1-year period.

Family therapy, on the other hand, is less standardized. In some cases, family therapy is used as one of the primary interventions throughout the treatment, as in the case that is discussed later. More frequently, however, family therapy is used at selected phases of substance abuse treatment, when it is thought to have the most impact. For example, a family-based intervention may be used to persuade a substance abuser to enter a formal treatment program or go to a self-help program such as Alcoholics Anonymous. In many treatment programs, two to four family sessions are scheduled during the rehabilitation process to help the family to pull together around the substance abuser's attempt at recovery. In other cases, recovery can lead to disruptions in patterns of functioning that were established while the substance abuser was actively using (Steinglass et al., 1987). Family members may learn that they now have to contend with a recovering member who wants to again assume responsibilities that others had taken over. Or, the family may discover that certain areas of functioning actually appear to be more difficult now that the substance abuser is abstinent (Steinglass et al., 1987). Relatively brief courses of family therapy further into the recovery process can be helpful for families dealing with these issues.

Working with Major Marital Problems

In marriages in which one or both partners are substance abusers, there are usually other problems that need to be addressed. Sometimes these are relatively mild and may even clear up if the substance abuser is able to stop using. In other cases, however, the problems may be much more serious. For example, it is not at all unusual for one or both partners to have lost their commitment to staying together. Other serious problems that may be present include violence, infidelity, and sexual dysfunction. When major marital problems are present, the therapist may need to focus on them immediately. If the substance abuser is violent toward other family members when intoxicated, the first order of business for the therapist is to take steps to increase the safety of these individuals. This could include getting the substance abuser into an inpatient program, helping the family to face the seriousness of the problem rather than avoiding it, helping family members to find another place to stay temporarily, or providing information about agencies that the family could contact. If problems such as lack of commitment and infidelity are present, therapists usually encourage couples to discuss these issues in therapy sessions but postpone making any major decisions about the relationship until they have had the chance to be in therapy together for awhile.

Working with Resistance

When family members agree to couple or family therapy, they make a commitment to attend the sessions. Therefore, failure to come to therapy sessions is the most obvious form of resistance. Therapists who work with families with substance abuse problems are all too frequently confronted with a situation in which some family members come to the office while other members are absent. Sometimes the explanations seem plausible; a child is sick or someone had to go out of town on business. In most cases, however, the real message is that the family is struggling in some way with the therapy. Members may object to what is being said, or they may be bored or frustrated over the slowness of the process. In these situations, the therapist first has to decide whether to cancel the session or proceed with the individuals who have come in. Either tactic is defensible; what is important is that the therapist and family decide on how these situations will be handled at the beginning of the therapy. In addition, the therapist should communicate to the family that when family members begin to miss sessions, it might be perceived as a sign of resistance and addressed accordingly. That way, family members will be clear from the beginning of therapy how missed sessions will be interpreted.

Matching Substance Abusers and Their Families to Proper Interventions

Family therapy is clearly not feasible when other family members either are unavailable or refuse to participate. However, even when other family members are willing to participate, family therapy may not always be the treatment of choice. In a recent study, improvements in family functioning during the course of treatment were correlated with better drinking outcomes for individuals with low autonomy scores but not for those with high scores (McKay et al., 1993a). The authors concluded that individuals with low autonomy scores were probably more affected by the behavior of others in their families; consequently, they were less likely to drink if family functioning improved and more likely to drink if family functioning worsened. It therefore seemed reasonable to assume that family therapy would be indicated for low-autonomy substance abusers. However, additional analyses demonstrated that family functioning improved to a greater degree when low-autonomy alcoholics were treated in individual therapy rather than in conjoint therapy with a significant other (McKay, Longabaugh, Beattie, Maisto, & Noel, 1993b).There was also some evidence that for high-autonomy patients, conjoint therapy led to greater improvements in family functioning than individually focused treatment. The authors offered the following interpretation of the results:

> Therapeutic approaches that challenge alcoholic patients' usual interactional styles may be useful for bringing about improvements in family functioning. The nonconjoint treatment may be helpful for low-autonomy alcoholics by directing them to focus on themselves and their own problems and fostering increased self-efficacy by teaching coping skills. . . . As these individuals begin to feel more capable of helping themselves, other family members might feel less pressure or responsibility for them, leading to improvements in the functioning of the family as a whole. Conversely, treating high-autonomy alcoholics with family members may help these individuals to moderate their counterdependence, thus allowing the family to function more effectively. (pp. 56–57)

Research has also shown that conjoint therapy leads to worse drinking outcomes if family members are not supportive of the patient's efforts to achieve and maintain abstinence (Longabaugh, Beattie, Noel, Stout, & Malloy, 1993).

These studies demonstrate that it is important for clinicians working with substance abusers to think carefully about the pros and cons of involving family members or significant others in the treatment process before recommending couple or family therapy. Will a family intervention clear up interpersonal problems that might make it more difficult for the patient to achieve abstinence or increase the risk of relapse, or will family therapy simply enable the substance abuser to avoid taking personal responsibility for his/her recovery? By considering the personality, defenses, and coping styles of the patient, as well as the family dynamics, the clinician can make an informed judgment concerning the advisability of conjoint interventions.

Addressing Other Forms of Psychopathology

Studies have consistently found that substance abusers are at higher risk than the general population for other forms of psychopathology, such as depression, anxiety, and antisocial personality disorder (Hesselbrock, Meyer, & Keener, 1985). When comorbidity is present, it is important for the clinician to elicit all family members' reactions to this other "problem" and inquire whether they think that it is related to the substance abuser's use of alcohol and/or drugs. For example, some family members may avoid confronting a depressed individual about his drinking for fear that he is too fragile. Or, family members may find that an individual with an anxiety disorder seems to worry less when drinking; hence, they are reluctant to urge the person to stop. Still other family members may become exasperated with an individual who is both depressed *and* drinking and may become highly critical or judgmental. These reactions may all get in the way of recovery and should therefore be addressed during couple or family sessions. In cases in which Axis I pathology is severe enough that medication is warranted, conjoint sessions can be used to educate family members about the potential risks and benefits of the medication, to explore any feelings of shame or embarrassment the substance abuser and other family members may have about medication, and to provide an opportunity for the family to show its support for the substance abuser's attempts to deal with both addiction and comorbidity.

Doing conjoint therapy with antisocial substance abusers and their significant others is considerably more difficult. These families tend to be chaotic; therefore getting all the appropriate family members into the same room at the same time is even more difficult than usual. Sessions themselves can be explosive; one of the main therapeutic tasks is to keep the sessions from deteriorating into shouting matches. Families such as this come by their pathology honestly; the members have often been badly hurt emotionally and/or physically by significant others and consequently they expect to be misunderstood, abandoned, deceived, or otherwise treated badly. In these cases, conjoint sessions can be useful if the substance abuser and family members can find a way to both express their negative expectations concerning interpersonal relations and listen to others do the same. Family sessions can also be used to come to some agreement on what constitutes appropriate behavior between family members.

Handling Relapse

When substance-abusing patients begin to drink and/or use drugs again after achieving abstinence for some length of time, the first task is to get them into a therapy session. This can be difficult, as patients are at increased risk to drop out of therapy following relapses. Family members can sometimes help to persuade the substance abuser to attend a therapy session. If the substance abuser is willing to come for a session, it is important for the therapist to elicit the details of the substance use episode. Specifically, patients should be queried about what was happening in their life prior to the relapse, what they were thinking and feeling, what happened immediately prior to the relapse, what they did after beginning to use, and so forth (Annis & Davis, 1989; Marlatt & Gordon, 1985). These details help the therapist, the identified patient, and the family to arrive at an understanding of the factors that triggered this particular episode of use.

Couple or family therapy can be particularly helpful around the time of a relapse because other family members can provide additional information about the events surrounding the substance use episode. For example, substance abusers frequently attribute their relapses to interpersonal factors or emotional arousal (Marlatt & Gordon, 1985). Although these factors can certainly be talked about in individual therapy sessions, it can be quite illuminating for the therapist, and often for the patient as well, to hear someone else's perspective on what happened before and during the relapse. Furthermore, in situations in which a relapse follows on the heels of interpersonal difficulties with a significant other, conjoint sessions can provide a relatively safe place for both partners to work on the relationship problems that may have contributed to the relapse.

At the same time, there is no guarantee that substance abusers and their significant others will initially agree on what caused the relapse or what needs to be done to avert another episode of use. Research has shown that male alcoholics tend to attribute their relapses to the behavior of their wives, whereas the wives seldom blame themselves for their husbands' relapses (Maisto, O'Farrell, & McKay, 1988). This difference in viewpoint appears to be particularly pronounced soon after a relapse event (McKay, O'Farrell, Maisto, Connors, & Funder, 1989). When there is a great deal of initial disagreement between family members about the causes of relapse, individuals are likely to feel criticized, abandoned, or misunderstood. These emotions create a climate within the family that may increase the risk of further episodes of drinking or drug use. In conjoint sessions, it is therefore important for both the substance abuser and significant others to talk about their perceptions of the relapse event and for each family member to be able to listen to what the others have to say about it.

Working with Self-Help Programs

Although some therapists are uncomfortable with aspects of 12-Step programs (e.g., the notion of complete powerlessness over alcohol and drugs), it is often considerably easier to work with substance abusers and their families if they are involved with self-help programs. First, substance abusers who are actively participating in self-help groups are less likely to relapse (McKay, Alterman, McLellan, & Snider, 1994; Moos, Finney, & Cronkite, 1990; Vaillant, 1983). Second, if relapses do occur, other self-help group members can provide considerable support to the substance abuser and other family members. One of the other major advantages of self-help programs is that they urge individuals to take responsibility for their own behavior and not be overly concerned about trying to change the behavior of others. This philosophy is nicely summed up by the self-help "Serenity Prayer." All the approaches to family therapy discussed in this chapter stress that it is important to straighten out problems with role functioning and boundaries, such as family members' tendencies to take on the responsibilities of the substance abuser. Therefore, the work that the family does in therapy can be reinforced and supported by self-help group participation.

Although some substance abusers and family members become active members of self-help programs, there are others who participate only infrequently or not at all. In these families, there can be tension when some members participate and others do not. It is therefore important to bring up the issue of self-help groups when working with either couples or families and explore each member's views on participation. In most cases, therapists should strongly urge the substance abuser to get involved with self-help groups (McCrady & Irvine, 1989). If there is resistance, other family members may be able to persuade the substance abuser to reconsider. The family therapy sessions can be a safe place in which to discuss these issues.

ADOLESCENTS AS THE IDENTIFIED PATIENTS

Although conjoint interventions are not recommended for all adult substance abuse patients (Longabaugh et al., 1993; McKay et al., 1993b), there is widespread agreement that family therapy of some sort should be considered for virtually all adolescent substance-abusing patients. This belief has grown out of the observation that whereas experimentation with alcohol and/or drugs during adolescence seems to be largely determined by peer group behavior, substance abuse appears to be more strongly associated with psychopathology and family dysfunction (Newcomb & Bentler, 1989). Some of the more popular approaches to family therapy for adolescents include psychodynamic (Shapiro, 1982b) and family systems (Fishman et al., 1982; Kaufman & Kaufmann, 1979) interventions. There is even a "family therapy" approach that involves treating only one member of the family (Szapocznik, Kurtines, Foote, Perez-Vidal, & Hervis, 1986). This section addresses issues that should be considered when treating adolescent substance abusers with family therapy: the age of the adolescent, treatment goals, comorbid psychiatric conditions, parenting issues, and the state of the relationship between the adolescent's parents.

Age

Although we frequently talk about adolescents as if they constitute a homogeneous group, they obviously do not. One major distinction with important clinical implications concerns the difference between younger and older adolescents. With older adolescents (e.g., 16–18 years old), substance abuse is often connected in some way to separation issues (Fishman et al., 1982; Kaufmann, 1979). As adolescents approach young adulthood, they are faced with negotiating the difficult task of separating to some degree from their family of origin. For some adolescents, the separation involves leaving home to go to college; others may choose to strike out on their own or live with a spouse, lover, or friend(s). Although the task of separation entails some struggle for almost all adolescents, it can be particularly difficult for some. These individuals may experience strong internal prohibitions about separating, which are likely connected to some sense that they will be abandoning their parents if they get on with their lives. These prohibitions may reflect old family dynamics that were internalized but are really no longer in operation, or they could stem from current behaviors of parents who consciously or unconsciously do not want the adolescent to grow up and leave. By getting involved with alcohol and drugs, the adolescent complies with the prohibition by sabotaging any real attempts to assume adult roles and responsibilities, while at the same time achieving a pseudoseparation by opting for a lifestyle that is very different from that of the parents. Therefore, with many older adolescents, one of the main tasks of family therapy is to uncover and address prohibitions within the adolescent and/or parents against the separation process that should occur in late adolescence.

In contrast to older adolescents, younger adolescent substance abusers are probably not struggling with separation issues. They are not at the developmental stage where they are preparing to leave their family of origin; indeed, they are at an age where it is appropriate for them to be quite dependent on parents. In some cases, substance abuse in early adolescence can reflect precocious development on the part of the adolescent, sometimes referred to as pseudomaturity or parentification. Unfortunately, substance abuse in this age group is generally more likely to be an indication that there are serious problems in either the adolescent or the family or both. For these adolescents, family therapy should focus on uncovering and addressing the dysfunction in the family.

Treatment Goals

When treating adolescent substance abusers with family therapy, it is useful to consider goals related specifically to substance use and goals related to other aspects of functioning. With any adolescent with a substance abuse problem, the optimal substance use goal, at least in the short run, is total abstinence. However, this may not be a very realistic goal. Many adolescents with substance abuse problems do not want to totally abstain from alcohol and drugs. They are in treatment because their parents or the courts (or both) have insisted on it, not because they want to quit. According to a stages-of-change model proposed by Prochaska and DiClemente (Prochaska, DiClemente, & Norcross, 1992), these adolescents are at the "precontemplation" or "contemplation" stages rather than the "preparation" or "action" stages. It may therefore be more useful to make risk reduction the primary substance use goal rather than total abstinence. This involves helping the adolescent learn to recognize and anticipate potential high-risk situations, such as heavy or binge drinking, drinking and driving, and substance use and violence. Another strategy is to advocate total abstinence for a period, during which the adolescent can see what it is like to experience life without using, think further about the role alcohol and drugs are playing in his/her life, and learn ways to limit alcohol and drug use should he/she decide to use again at some future point. Obviously, the age of the adolescent needs to be considered when setting substance use goals. Whereas some experimentation is to be expected with older adolescents, any substance use can pose serious problems for younger adolescents. For adolescents under 16, it is therefore important to stick to a goal of total abstinence.

The other goals of family therapy often pertain to resolving communication problems, problematic relationships, and boundary issues within the family. In many cases, adolescent substance abusers are much closer to one parent, usually the mother, than to the other parent (Fishman et al., 1982; Kaufman & Kaufmann, 1979). This can be the case in families with two parents as well as in families with divorced or single parents. In family systems therapy, the therapist attempts to strengthen the bond between the parents and help them to function as a unit, while at the same time taking steps to decrease the strength or intensity of the connection between the adolescent and parent.

Comorbidity

In many cases, adolescent substance abusers are also struggling with other Axis I problems, such as anxiety, depression, or attention-deficit disorder, or some form of conduct disorder or anti-social personality disorder (Bukstein, Brent, & Kaminer, 1989; Donovan & Jessor, 1985). In fact, it is often behaviors associated with these other disorders, such as suicidality, violence, or criminal activity, that cause parents to bring adolescents to treatment. It is therefore important when treating adolescent substance abusers with family therapy also to have the adolescent undergo a thorough evaluation to determine whether other disorders are present. For most substance-abusing adolescents with a comorbid disorder, individual therapy is recommended in addition to family treatment. Adolescents who are depressed or have attention deficit disorder may also benefit considerably from medication.

Parenting Issues and Marital Problems

In families with a substance-abusing adolescent, there are frequently issues between the parents that need to be addressed because they have an impact upon the adolescent. Some parents have difficulty with basic parenting issues, such as setting limits and monitoring the activities and whereabouts of their adolescent (Dishion, Pattison, & Reid, 1988). In single-parent families and families in which both parents are working full time, it can also be difficult for parents to provide structure and supervision for their adolescents. In some cases there may be serious problems between parents or between a single parent and a significant other. When these issues surface in family therapy sessions, the therapist has to decide whether to address them during the session. Problems between the parents that have to do with parenting issues, such as who is supposed to be monitoring the whereabouts of the adolescent and parents' difficulties in presenting a united front when dealing with the adolescent, should generally be addressed in family therapy sessions. However, problems between parents that concern their relationship should not be discussed when the adolescent is present, as this can reinforce the tendency for substance-abusing adolescents to be overinvolved with one parent (Fishman et al., 1982).

CASE ILLUSTRATION

In this section, a family therapy case is presented. The identified patient, Mike S, was a 16-year-old adolescent boy with substance abuse and other forms of conduct disorder. Substance abuse was also a major issue for the parents. Mike's mother was a recovering alcoholic who had been sober for several years. Mike was an inpatient on a long-term, open-door adolescent unit that required a high level of family participation in the treatment process. Family therapy sessions were co-led by the adolescent's individual therapist and the parents' couple therapist. Treatment on the unit focused on helping adolescents make connections between their feelings and behaviors and helping the families to understand how the dynamics of the family affected the adolescents. The unit is described in detail in Shapiro (1982b).

Mike was an adopted white adolescent boy, the only child of Mr. and Mrs. S. His behavior prior to coming into the hospital and the results of psychological testing indicated he had a borderline personality disorder; he also met diagnostic criteria for conduct disorder. Mike was admitted to the hospital after a weekend in which he vandalized a neighbor's house and smashed a window at home and threatened to castrate his father with a shard of glass. Mike reported he had been drinking and smoking marijuana throughout the weekend.

Mike spent the first 9 months of his life with the family of his mother, an unmarried woman in her teens. Over the next 2½ years, he was placed in seven foster homes before being adopted by Mr. and Mrs. S, who were unable to have children of their own. From the beginning Mr. and Mrs. S found Mike to be an extremely difficult child. He was aggressive, hyperactive, and demanding, and his behavioral problems became worse once he began school. After a period of increasing violence and threats toward his parents, particularly his mother, Mike was hospitalized at age 14. After a 4-month stay in the hospital, Mike did reasonably well for several months at home. He began to have frequent angry outbursts at school, however. A similar escalation followed at home, this time with the brunt of Mike's anger directed at his father.

Mike's adoptive parents were inhibited, distant people who were frequently described as "lifeless" by the unit staff. They experienced each other as cold and rejecting. Their 20-year marriage had been a difficult one and they had considered divorce many times, including while Mike had been hospitalized the first time. When Mike was 4, his mother began to drink heavily at home in the late afternoons and evenings. During this period, Mr. S essentially ignored her drinking. Mrs. S was able to stop drinking 6 years later, when Mike was 10, through the help of Alcoholics Anonymous. At first, Mrs. S was reluctant to discuss her alcoholism in family therapy. Furthermore, whenever the therapists brought up the issue, Mike became angry and asserted that his mother's drinking had had no effect on him. "I don't remember ever seeing her drunk," he claimed.

Later in the hospitalization, two disclosures made by Mrs. S about her alcoholism had a profound effect on the treatment.

Soon after coming to the hospital Mike reported that when he was around 8 he was frequently beaten up by a group of older boys in front of his house after school. This went on for several years. Mike said that his mother often saw what was happening through a window in the front door, but that she had never done anything to stop it. She had, in fact, sometimes locked the door so that he was caught outside the house. When Mike first brought up this issue in family therapy, his mother offered a vague explanation for her behavior that really made no sense. Mike did not challenge her explanation; instead, he became sullen and withdrawn. The therapists expressed their own confusion over Mrs. S's explanation, and urged her to be more specific. Initially, she was unable to do so. In the next individual therapy session, Mike's therapist tried to elicit Mike's real feelings about his mother's failure to protect him. Eventually, Mike was able to say that he was hurt and angry and also confused about why his mother had abandoned him.

In the next family therapy session, Mike confronted his mother and demanded to know why she had not protected him. At first Mrs. S continued to try to avoid the issue by claiming that she really did not remember what had happened. When the therapists began to push her to remember why she had not come to her son's aid, Mike became increasingly agitated and began disrupting the session. In a case discussion after this family session, the therapists decided that it made more sense to explore Mrs. S's resistance in a couple session. In couple treatment, she was finally able to admit that on those afternoons, she had been either drunk or badly hung over and had been too confused to be of any help to Mike. The therapist told her that although he could certainly understand why she was reluctant to tell Mike about this, her refusal to do so helped support his belief that her drinking problem had not affected him. The next time Mike confronted his mother in family therapy, she told him why she had not come to his aid. Initially he was very angry at her but soon appeared to be quite relieved. The therapist commented to the family that because Mike now knew that his mother's failure to protect him had been due to her alcoholism, perhaps he could trust that his mother would not abandon him again now that she was no longer drinking.

In subsequent family therapy sessions, the therapists continued to support Mrs. S's efforts to discuss the ways in which her drinking had caused problems for her and other family members. Mrs. S revealed that she had once broken her arm by falling down the stairs when drunk. Mike immediately burst into tears and cried out, "You told me you tripped on a toy I had left on the stairs!" In past family therapy sessions, Mike had

had frequently expressed his disappointment in his parents by screaming insults and obscenities at them and storming out of the room. This time, however, he simply sat and cried. At the end of the session, the therapist told the family that Mrs. S's willingness to face the consequences of her behavior had helped Mike to make important progress. He was beginning to be able to experience painful feelings without having to immediately lash out at his parents or engage in self-destructive behavior.

Because he had not understood that his mother was alcoholic, Mike had come to blame himself for these two situations. He had broken his mother's arm and had not been worthy of any protection. Although he knew about his mother's alcoholism and recovery prior to his second hospitalization, he had clung to his belief that her drinking had had no effect on him. It was only when his mother explicitly connected her drinking with these two important events that he was able to experience his profound sadness and rage over her abandonment of him. Mr. S was also able to acknowledge for the first time his anger at Mrs. S for abandoning him through her drinking. Mike began to make real progress in treatment and he also became willing to discuss his own substance abuse. The therapists facilitated this process by not participating in the family's attempts to deny or ignore problems in the marital relationship and in parenting behaviors by focusing only on Mike's acting out. When family members were vague or avoidant, the therapists asked for details and clarification or offered interpretations designed to call attention to what was happening in the therapy session.

This case provides an illustration of some of the family processes described earlier in the chapter. From a family systems perspective, Mike's substance abuse and acting-out behavior can be understood as a symptom designed to distract his parents from their marital difficulties, thereby preventing a divorce. From a psychodynamic perspective, Mike's assertions that he was not upset or bothered by his mother's drinking problem can be seen as examples of how family members tend to support each other's defensive structures. For example, Mike's mother had been able to face her drinking problem and achieve abstinence, but she was not yet ready to fully acknowledge the ways in which her drinking had hurt her husband and son. Mike supported her defensive organization (i.e., denial) by insisting that he had not been affected by her drinking and blaming himself for her mistakes. Mike's mother needed the structure of family therapy sessions and the support provided by therapists to face aspects of herself that she had formerly denied. By doing this with Mike present, she let him know that she no longer needed him to support her defensive organization. Mike's fear of being abandoned diminished, and he was able to experience and express genuine feelings associated with his mother's alcoholic behavior. Although parents may be able to do this sort of work in couple or individual therapy, the adolescent must be involved as well at some point in the process in order for treatment to progress.

CONCLUSIONS

The family-based interventions that have been discussed in this chapter can be effective tools for decreasing alcohol and drug use and maintaining such improvements over time. Furthermore, these interventions can also have positive effects on the overall functioning of the couple or family. At the same time, family therapy is not possible in some cases (e.g., when other family members are not available or refuse to participate) and may not be appropriate in others (e.g., when family members are not supportive of abstinence). Even when family therapy is appropriate, it can be difficult to initiate and sustain. Some family members may express their resistance by missing sessions or dropping out altogether. In extremely disturbed or chaotic families (see, e.g., the case illustration described earlier), it may be possible to conduct family therapy only during an inpatient hospitalization.

In each family therapy approach discussed in this chapter, certain techniques and maneuvers are thought to promote change. With the exception of the behavioral approach, however, little research has been done to either support or refute these assertions. Therefore, we do not really know which techniques are most effective in the psychodynamic, family systems, or family disease approaches. Additional research may help to identify the "active ingredients" in these approaches that lead to decreases in substance use and improvements in interpersonal functioning. Another unresolved question is whether family therapy is more effective when therapists make use of techniques from one approach only, rather than employing techniques from different approaches when they seem appropriate. Further research is also needed to identify characteristics of substance abusers and their families that predict better outcomes in each of the approaches discussed in this chapter. This would make it possible to better match families to treatments.

There is also a need for more research on the timing of conjoint interventions with substance abusers and their family members. Is it important to involve family members at the beginning of treatment, or are family sessions more effective after the substance abuser has achieved abstinence? Another area in need of research concerns which family members should be involved in the treatment process. With adult substance abusers, for example, is it more effective to involve the entire family or only the spouse? Perhaps couple treatment, along with several sessions that involve the whole family, would be the most effective approach.

A number of manuals have been developed for behavioral marital therapy that provide specific directions for the proper implementation of the treatments (McCrady, 1982; O'Farrell, 1993). In most cases, these manuals spell out what is to be accomplished in each session. This has made it possible to standardize BMT treatments across different settings and providers. Furthermore, the manuals have greatly simplified the process of teaching BMT. Specific techniques for psychodynamic family therapy and family systems therapy have been described. However, detailed manuals that outline how these techniques are to be implemented on a session-by-session basis have not been developed. Given the nature of these treatments and the fact that families rather than couples are involved, it is probably not possible to develop detailed, session-by-session descriptions of the interventions. At the same time, the development of treatment manuals for these family interventions that provide more information on proper techniques and goals for each phase of the treatment would be a significant advance in the field. For example, Luborsky's (1984) description of short-term psychodynamic, supportive–expressive therapy is a good example of how dynamic treatments can be manualized.

ACKNOWLEDGMENT

Preparation of this chapter was supported by National Institute on Drug Abuse grants DA08399, to James R. McKay, Ph.D., and DA05186, to Charles P. O'Brien, M.D., Ph.D.

REFERENCES

Annis, H. M., & Davis, C. S. (1989). Relapse prevention. In R. K. Hester & W. R. Miller (Eds.), *Alcoholism treatment approaches* (pp. 170–1182). New York: Pergamon Press.

Azrin, N. H. (1976). Improvements in the community-reinforcement approach to alcoholism. *Behavior Research and Therapy, 14,* 339–348.

Billings, A. G., Kessler, M., Gomberg, C. A., & Weiner, S. (1979). Marital conflict resolution of alcoholic and nonalcoholic couples during drinking and non-drinking sessions. *Journal of Studies on Alcohol, 40,* 183–195.

Brown, S. (1988). *Treating adult children of alcoholics: A developmental perspective.* New York: Wiley.

Bukstein, O. G., Brent, D. A., & Kaminer, Y. (1989). Comorbidity of substance abuse and other psychiatric disorders in adolescents. *American Journal of Psychiatry, 146,* 1131–1141.

Dishion, T. J., Patterson, G. R., & Reid, J. R. (1988). Parent and peer factors associated with drug sampling in early adolescence: Implications for treatment. In E. R. Rahdert & J. Grabowski (Eds.), *Adolescent drug abuse: Analysis of treatment research* (NIDA Research Monograph 77, pp. 69–93). Rockville, MD: National Institute on Drug Abuse.

Donovan, J. E., & Jessor, R. (1985). Structure of problem behavior in adolescence and young adulthood. *Journal of Consulting and Clinical Psychology, 53,* 890–904.

Fishman, H. C., Stanton, M. D., & Rosman, B. L. (1982). Treating families of adolescent drug abusers. In M. D. Stanton, T. C. Todd, & Associates, *The family therapy of drug abuse and addiction* (pp. 335–357). New York: Guilford Press.

Hesselbrock, V., Meyer, R., & Keener, J. (1985). Psychopathology in hospitalized alcoholics. *Archives of General Psychiatry, 42,* 1050–1055.

Holder, H. D., Longabaugh, R., Miller, W. R., & Rubonis, A. (1991). The cost effectiveness of treatment for alcohol problems: A first approximation. *Journal of Studies on Alcohol, 52,* 517–540.

Jacob, T., Richey, D., Cvitkovic, J. F., & Blane, H. T. (1981). Communication styles of alcoholic and nonalcoholic families when drinking and not drinking. *Journal of Studies on Alcohol, 42,* 466–482.

Johnson, V. E. (1986). *Intervention: How to help those who don't want help.* Minneapolis, MN: Johnson Institute.

Kaufman, E. (1985). Family therapy in the treatment of alcoholism. In E. T. Bratter & G. G. Forrest (Eds.), *Alcoholism and substance abuse: Strategies for clinical intervention* (pp. 376–397). New York: Free Press.

Kaufman, E., & Kaufmann, P. (1979). From a psychodynamic orientation to a structural family therapy approach in the treatment of drug dependency. In E. Kaufman & P. Kaufmann (Eds.), *Family therapy of drug and alcohol abuse* (pp. 43–54). New York: Gardner Press.

Kaufman, E., & Pattison, E. M. (1981). Differential methods of family therapy in the treatment of alcoholism. *Journal of Studies on Alcohol, 42,* 951–971.

Kaufmann, P. (1979). Family therapy with adolescent substance abusers. In E. Kaufman & P. Kaufmann (Eds.), *Family therapy of drug and alcohol abuse* (pp. 71–79). New York: Gardner Press.

Longabaugah, R., Beattie, M. C., Noel, N., Stout, R., & Malloy, P. (1993). The effect of social investment on treatment outcome. *Journal of Studies on Alcohol, 54,* 465–478.

Luborsky, L. (1984). *Principles of psychoanalytic psychotherapy.* New York: Basic Books

Maisto, S. A., O'Farrell, T. J., Connors, G. J., McKay, J. R., & Pelcovits, M. (1988). Alcoholics' attributions of factors affecting their relapse to drinking and reasons for terminating relapse events following marital therapy. *Addictive Behaviors, 13,* 79–82.

Maisto, S. A., O'Farrell, T. J., & McKay, J. R. (1988). Alcoholic and spouse concordance on attributions about relapse to drinking. *Journal of Substance Abuse Treatment, 5,* 179–181.

Marlatt, G. A., & Gordon, J. R. (Eds.). (1985). *Relapse prevention: Maintenance strategies in the treatment of addictive behaviors.* New York: Guilford Press.

McCrady, B. S. (1982). Conjoint behavioral treatment of an alcoholic and his spouse. In W. M. Hay & P. E. Nathan (Eds.), *Clinical case studies in the behavioral treatment of alcoholism* (pp. 127–156). New York: Plenum Press.

McCrady, B. S. (1986). The family in the change process. In W. R. Miller & N. Heather (Eds.), *Treating addictive behaviors: Processes of change.* New York: Plenum Press.

McCrady, B. S., Dean, L., Dubreuil, E., & Swanson, S. (1985). The Problem Drinkers Project: A programmatic application of social learning based treatment. In G. A. Marlatt & J. R. Gordon (Eds.), *Relapse prevention: Maintenance strategies in the treatment of addictive behaviors* (pp. 417–471). New York: Guilford Press.

McCrady, B. S., & Irvine, S. (1989). Self-help groups. In R. K. Hester & W. R. Miller (Eds.), *Alcoholism treatment approaches* (pp. 153–169). New York: Pergamon Press.

McKay, J. R., Alterman, A. I., McLellan, A. T., & Snider, E. (1994). Treatment goals, continuity of care, and outcome in a day hospital substance abuse rehabilitation program. *American Journal of Psychiatry, 151,* 254–259.

McKay, J. R., Longabaugh, R., Beattie, M. C., Maisto, S. A., & Noel, N. (1992). The relationship of pretreatment family functioning to drinking during follow-up by alcoholic patients. *American Journal of Drug and Alcohol Abuse, 18,* 445–460.

McKay, J. R., Longabaugh, R., Beattie, M. C., Maisto, S. A., & Noel, N. (1993a). Changes in family functioning during treatment and drinking outcomes for high and low autonomy alcoholics. *Addictive Behaviors, 18,* 355–363.

McKay, J. R., Longabaugh, R., Beattie, M. C., Maisto, S. A., & Noel, N. (1993b). Does adding conjoint therapy to individually-focused alcoholism treatment lead to better family functioning? *Journal of Substance Abuse, 5,* 45–60.

McKay, J. R., Maisto, S. A., Beattie, M. C., Longabaugh, R., & Noel, N. (1993). Differences between alcoholics and significant others in their perceptions of family functioning. *Journal of Substance Abuse Treatment, 10,* 17–21.

McKay, J. R., Murphy, R. T., Rivinus, T. R., & Maisto, S. A. (1991). Family dysfunction and alcohol and drug use in adolescent psychiatric inpatients. *Journal of the American Academy of Child and Adolescent Psychiatry, 30,* 967–972.

McKay, J. R., O'Farrell, T. J., Maisto, S. A., Connors, G. T., & Funder, D. C. (1989). Biases in relapse attributions made by alcoholics and their wives. *Addictive Behaviors, 14,* 513–522.

Meeks, J. E. (1988). Adolescent chemical dependency. In S. Feinstein (Ed.), *Adolescent psychiatry: Developmental and clinical studies* (Vol. 15, pp. 509–521). Chicago: University of Chicago Press.

Minuchin, S. (1974). *Families and family therapy.* Cambridge, MA: Harvard University Press.

Minuchin, S., & Fishman, H. C. (1981). *Family therapy techniques.* Cambridge, MA: Harvard University Press.

Modell, A. H. (1975). A narcissistic defense against affects and the illusion of self-sufficiency. *International Journal of Psychoanalysis, 56,* 275–282.

Moos, R. H., Finney, J. W., & Cronkite, R. C. (1990). *Alcoholism treatment: Context, process, and outcome.* New York: Oxford University Press.

Moos, R. H., & Moos, B. (1984). The process of recovery from alcoholism III. Comparing functioning in families of alcoholics and matched control families. *Journal of Studies on Alcohol, 45,* 111–118.

Newcomb, M. D., & Bentler, P. M. (1989). Substance use and abuse among children and teenagers. *American Psychologist, 44,* 242–248.

O'Farrell, T. J. (1993). A behavioral marital therapy couples group program for alcoholics and their spouses. In T. J. O'Farrell (Ed.), *Treating alcohol problems: Marital and family interventions* (pp. 170–209). New York: Guilford Press.

O'Farrell, T. J., Choquette, K. A., Cutter, H. S., Brown, E. D., & McCourt, W. F. (1993). Behavioral marital therapy with and without additional couples relapse prevention sessions for alcoholics and their wives. *Journal of Studies on Alcohol, 54,* 652–666.

O'Farrell, T. J., & Cowles, K. S. (1989). Marital and family therapy. In R. K. Hester & W. R. Miller (Eds.), *Alcoholism treatment approaches* (pp. 183–205). New York: Pergamon Press.

O'Farrell, T. J., Cutter, H. S., & Floyd, F. J. (1985). Evaluating behavioral marital therapy for male alcoholics: Effects on marital adjustment and communication from before to after therapy. *Behavior Therapy, 16,* 147–167.

Prochaska, J. O., DiClemente, C. C., & Norcross, J. C. (1992). In search of how people change: Applications to addictive behaviors. *American Psychologist, 47,* 1102–1114.

Shapiro, E. R. (1982a). On curiosity: Intrapsychic and interpersonal boundary formation in family life. *International Journal of Family Psychiatry, 3,* 69–89.

Shapiro, E. R. (1982b). The holding environment and family therapy with acting out adolescents. *International Journal of Psychoanalytic Psychotherapy, 9,* 209–226.

Stanton, M. D., Todd, T. C., & Associates. (1982). *The family therapy of drug abuse and addiction.* New York: Guilford Press.

Steinglass, P., Bennett, L. A., Wolin, S. J., & Reiss, D. (1987). *The alcoholic family.* New York: Basic Books.

Stolorow, R. D., & Brandchaft, B. B. (1987). Developmental failure and psychic conflict. *Psychoanalytic Psychology, 4,* 241–253.

Szapocznik, J., Kurtines, W. M., Foote, F., Perez-Vidal, A., & Hervis, O. (1986). Conjoint versus one-person family therapy: Further evidence for the effectiveness of conducting family therapy through one person with drug-abusing adolescents. *Journal of Consulting and Clinical Psychology, 54,* 395–397.

Vaillant, G. E. (1983). *The natural history of alcoholism.* Cambridge, MA: Harvard University Press.

Zinner, J., & Shapiro, R. (1972). Projective identification as a mode of perception and behavior in families of adolescents. *International Journal of Psycho-Analysis, 53,* 523–530.

CHAPTER 7

Behavioral Theory of Substance Abuse Treatment: Bringing Science to Bear on Practice

FREDERICK ROTGERS

Behavioral theories of treatment for psychoactive substance use disorders (PSUDs) are based on principles of learning and behavior change in both animals and humans that have been delineated by experimental psychologists (Eysenck, 1982). They are a part of the larger group of behavior change techniques that fall under the rubric of behavior therapy. This chapter reviews the current status of behavioral theory of substance abuse treatment, beginning with a delineation of basic assumptions followed by a brief outline of the processes presumed to operate in treatment of PSUDs and behavior change efforts in general. This review is followed by a consideration of the etiology, maintenance, and individual client characteristics in treating PSUDs within a behavioral framework. Discussion then proceeds to the tasks behaviorally oriented clinicians attempt to accomplish in treatment and what behavioral theory has to say about the issue of treatment goal selection. The chapter concludes with a review of the advantages and disadvantages of behavioral theories of PSUDs.

BASIC ASSUMPTIONS

Behavioral theories are based on psychological learning principles as delineated in animal and human experiments during the course of the last 75 years. With the recent advent of the "cognitive revolution" in psychology (Baars, 1986), additional components have been added to the theoretical armamentarium. For the sake of convenience I use the term "behaviorist" to refer to anyone who adopts a theory of treatment based on the theoretical principles outlined below, be they classical conditioning, operant conditioning, cognitive theory, or social learning theory (SLT). These microtheories of behavior change differ from each other somewhat in the aspects of the person–environment interactions on which they focus. Nonetheless, regardless of the particular microtheory of behavior and behavior change on which a set of behavioral techniques is based, all share seven basic assumptions that characterize a behavioral approach to therapeutic change. These assumptions are outlined in Table 7.1.

First and most fundamental of these assumptions is that despite some evidence for biological or genetic components, human behavior is largely learned. Behaviorists (Bandura, 1977; Eysenck, 1982) assume that biological factors form a substrate on which a person's experiences build in producing individual patterns of behavior. Learning is thus the result of person–environment interactions. While the process of learning may vary depending on the particular behavior at issue, biological and genetic

TABLE 7.1. Basic Assumptions of Behavioral Theories of PSUDs and Their Treatment

1. Human behavior is largely learned rather than being determined by genetic factors.
2. The same learning processes that create problem behaviors can be used to change them.
3. Behavior is largely determined by contextual and environmental factors.
4. Covert behaviors such as thoughts and feelings are subject to change through the application of learning principles.
5. Actually engaging in new behaviors in the contexts in which they are to be performed is a critical part of behavior change.
6. Each client is unique and must be assessed as an individual in a particular context.
7. The cornerstone of adequate treatment is a thorough behavioral assessment.

factors are presumed by most behavioral theorists to take a backseat in the formation and change of behavior. Behaviorists tend to believe that biological and genetic factors are largely immutable given our current level of knowledge, and that change efforts are better focused on a higher-order level: that of behavior itself.

A corollary to the first assumption is that the same processes by which behavior develops can be harnessed in helping a person change unwanted or undesirable behavior (Krasner, 1982). A sophisticated technology has been developed, and is described in more detail in the companion chapter (Morgan, Chapter 8, this volume), based on the notion that any behavior that is shaped by learning can be reshaped, reduced, or even eliminated by learning.

A third assumption is that contextual and environmental factors are significant in the initiation, maintenance, and change of behavior. Consistent with the focus of behavioral theories on person–environment interactions, many behavioral techniques focus explicitly on altering aspects of this interaction as a means of changing behavior. The degree to which importance is placed on changing environment versus changing individual reactions to the environment varies from microtheory to microtheory. Techniques such as the community reinforcement approach of Azrin and Sisson (Azrin, Sisson, Meyers, & Godley, 1982), based explicitly on operant learning theory, rely heavily on environmental changes to promote changes in behavior. In contrast, more cognitive theories, such as those of Ellis (Ellis, McInerney, DiGiuseppe, & Yeager, 1988) and Beck (Beck, Wright, Newman, & Liese, 1993), place a greater emphasis on changing individual reactions to the environment. All, however, recognize the importance of context and environment in both the origins and treatment of PSUDs.

The fourth assumption common to behaviorist approaches is that behaviors that appear to be internal or covert (e.g., thoughts, feelings, and physiological changes) are all susceptible to change through the application of learning theory principles. This assumption has been borne out in numerous studies of the changes in internal processes that occur in response to treatment of a variety of disorders other than PSUDs. Specifically, there is substantial evidence from research on anxiety disorders and depression, among other disorders, that the application of learning theory-based approaches to clients brings about changes in internal processes in addition to changes in overt, observable behavior.

The fifth basic assumption is that techniques should emphasize actually engaging in new behaviors in the contexts that are problematic for clients. Whereas the practice of new skills and behaviors in the office setting is helpful as a first step in changing behavior, actual confrontation of problem situations in the real world is considered to be a more effective way of promoting lasting behavior change.

Sixth, behaviorists assume that although general principles of behavior change can be applied to any client's circumstance, each client is a unique case which requires a thorough understanding within a behavioral framework in order for treatment to be successfully accomplished. Behaviorists approach each new client as a unique entity and attempt to delineate the particular and specific configuration of forces in that client's life that produce and maintain the behavior that is the target of change efforts. Thus, while a cognitive behaviorist may believe that there are certain identifiable, common errors in thinking and reasoning that produce or maintain substance use, each individual is still presumed to suffer from a combination of those errors that is unique to that person.

The previous assumption leads logically into the seventh assumption: that treatment within a behavioral context must be preceded by a thorough, rigorous assessment of the client's behavior (Donovan, 1988). Without a complete, thorough initial assessment that focuses on delineating how specific learning processes operate in a particular client's case, therapy and consequent behavior change are bound to fail.

In addition to adherence to these basic assumptions about the nature of PSUDs and the process of treatment and behavior change, behavioral theorists also place a heavy emphasis on empirical validation of the efficacy of their techniques. As noted earlier, behavioral theory of substance abuse treatment is a form of behavior therapy. Although behavior therapy has often been equated with a rigid, mechanistic, and authoritarian approach to behavior change, nothing could be further from the truth in practice. Behavior therapists, and those who adhere to a behavioral theory of substance abuse treatment, by and large adopt an approach to the therapeutic enterprise that insists on rigorous, but humanistically based, application of well-validated principles in the interest of helping people change unwanted behavior that is standing in the way of a more fulfilling life.

With the basic assumptions of behavioral theory as background, let us now turn to a consideration of the processes behavioral theorists view as central to the initiation, maintenance, and change of PSUDs. The discussion that follows is brief and presents only a bare outline of each process. (For more specific information about how these processes are applied to form a detailed theory of the development of PSUDs, see Abrams & Niaura, 1987.) Although focused on alcohol and alcoholism, this chapter provides an excellent framework for the application of behavioral theory to PSUDs in general.

BASIC BEHAVIORAL PROCESSES
AND MODELS OF PSUDs

There are three basic learning theory processes that contribute to the initiation, maintenance, and change of behavior: classical conditioning, operant conditioning, and psychological modeling. These three processes form the core of most behavioral theories of substance abuse treatment. In addition, since the advent of the cognitive revolution in psychology, increasing emphasis is being placed by some theorists (notably those who adopt Bandura's [1977] social learning models and followers of Ellis et al.'s [1988] and Beck et al.'s [1993] cognitive approaches) on the role of cognitive processes in the initiation and maintenance of behavior. Nonetheless, the basic processes of classical and operant conditioning and modeling are still presumed to operate within cognitive models. In the sections that follow, I outline classical and operant conditioning and modeling formulations of various aspects of PSUDs. I then discuss cognitive factors in substance abuse and its treatment as presented in SLT and cognitive-behavioral theories. The focus in the following sections is on how basic learning and cognitive processes are presumed to operate in substance abuse and can be brought to bear on changing substance use behavior.

Classical Conditioning

Classical conditioning is a basic learning process that was first intensively studied experimentally and systematically by the Russian physiologist Ivan Pavlov (1927) and the American psychologist J. B. Watson (1919) around the turn of the century. In a typical classical conditioning paradigm, presentation of a stimulus (the conditioned stimulus [CS]) that has previously been neutral—that is, it does not elicit the particular response of interest (the unconditional or unconditioned response [UCR])—is repeatedly paired in time and location with another stimulus (the unconditioned stimulus [UCS]) that innately elicits the response of interest. With repeated pairings with the UCS, the CS comes to elicit a response that is highly similar to the response of interest. However, this new response (the conditional or conditioned response [CR]) typically differs somewhat in magnitude and character from the UCR.

Learning via classical conditioning affects both consciously controlled behaviors and involuntary ones. Processes of physiological arousal can be conditioned to occur in response to external cues, often symbolic ones such as the sight of money that might be used to purchase drugs or alcohol. Whether a cue elicits the CR depends, among other factors, on the frequency with which the UCS and CS have been paired, the intensity of the CS when it is presented, and the physiological and psychological motivational state of the organism at the time the CS is presented. Thus, in a hungry person, the mere sight of a picture of a Big Mac, without any of the associated cues of smell and taste, may elicit a salivation response or a subjective feeling of desire or craving to go out and buy lunch.

Classical conditioning has been most often invoked as the primary process by which environmental cues come to elicit urges or cravings to use psychoactive substances. In the 1960s, Wikler, working at the U.S. Public Health Service Hospital in Lexington, Kentucky, discovered that some of the chronic heroin users being treated experienced what appeared to be withdrawal symptoms when merely viewing the paraphernalia associated with heroin use. In a series of studies, Wikler and others (outlined in Wikler, 1965, 1973) provided addicts with paraphernalia and an opportunity to engage in the ritual of preparing and injecting heroin but with an inert solution in fact being injected. In many of the subjects, the sight of the paraphernalia elicited physiological and subjective signs of withdrawal, which Wikler began to view as conditioned withdrawal phenomena. When presented with the opportunity to "use" what they thought was heroin, these individuals often experienced a "high" even when the substance they injected was merely an inert solution that resembled heroin in appearance.

According to a classical conditioning model, in Wikler's studies the UCS was heroin, the UCR the withdrawal symptoms and subsequent high that the user experienced upon injection of heroin. The CS was the paraphernalia associated with heroin preparation and use and the CR was the pseudowithdrawal and high experienced by the experimental subjects when preparing and injecting an inert solution. Based on these findings, classical conditioning theorists postulate that substance users actually condition many stimuli in the environment to the rituals, paraphernalia, and use of their drug of choice by repeatedly using the drug in specific settings, with specific people, and according to a specific ritual. The types and variety of cues that become CSs for substance users are vast, and the specific cues are unique to each individual's experience and substance use pattern.

Classical conditioning theory has formed the basis for at least four prominent procedures in the treatment of PSUDs: cue exposure treatments (e.g., Childress et al., 1993; McLellan, Childress, Ehrman, & O'Brien, 1986), stimulus control techniques (e.g., Bickel & Kelly, 1988), relaxation training (e.g., Monti, Abrams, Kadden, & Cooney, 1989), covert sensitization and other aversion therapy techniques (Rimmele, Miller, &

Dougher, 1989). In addition, they form a part of the theoretical basis for teaching drink refusal skills (Monti et al., 1989) Other than aversion therapy, all these procedures attempt, at least in part, to break the conditioned connection between particular aspects of the client's environment and the conditioned withdrawal or cravings presumed to form the motivational basis for substance seeking and subsequent use. Aversion therapy and its variant covert sensitization apply classical conditioning theory in a different fashion by attempting to condition a new, aversive response to substance use and the cues associated with it.

Operant Conditioning

Operant conditioning is the form of learning most associated with the work of B. F. Skinner (1953). Operant conditioning occurs primarily with respect to voluntary behaviors that are increased or decreased in frequency depending on the environment's response to them (contingencies). Learning occurs through operant conditioning when a person's behavior, either overt such as pouring a drink or covert such as a thought ("I need a drink"), is followed by either a subjectively positive stimulus from the environment or a subjectively negative stimulus from the environment. Any environmental stimulus that increases the frequency of a behavior it follows is called a reinforcer. In contrast, any stimulus that decreases the frequency of a behavior it follows is called a punisher. Reinforcement can occur either by presentation of a subjectively positive stimulus (positive reinforcement) or by removal of a subjectively negative one (negative reinforcement). Both increase the frequency of a desired behavior. Punishment can occur either by presentation of a subjectively negative stimulus or by removal of a subjectively positive one. Punishment reduces the frequency of undesired behavior.

In applying operant theory to PSUDs, theorists have typically focused on the reinforcing properties of psychoactive substances as a primary factor that determines continued use. For many persons, substance use carries with it powerful innate positive effects, whereas for many persons it also removes many subjectively negative effects. For example, the alcoholic who drinks in the morning to curtail early withdrawal symptoms may experience both the positive reinforcement of the relaxing qualities associated with alcohol as a pharmacologic agent and also the negative reinforcement of removal of withdrawal symptoms. For this person, drinking in the morning is doubly reinforced each time it occurs.

Operant theory provides a framework within which to understand what drives persons suffering from PSUDs to continue substance use despite many negative or punishing consequences that may result. Operant researchers have found that reinforcers that are closer in time to the behavior one wants to influence, even though the reinforcer may be small in magnitude, exert greater control over behavior than do reinforcers or punishers that occur at a more distant point in time. To continue the analogy with the alcoholic previously cited, alcohol exerts a stronger effect as a reinforcer maintaining drinking behavior when taken in the morning to alleviate withdrawal than does the later punishing stimulus of being chewed out by one's boss for coming to work intoxicated simply because the reinforcing effect of alcohol occurs closer in time to drinking than does the boss's scolding.

Reinforcing stimuli affect not only overt behavior but also thoughts and feelings. In addition to reinforcing our alcoholic's drinking behavior in the example above, the effects of alcohol can also reinforce thoughts that accompany drinking ("I need a drink, now"), as well as expectancies of alcohol's effects that may produce a strong positive subjective response even though the alcohol has not yet had time to exert its pharmacologic effect. Thus, an alcoholic, like an addict who has become classically conditioned to cues associated with substance use, may experience a strong feeling of relaxation immediately following a drink even though the alcohol has not yet been absorbed into the blood stream. The expectation of relief from withdrawal through drinking is strengthened along with the propensity to engage in the drinking behavior itself.

From an operant perspective, treatment involves the rearrangement of environmental responses to drinking (contingencies) so that the reinforcement for engaging in behavior other than drinking becomes more immediate and obvious to the client and thereby begins to replace the reinforcement associated with substance use as a controller of behavior. Operant theory has led to the development of at least one specific procedure for treating substance abuse: the community reinforcement approach (CRA) of Azrin and Sisson (Azrin et al., 1982). Thinking in operant terms leads to the idea of rearranging one's environment to shift reinforcement contingencies more toward punishing contingencies for substance use and more toward reinforcing contingencies for nonuse. CRA attempts to do exactly that.

Operant thinking also leads to the notion that clients can reinforce themselves for behaviors that are incompatible with substance use and can implement punishing contingencies for any substance use (cf. Miller & Munoz, 1982; Monti et al., 1989). Operant theory is clear, however, that for most behavior change, emphasis on increasing reinforcement for desired behaviors, rather than punishing undesirable ones, is likely to be the best strategy for two reasons. First, punishment tends to elicit negative feelings and often retaliatory behavior from the client that may interfere with the behavior change process. Second, programs that rely largely on punishment tend to experience very high dropout rates, quite obviously a hindrance to treatment success.

Modeling

Modeling (Bandura, 1977) is the third basic learning process that has been used in developing behavioral theories of substance abuse treatment. Of the three basic learning processes, modeling is the one that appears to be most efficient and most rapid in producing new learning. Modeling involves, as its name implies, observation of another's behavior and then performance of that behavior given appropriate reinforcement contingencies. Modeling is efficient and rapid as a means of learning new behaviors because many, often complex behaviors can be learned by humans with very few observations. Many complex behaviors can be learned and accurately performed with only a single observation.

The modern theory of modeling began with the work of Albert Bandura (1977), also one of the founders of SLT. He and his coworkers mapped out the parameters of modeling as a learning process. Modeling involves two subprocesses: observational learning and performance. Learning can occur by observation, and the newly learned behavior can be reproduced quite accurately without any prior practice. Bandura postulates that a process of cognitive mapping occurs at this stage in which the individual stores aspects of the behavior that are later reproduced from this cognitive map. The adequacy with which this cognitive representation of the modeled behavior occurs depends on, among other factors, the degree to which the observer was attentive to this aspect of the model's behavior and the process of encoding the modeled behavior (verbal, visual, tactile, etc.). The more modalities (e.g., sensory aspects and links with other previously learned behaviors) through which a modeled behavior is encoded, the more efficiently will the behavior be learned. Thus, when sensory, emotional, cognitive, and motor modalities are all engaged in encoding newly modeled behavior, that behavior will be most efficiently stored and retrieved.

Whether behavior learned by observation will actually be performed depends on factors beyond the adequacy with which a cognitive map of the behavior is formed. The actual performance of the behavior depends on characteristics of the model (e.g., the degree to which the observer holds the model in esteem and a person to be imitated), whether the model is seen as being reinforced or punished for engaging in the behavior, whether the observer has an incentive to perform the modeled behavior, and whether the observer expects to be reinforced in a similar fashion to the model if the behavior is performed.

Modeling processes have been strongly implicated in the development of PSUDs in adolescence. Adolescents who observe substance-using peers with whom they wish to relate, or the behavior of persons whom they view as powerful or popular and who use alcohol or drugs, may both learn and perform those behaviors quite rapidly. Modeling also influences the maintenance of PSUDs in that people will often engage in behaviors that members of their peer group engage in as a means of ensuring continuing inclusion in the group.

The efficiency of modeling as a learning process (it can occur in only a few trials, without the necessity of repeated experiences, as is the case in both classical and operant learning) has led to its utilization as a major process in behavioral treatment of PSUDs. Persons with PSUDs often lack behavioral skills that would enable them to cope with situations that presently evoke substance use. Persons who lack assertiveness or refusal skills or who are prone to inappropriate thought processes that lead to substance use can be taught new skills and thought processes by observing skilled others modeling those processes and behaviors. Thus, modeling theory provides the theoretical basis for social skills approaches to the treatment of PSUDs, as well as forming a component of the teaching of other intrapersonal skills such as relaxation, coping self-statements, and anger management. Almost any new behavior that does not rely directly on repeated pairings of environmental stimuli with client responses can be taught or its teaching enhanced by inclusion of modeling processes.

Cognitive Mediation of Behavior

Cognitive mediation of behavior is the fourth basic process that behavioral theorists have integrated into their thinking about PSUDs, particularly since the 1970s. Several theoretical behavioral accounts of PSUDs heavily emphasize the roles of various cognitive processes in the initiation, maintenance, and change of substance use behavior (e.g., Abrams & Niaura, 1987; Goldman, Brown, & Christiansen, 1987; Sher, 1987). These cognitive theories vary in the emphasis placed on cognitive mediators, but all imply a heavy reliance on behavior change processes based on the three basic learning processes for promoting behavior change in treatment.

SLT represents an extension of the theories of classical conditioning, operant conditioning, and modeling just discussed with the addition of cognitive mediational processes as a central feature presumed to regulate the operation of psychological processes resulting from basic learning. Primarily associated with the work of Bandura (1977), SLT is a comprehensive theory of the development, maintenance, and change of learned behavior. While firmly rooted in the animal experimental literature, SLT research has focused largely on humans. In a nutshell, SLT postulates that human behavior develops by a combination of classical conditioning, operant conditioning, and modeling, which not only produce overt behaviors but lead to the development of patterns of thought and emotion that, themselves, guide and shape behavior.

A central concept in SLT is reciprocal determinism, which states that people both influence and are influenced by their environments. This implies that behavior change can be brought about by changing a person's environment, but it also implies that behavior change can be engineered by the person him/herself through a planned process of self-control and changes in his/her environment. This "self"-control is a central feature of SLT-based approaches to treatment of PSUDs.

In addition to postulating a reciprocally determined relationship between environment and behavior, SLT emphasizes the role of cognition in the control and performance of behavior. A person's thoughts, feelings, and expectations with regard to whether a particular behavior will be reinforced and his/her confidence about the adequacy with which potentially reinforced behavior can be performed, as well as the level of behavioral skill that person can bring to bear to cope with problematic situations, all influence the coping strategies and behaviors he/she will use in navigating through life. The interaction of expectations and skill levels is encapsulated in the notion of self-efficacy, a central concept of SLT. Self-efficacy refers to the person's expectations that he/she will be able to perform a coping response in a given situation, coupled with the expectation that performance of that response will be reinforced. The extent to which a person lacks requisite coping skills, or views his/her ability to execute those skills as being deficient, contributes to the person's self-efficacy expectations for coping in a given situation. According to SLT, self-efficacy expectations are primary cognitive mediators that determine whether or not a person will engage in a particular coping response. When self-efficacy regarding an appropriate coping skill is high, the person will be more likely to enact that skill in an attempt to cope with life. When self-efficacy is low with regard to a particular skill, the person will likely choose some other skill or coping strategy with which he/she feels more comfortable.

SLT views PSUDs as basically a failure of coping (Abrams & Niaura, 1987). This failure may be due to any combination of inappropriate conditioning, reinforcement contingencies, modeling of inappropriate behaviors, failure to model appropriate coping skills, and reduced self-efficacy with regard to behaviors that not only enhance coping but are also widely reinforced. Failure to perform skills one already knows may also be the result of reduced self-efficacy or outcome expectations or be due to physiological, emotional, or other cognitive factors that interfere with effective skill performance.

Following logically from this view of PSUDs, SLT-based approaches to treatment of PSUDs emphasize skills training and practice. In addition, SLT approaches seek not only to teach skills for coping with known stresses or problems but to enhance the possibility of future avoidance of substance use by helping the client anticipate situations in which he/she either lacks appropriate coping skills or has low self-efficacy with regard to performance of those skills. This process, coupled with teaching clients to address the cognitive aspects of relapse (e.g. how to cope with the abstinence violation effect that results from a slip back to use after a period of abstinence) forms the core of relapse prevention approaches to PSUDs (Marlatt & Gordon, 1985). Treatments within this framework are initiated following a thorough functional analysis of substance use behavior to determine whether substance use is maintained because the person lacks other coping skills, because the person has adequate coping skills but low self-efficacy expectations with regard to using those skills, or because the person expects that using the available coping skills will be ineffective. The client is also assessed with regard to physiological or emotional factors that may be interfering with skill performance (e.g., high levels of anxiety, depression, or anger) or which may themselves drive substance use. Assessment of skills and expectations continues throughout treatment in order to measure progress toward adequate, substance-free coping.

Treatments that have been developed within an SLT framework include social and communication skills training, assertiveness training, anger and stress management training, self-control training, and relapse prevention training following a model developed by Marlatt (Marlatt & Gordon, 1985). Marital and family approaches to treatment have also been developed from an SLT perspective (see McCrady & Epstein, Chapter 5, this volume).

Two other cognitive theories of treatment bear mention. These have grown primarily out of the work of two theorists: Ellis, the founder of rational–emotive therapy (RET), and Beck, the founder of cognitive therapy (CT). Although differing somewhat in their details, both of these cognitive theories view thought (cognition) as a primary causal factor in emotion and substance use and abuse primarily as an effort to cope with negative emotional states that arise as a result of illogical or distorted thinking.

Ellis's RET approach (Ellis et al., 1988) is an excellent example of how a cognitive framework addresses the role of cognition (thoughts) in the development of emotional disturbance and the consequent development of PSUDs in some people as a means of coping with negative emotions. Ellis has developed what he calls the A-B-C model of emotion. According to the A-B-C model of emotion, the events or situations a person encounters do not, in and of themselves, create negative emotions. Rather, the person's assessment or interpretation of the meaning of events based on his/her beliefs is what creates the negative emotion. In order for change in emotions to occur, the client must learn this and begin to identify and challenge the thoughts occurring at B through a process of rational disputation. Ellis has identified a variety of irrational beliefs that, coupled with what he views as the addict's inability to tolerate frustration or other negative emotions, are believed to set the stage for use of drugs or alcohol as a means of coping with negative emotions. According to Ellis, a further factor that triggers alcohol or drug use to cope with emotions is poor ability to tolerate negative affect. This results in a belief that Ellis calls "I-can't-stand-it-itis." This belief prompts people suffering from PSUDs to react impulsively in order to alleviate negative emotions immediately. Ellis refers to this tendency as low frustration tolerance and believes that this additional set of beliefs must be addressed for substance abuse to be successfully treated.

Beck (Beck, Rush, Emery, & Shaw, 1979; Beck et al., 1993) has also articulated a complex theory of negative emotion based on an inventory of illogical or irrational reasoning processes which he terms "core beliefs." These beliefs are often commonly held, but irrational, ideas about the nature of the world or what a person needs in order to lead a more contented life. When the person faces a problematic situation or other activating cues or stimuli, these core beliefs are activated as a way of construing the experience the person is having and of generating coping responses. Because these core beliefs are maladaptive or illogical the coping responses they trigger are often illogical, or maladaptive. Coupled with these core beliefs are highly stereotyped "automatic" thoughts, which are similar to the "B" component of Ellis's A-B-C model of emotion. The occurrence of these automatic thoughts is presumed to activate urges or cravings to use drugs or alcohol to alleviate negative emotions produced by the automatic thoughts. Action on urges or cravings in substance abusers is presumably triggered by additional thoughts or beliefs, which Beck terms "facilitating beliefs." Facilitating beliefs are, in Beck's model, the proximate cause of drug- and alcohol-seeking behavior in an addicted person faced with problematic situations or emotions.

Despite their emphasis on cognitive processes, cognitive therapies rely heavily on techniques based on SLT to facilitate the changes in cognition that are viewed as being crucial to the treatment of PSUDs. Cognitive theorists do, however, believe that lasting behavior change is difficult to achieve without changing the underlying faulty patterns of thinking that they believe lie at the root of most emotional upsets and thereby trigger substance use.

Techniques for treating PSUDs that derive wholly or in part from cognitive theories are anger management training, rational disputation of positive thoughts about alcohol/drug use, and rational disputation of thoughts linking substance use to alleviation of negative emotional states. Techniques based on cognitive theory tend to blend quite nicely with SLT-based techniques, and current research aimed at enhancing aspects of techniques based on other behavioral theories (e.g., cue-exposure based on classical conditioning theory) is beginning to incorporate explicit cognitive strategies into treatment. With its flexibility and inclusiveness, SLT has emerged in the last two decades as the predominant behavioral theory of addictions origin and treatment.

With this brief overview of behavioral theories of substance abuse treatment in mind, let us now turn to a discussion of critical issues in treating substance abusers as viewed through the lens of behavioral theory. These issues are discussed from the perspective of SLT because that theory provides the most comprehensive behavior theoretical framework currently available.

CRITICAL ISSUES IN SUBSTANCE ABUSE TREATMENT

Etiology and Maintenance of Substance Use

Behavioral theories view PSUDs as resulting from a combination of factors presumed to interact in different ways to produce PSUDs depending on each individual's unique characteristics and environment. Although explicitly endorsing a "biopsychosocial" perspective from which to view the origins of PSUDs, behavioral theories tend to minimize the causal role of genetic factors while placing a heavier emphasis on the interacting influences of an individual's environment, innate biological makeup or temperament, and learning processes. These factors are presumed to interact with each other in individual-specific fashion to produce PSUDs.

Behavioral theories view the initiation of substance use as primarily due to a combination of environmental factors (particularly substance availability and peer group norms) and individual physiological responses to initial use, resulting in substance use being either reinforcing or punishing for the individual. Whether substance use will be initiated and continued depends on whether the individual lives in a place where substances are available, peer group behavior and norms with respect to substance use, degree of importance of the peer group in the individual's life, and whether or not initial use of the substance is pleasurable. Parental attitudes and behaviors also play a role, with parental behavior being more likely to be modeled than parental dictates followed, especially if other factors (e.g., substance availability or peer group norms) favor substance use. These factors combined result in the development of drinking and drug use outcome expectancies that appear to play an important role in the initiation and maintenance of early drinking (Christiansen, Smith, Roehling, & Goldman, 1989).

For persons who develop PSUDs, behavioral theories postulate that the pharmacologic and social reinforcements attendant on initial use increase the probability of substance use behavior. With increased use, the person begins to recognize the role that drugs or alcohol can play in reducing negative emotions and may fail to learn alternative coping responses. In a somewhat different fashion, persons who have failed to learn adequate coping skills prior to the onset of substance use may begin to use drugs or alcohol as a means of compensating for the lack of those skills. Finally, some substance users may, by virtue of temperamental factors such as sensation seeking and impulsivity, use alcohol or drugs initially for their excitement-producing properties rather than as a means of coping.

The processes presumed to operate in the development of PSUDs at the earliest, or less severe, stages are largely modeling, operant conditioning (reinforcement of substance use), and cognitive mediators such as expectancies that substance use will result in highly positive outcomes. With repeated substance use and at more severe stages of dependence, classical conditioning factors begin to play a more prominent role in the development of PSUDs, with both conditioned craving and withdrawal playing an important part in production of severe dependence in some individuals. There is also evidence that tolerance is, at least to some extent, a learned phenomenon (Vogel-Sprott, 1992). At severe levels of dependence, use is often driven by the reinforcing value of avoiding withdrawal (negative reinforcement) rather than the pleasurable effects of use. It is clear, at more severe levels of dependence, that the person's body has adapted to the continuing presence of alcohol or drugs, and that these physiological changes play an important role in shifting the reinforcing contingencies of substance use. At this latter stage, behavioral theories of treatment shift the focus of treatment somewhat toward coping with the effects of these physiological changes, particularly withdrawal symptoms that may trigger a return to use following brief abstinence. Nonetheless, the basic processes by which treatment proceeds remain the same and involve implementation of learning strategies to cope with the long-term effects of substance use.

As substance use begins to assume a greater role in the individual's life, negative consequences of use may begin to increase. These consequences are often unique to the individual and may require active coping responses. Coping skill deficits again begin to assume importance as the individual may be unable to cope with the problems associated with substance use itself (e.g., family, work, or legal problems) and begins to use substances more in an effort to cope with increasingly frequent negative emotions. The immediate reinforcing value of substance use assumes a prominent role in the maintenance of substance use in the face of negative consequences because use produces immediate reinforcement whereas the punishment of negative consequences is often quite removed in time from substance use behavior.

As the severity of an individual's PSUD increases, several things may happen depending on the particular individual. Often substance use itself becomes stereotyped and limited to certain situations. These settings and the associated stimuli may become conditioned to substance use and come to elicit physiological or psychological responses that prompt drug use. With increasingly complex problems to face, the individual's coping skills may be overwhelmed and substance use increased as a means of alleviating the negative emotions that stem from failure to cope adequately.

Associations with peer groups whose members are, themselves, substance users may exert pressure on the individual to maintain substance use as a means of interaction with peers or of retaining the reinforcement of group membership. Peers may also reinforce unrealistic positive expectancies for drug or alcohol effects by their own behavior under the influence.

Consistent with natural history studies of the development of PSUDs, behavioral theories suggest that although the nature and quality of reinforcement for substance use may change over the course of a particular individual's substance use, principles of classical conditioning, operant conditioning, modeling, and cognitive mediation of behavior still operate in the maintenance of substance use behavior. In the many cases now being documented in which persons suffering from PSUDs stop using drugs or alcohol on their own without any treatment, a combination of shifting reinforcement contingencies and cognitive changes appears to explain the change in behavior (Sobell, Sobell, Toneatto, & Leo, 1993).

Homogeneity/Heterogeneity of Persons with PSUDs

Behavioral theories are entirely consistent with current views of substance use as falling along a continuum ranging from no use at all to severely dependent use (Institute of Medicine, 1990). Behavioral theories view each individual as forming a unique constellation of biological bases, learning history, and current environment. In spite of the uniqueness of every individual's history and development of substance use and problems surrounding substance use, behavioral theories believe that there are also commonalities among substance users and abusers. Nonetheless, behavioral theories tend to minimize the importance of global subtyping or labeling of individuals in treatment. Although guided by empirical evidence that suggests differences in treatment outcomes and the advisability of various treatment goals among persons with PSUDs who have particular genetic backgrounds, personality makeup, and environments, behavioral theorists tend to use these data as guidelines for how to proceed in treatment rather than as strict determinants of treatment.

In essence, although broad groups of PSUDs who suffer from personality disorders, depression, or anxiety are recognized by behavioral theorists, thorough assessment and treatment are based on an individualized behavioral analysis rather than on assumptions about particular individuals based on their membership in identifiable subtypes or groups. Behavioral theories of treatment emphasize the matching of treatment procedures and goals to patient needs to a greater extent than do other theories of treatment. Although the therapist's armamentarium of techniques is relatively constant, the application of those techniques is based on individual analyses of a particular client's skill assets and deficits.

Role of Genetics/Biological Factors in PSUDs

It would be foolish to deny that human beings are to some extent the product of their biology. All behavior at the levels at which therapy tasks place (e.g., the overtly or subjectively observable) ultimately has a biological substrate. All learning, at bottom, involves changes at the neuronal level, if not change at a molecular level. The role of genetics in human behavior is not clearly specified, and at the present time the genetic substrate of human behavior is immutable by available methods. Thus, while biological and genetic factors are viewed as risk factors that must be taken into account in one's analysis of a particular individual's substance use patterns and addressed in the selection of treatment goals, they do not play a significant role in treatment itself.

Behavioral theorists believe that changes in behavior require something more than changes in a person's biological or neurochemical functioning. This belief rests on the assumption that environmental contingencies play a key role in the cause and control of behavior, as well as on the notion that skill assets and deficits are important contributors to the development, maintenance, and change of PSUDs.

Behavioral theories of change emphasize helping the client to learn coping skills that will be more effective in managing day-to-day life without using drugs or alcohol. While not rejecting the potential role of pharmacotherapeutic interventions, behavioral theorists point out that although some effective pharmacotherapeutic measures exist for helping some persons with PSUDs (e.g., disulfiram [Antabuse] for alcoholics [Fuller, 1989] and naltrexone for alcoholics [Volpicelli, Alterman, Hayashida, & O'Brien, 1992] and opiate addicts), these approaches have not yet made a wide impact on the treatment of PSUDs. The minimal impact of pharmacologic interventions on the treatment of substance abuse to date is most likely due to difficulties in persuading persons with PSUDs to take these medications reliably, and to a lack of knowledge as to which clients will respond best to pharmacologic interventions. This sort of client–treatment matching is an issue that behavioral treatment techniques are uniquely equipped to address.

Tasks of Treatment

Behavioral theories typically view treatment as needing to accomplish several tasks in order to be successful.

As with all psychosocial treatment approaches, the first task in treatment, if necessary, is to detoxify the client from hazardous or potentially life-threatening levels of substance use, preferably to a level of temporary abstinence, although behavioral theories do not usually make total abstinence a precondition for treatment, or even a necessary treatment goal for some clients.

Once detoxification has been accomplished, the therapist must conduct, in collaboration with the client, a thorough functional analysis of substance use behavior and its triggering and maintaining factors. This analysis should focus both on skill deficits and on the client's environment, with a particular emphasis on identifying those factors in the person (e.g., emotional states and thoughts) and his/her environment that are highly associated with, or perhaps trigger, substance use. These high-risk situations, which may be both internal or external, need to be addressed in order for treatment to succeed and treatment gains to be maintained. Without this thorough assessment, treatment cannot proceed and is likely to fail.

Following a functional analysis, work then proceeds on teaching the client a specifically tailored menu of techniques and strategies aimed at intervening in the problems identified in the assessment. In behavioral treatments, assessment and treatment are closely linked, and assessment is reiterated throughout the process of treatment in order to gauge progress and identify continuing problem areas and behaviors. The fact that problems may continue to emerge during treatment reinforces the importance of ongoing client assessment.

The final task of behavioral treatments is to assist the client in identifying and planning strategies for coping with high-risk situations that may occur in the future. This task is designed to provide the client with the tools necessary to prevent relapse to substance use—the core of behavioral notions of relapse prevention. Clients are also taught how to cope with slips into substance use or relapses, should they occur, in ways that will shorten the length and intensity of any future return to substance use.

The three core tasks of treatment from a behavioral perspective—functional analysis, skills training, and relapse prevention—are accomplished both by individual work with the client and by helping the client make active attempts to change environmental factors that may be triggering or maintaining substance use. Thus, clients may be encouraged to make significant lifestyle changes, or changes in their daily routine or interactions with family and friends, that the functional analysis suggests might enhance the client's ability to cope without use of drugs or alcohol. Although not always explicitly addressed, the key role of the environment in PSUDs is always a factor in guiding treatment.

Treatment Goals

Behavioral approaches to treatment of PSUDs, by their very nature and heavy emphasis on matching treatment to specific client characteristics and needs, imply flexibility in the selection of treatment goals. Unlike other theoretical positions that insist on abstinence from psychoactive substances as the only legitimate goal of treatment, and that often make abstinence a prerequisite for treatment entry, behavioral theories allow for a more flexible and incremental approach to substance use reduction that is often more attractive to clients who might otherwise avoid more traditional treatments.

Although individual therapists may vary in the degree to which they insist on an abstinence goal for all clients, there is a substantial body of literature suggesting that many persons with PSUDs, particularly those with less severe dependence, can and do become moderate users, often without any treatment at all (Booth, Dale, Slade, & Dewey, 1992; Duckert, Amundsen, & Johnsen, 1992; Sobell et al., 1993). Many persons who have been treated for PSUDs in abstinence-oriented programs become moderate users, and many persons who set out to achieve only a reduction in substance use ultimately become abstinent. There appear to be cognitive variables that have an impact upon the decision to change substance use behavior and to what degree to change. There are now data to suggest that a particular individual's stage of readiness to change (Prochaska, DiClemente, & Norcross, 1992) strongly influences the process of treatment participation and commitment.

Being guided by the scientific literature, behaviorally oriented therapists will typically work with a client incrementally toward abstinence and its maintenance, if that is what the client insists on, and if the client's level of substance use at treatment entry does not carry with it the risk of immediate catastrophic consequences if some level of use continues. The process of goal determination is one of negotiation rather than therapist insistence, consistent with the notion that the more committed the client is to the particular treatment goal, the greater the likelihood of reaching it.

Recently, another approach to treatment goals has emerged that has been termed "harm reduction" (Marlatt & Tapert, 1993). The harm reduction approach attempts to reflect the realities of treating persons with PSUDs in recognizing that complete, lifelong abstinence is often extremely difficult to accomplish, even though that is the healthiest goal for a particular client, even when a client is committed to abstinence. When immediate cessation of substance use is not likely or does not occur (due, perhaps, to severity of the individual's PSUD), taking a harm reduction approach leads to working in an incremental fashion, in smaller steps, toward an ultimate goal of abstinence. The ultimate aim of harm reduction is to enhance health by minimizing or reducing the impact of behaviors or factors that threaten health. From this perspective, any change in the environment or client behavior that leads to reduced substance use is one that should be promoted.

Empirical Research and Behavioral Theory

Of all the approaches presented in this book, with the exception of motivational and pharmacotherapeutic approaches, behaviorally based approaches are the most closely linked with existing scientific knowledge of PSUDs. Empirical validation of treatment techniques has been an integral part of behavioral theory of treatment from the beginnings of the behavior therapy movement in the early 1950s. Behaviorally based therapists view each client and his/her treatment as, in a sense, a minilaboratory within which the therapist and client collaborate to assess client needs and apply and evaluate the effect of various treatment technologies.

Not only are behaviorally based treatments open to scientific scrutiny, they insist on it. Without well-designed experimental studies of treatments and their outcomes, behavioral theorists believe that no progress can be made toward resolving the most difficult issue treating PSUDs: what treatments work best under what conditions with what clients. This is the crux of the patient–treatment-matching research currently being conducted under the auspices of the National Institute on Alcohol Abuse and Alcoholism (Donovan & Mattson, 1994). The behavior therapy movement, from which behavioral theories of treating PSUDs are derived, insists on empirical validation of the techniques used to treat clients as a cornerstone of ethical professional practice. To apply scientifically untested or untestable techniques routinely, solely on the basis of single case histories or client testimonials, is considered by most behavioral therapists to be unethical practice, especially when empirically validated techniques exist and could be widely used were more practitioners aware of them.

ADVANTAGES AND DISADVANTAGES
OF BEHAVIORAL APPROACHES

Advantages of Behavioral Approaches

Approaches to treating PSUDs based on behavioral theory have a number of advantages over other currently available approaches to treatment. That this is the case can be seen by the extent to which concepts that were originally developed by behavioral theorists (e.g., Marlatt's relapse prevention concept) have begun to be incorporated, although often in altered form, into the practice of therapists trained in other approaches (Morgenstern & McCrady, 1992; Rotgers & Morgenstern, 1994). There are seven clear-cut advantages to adopting a behavioral view of PSUDs and their treatment. These are outlined briefly in Table 7.2.

TABLE 7.2. Advantages of Behavioral Theories of PSUDs and Their Treatment

1. Flexibility in meeting specific client needs.
2. Readily accepted by clients due to high level of client involvement in treatment planning and goal selection.
3. Soundly grounded in established psychological theory.
4. Emphasis on linking scientific knowledge to treatment practice.
5. Clear guidelines for assessing treatment progress.
6. Empowerment of clients in making their own behavior change.
7. Strong empirical and scientific evidence of efficacy.

Flexibility in Tailoring Treatment to Client Needs

Because behavioral approaches eschew global labeling and place a heavy emphasis on individualized assessment, they are ideally suited to matching treatments to client needs. This flexibility extends to treatment goal selection as well as to selection of the particular interventions to be used with a given client. Behavioral theory allows for specific matching of client problems, client goals, client readiness for change, and selection of treatment interventions.

Ready Acceptance by Clients through Avoidance of Labeling and Goal Imposition

Behaviorally based treatments for PSUDs are readily accepted by clients. This is because therapists operating within this perspective adopt a collaborative rather than confrontational stance with clients and avoid labeling clients with terms that, in our society, carry strong pejorative connotations. Behaviorally based approaches are explicitly carried out in a collaborative fashion in which client input is given a high level of attention and consideration. Clients are not forced to accept a unitary explanation of their behavior as a precondition for their behavior change efforts. Behavioral theory allows for a high degree of individualization of treatment, in contrast to other approaches that attempt to apply a similar formula for recovery to all clients.

Within traditional approaches, if a client rejects that approach's conception of PSUDs and what is necessary to bring about change, treatment is likely to fail. The therapist is then often left with only two alternatives if he/she wishes to remain within the constraints of the approach: to continue to attempt to convince the client of the validity of the approach or to terminate the client from treatment. If the therapist adopts the first approach, the results are often countertherapeutic due to the elicitation of strong reactance on the part of the client against the therapist's views. This is likely to lead to treatment dropout and may become a barrier to that client seeking treatment elsewhere.

Sound Basis in Psychological Theory

Unlike other widely used approaches, behavioral approaches have a clear, coherent, well-tested theoretical basis that is rooted in scientific psychology. Having a clear, coherent theory of behavior change has been cited as a factor in treatment success (Onken, 1991) in substance abuse treatment.

Emphasis on Linking Science to Treatment

A corollary to behavioral theory's sound basis in psychological science is its strong emphasis on linking science to treatment. Scientific evaluation and knowledge are important both at the individual client–therapist level and at the systemic or treatment system level. In the client–therapist relationship the emphasis on continuous testing of assessment hypotheses and technique success is integral to the achievement of behavior change. At the systemic level, scientific evaluation of techniques derived from behavioral theory plays an integral role in ensuring that consumers of behaviorally based treatments get the best available treatment and in providing the scientific knowledge that can lead to development of more efficient and more effective treatments in the future.

Clear Guidelines for Assessing Treatment Progress

By focusing on continued assessment of the factors contributing to a particular client's substance use, as well as the degree to which clients are learning and implementing new coping skills and lifestyle changes, behaviorally based approaches provide clear milestones for evaluating individual treatment progress, or lack thereof. Knowing whether and how well a client is progressing is essential both to altering treatment strategies that may be ineffective and to determining when it is appropriate to terminate treatment with a particular client. Because treatment goals are mutually agreed on by client and therapist at the beginning of treatment, progress toward treatment termination is more easily assessed. This allows the length of treatment to be tailored explicitly to client needs on the basis of definable criteria.

Empowerment of Clients as Effective Agents in Changing Their Own Behavior

In contrast to traditional approaches that emphasize, in somewhat paradoxical (and often puzzling to clients) fashion, clients' powerlessness over their addiction, behaviorally based approaches explicitly attempt to enhance clients' sense of personal efficacy and problem-solving ability. By attempting to teach clients not only that they can be effective problem-solvers without using alcohol or drugs to cope but that they can learn skills necessary to solve new, unforeseen problems in the future, behaviorally based techniques accomplish two major functions: they destigmatize addiction and help enhance self-efficacy and self-esteem of clients, people on whom other approaches often place labels that carry with them strong pejorative connotations. They attempt to reduce the need for future treatment by teaching clients the skills to analyze problems themselves and develop effective coping. Behaviorally based approaches are consistent with the old adage that "when you give a man a fish, you feed him for a day, teach him to fish, and you feed him for a lifetime."

Empirical Evidence of Efficacy

In contrast to most other currently available treatment approaches, approaches based on behavioral theory have garnered some scientific evidence of efficacy in controlled clinical trials (Holder, Longabaugh, Miller, & Rubonis, 1991). A particular advantage is evidence that behaviorally based approaches may be more effective than other approaches with a group of clients that have generally poor prognosis: those that suffer from antisocial personality disorder (Kadden, Cooney, Getter, & Litt, 1989). Given evidence that a very high percentage of clients with PSUDs also suffer from antisocial personality disorder (Regier et al., 1990; Ross, Glaser, & Germanson, 1988), this finding of relative efficacy of behavioral techniques with this group is a strong reason to adopt a behaviorally based treatment approach.

Disadvantages of Behavioral Approaches

Despite the numerous advantages just presented, behavioral approaches as they currently exist have several disadvantages. These disadvantages have more to do with the current state of scientific knowledge than with any inherent difficulties with behaviorally based approaches. As scientific knowledge accumulates, it is likely that these disadvantages will disappear. As it now stands, these disadvantages could more reasonably be termed "limitations" of the approach.

First, while there is evidence of differential effectiveness for behaviorally based approaches, the exact reason for this is unclear. For example, the extent to which clients actually use the skills they are taught in treatment and the relationship of skill use to relapse or maintenance of change, are unclear.

Second, there is a distinct, and surprising lack of empirical support for the advantage of adding relapse prevention procedures to treatment as a means of enhancing long-term outcomes. Although some data suggest that those who learn relapse prevention techniques are able to curtail the length and severity of the relapses, the overall advantage predicted to accrue to clients as a result of the introduction of relapse prevention technologies has not been strongly validated empirically (Wilson, 1992).

Third, and unrelated to the scientific basis of behavioral techniques, is the fact that few treatment providers are well trained in these techniques, and that some aspects of behavioral practice are rejected out of hand by some therapists working with a more traditional perspective. Specifically, some within the traditional perspective reject the possibility of moderated use as a treatment goal without qualification in spite of empirical evidence that moderated use under certain circumstances is at least as common a treatment outcome overall as abstinence.

The lack of emphasis on a spiritual aspect to PSUDs is also disturbing to some practitioners, particularly ones who have themselves benefited from more traditional, 12-Step-based approaches to treatment, predominantly a reflection of the Alcoholics Anonymous philosophy. Although a behavioral approach is not inherently antithetical to a spiritual notion of PSUDs, the notion of powerlessness often associated with spirituality in addictions treatment is. For those who rely more strongly on personal belief rather than on scientific evidence to guide their practice, this may be an unbreachable barrier to the use of behaviorally based techniques in practice. For patients who reject the spiritual aspects of Alcoholics Anonymous there are a number of alternative self-help approaches (McCrady & Delaney, 1995), some, such as Rational Recovery (Trimpey, 1992), based directly on cognitive-behavioral approaches to recovery.

CONCLUSION

Behavioral theories have been among the most productive of the last quarter century with respect to advancement of empirically validated knowledge of the origins and treatment of PSUDs. The notion of basing treatment technology solidly on our knowledge of psychological processes in human behavior that originated with behavioral theorists has led to the development of a variety of new, demonstrably effective treatment technologies. Marital/family and motivational approaches (discussed elsewhere in this volume) are based largely in the work of behavioral theorists, although substantial progress beyond basic behavioral theory characterizes those approaches as well.

Although behaviorally based treatments still do not reliably and predictably produce the sorts of treatment outcomes all therapists desire (e.g., long-lasting, positive behavior change), they offer some of the most promising approaches currently available to therapists treating PSUDs. They also hold the promise, based on the strong emphasis by behaviorally oriented therapists on scientific study of both the efficacy and process of behavior change in addictions, of advancing our knowledge of how best to treat these difficult and socially costly problems.

REFERENCES

Abrams, D. B., & Niaura, R. S. (1987). Social learning theory. In H. T. Blane & K. E. Leonard (Eds.), *Psychological theories of drinking and alcoholism*. New York: Guilford Press.

Azrin, N. H., Sisson, R. W., Meyers, R., & Godley, M. (1982). Alcoholism treatment by disulfiram and community reinforcement therapy. *Journal of Behavior Therapy and Experimental Psychiatry, 13*, 105–112.

Baars, B. J. (1986). *The cognitive revolution in psychology*. New York: Guilford Press.

Bandura, A. (1977). *Social learning theory*. Englewood Cliffs, NJ: Prentice Hall.

Beck, A. T., Rush, A. J., Shaw, B. F., & Emery, G. (1979). *Cognitive therapy of depression*. New York: Guilford Press.

Beck, A. T., Wright, F. D., Newman, C. F., & Liese, B. S. (1993). *Cognitive therapy of substance abuse*. New York: Guilford Press.

Bickel, W. K., & Kelly, T. H. (1988). The relationship of stimulus control to the treatment of substance abuse. In B. A. Ray (Ed.), *Learning factors in substance abuse* (NIDA Research Monograph 84). Washington, DC: U.S. Government Printing Office.

Booth, P. B., Dale, B., Slade, P. D., & Dewey, M. E. (1992). A follow-up study of problem drinkers offered a goal choice option. *Journal of Studies on Alcohol, 53*, 594–600.

Childress, A. R., Hole, A. V., Ehrman, R. N., Robbins, S. J., McLellan, A. T., & O'Brien, C. P. (1993). Cue reactivity and cue reactivity interventions in drug dependence. In L. S. Onken, J. D. Blaine, & J. J. Boren (Eds.), *Behavioral treatments for drug abuse and dependence* (NIDA Research Monograph 137). Washington, DC: U.S. Government Printing Office.

Christiansen, B. A., Smith, G. T., Roehling, P. V., & Goldman, M. S. (1989). Using alcohol expectancies to predict adolescent drinking behavior after one year. *Journal of Consulting and Clinical Psychology, 57*, 93–99.

Donovan, D. M. (1988). Assessment of addictive behaviors: Implications of an emerging biopsychosocial model. In D. M. Donovan & G. A. Marlatt (Eds.), *Assessment of addictive behaviors*. New York: Guilford Press.

Donovan, D. M., & Mattson, M. E. (Eds.). (1994, December). Alcoholism treatment matching research: Methodological and clinical approaches. *Journal of Studies on Alcohol* (Suppl. No. 12).

Duckert, F., Amundsen, A., & Johnsen, J. (1992). What happens to drinking after therapeutic intervention? *British Journal of Addiction, 87*, 1457–1467.

Ellis, A., McInerney, J. F., DiGiuseppe, R., & Yeager, R. J. (1988). *Rational–emo-*

tive therapy with alcoholics and substance abusers. New York: Pergamon Press.

Eysenck, H. J. (1982). Neobehavioristic (S–R) theory. In G. T. Wilson & C. M. Franks (Eds.), *Contemporary behavior therapy: Conceptual and empirical foundations.* New York: Guilford Press.

Fuller, R. K. (1989). Antidipsotropic medications. In R. K. Hester & W. R. Miller (Eds.), *Handbook of alcoholism treatment approaches: Effective alternatives.* New York: Pergamon Press.

Goldman, M. S., Brown, S. A., & Christiansen, B. A. (1987). Expectancy theory: Thinking about drinking. In H. T. Blane & K. E. Leonard (Eds.), *Psychological theories of drinking and alcoholism.* New York: Guilford Press.

Holder, H. D., Longabaugh, R., Miller, W. R., & Rubonis, A. V. (1991). The cost effectiveness of treatment for alcoholism: A first approximation. *Journal of Studies on Alcohol, 52,* 517–540.

Institute of Medicine. (1990). *Broadening the base of treatment for alcohol problems: Report of a study by a committee of the Institute of Medicine, Division of Health and Behavioral Medicine.* Washington, DC: National Academy Press.

Kadden, R. M., Cooney, N. L., Getter, H., & Litt, M. D. (1989). Matching alcoholics to coping skills or interactive therapies: Posttreatment results. *Journal of Consulting and Clinical Psychology, 57,* 698–704.

Krasner, L. (1982). *Behavior therapy: On roots, contexts and growth.* In G. T. Wilson & C. M. Franks (Eds.), *Contemporary behavior therapy: Conceptual and empirical foundations.* New York: Guilford Press.

Marlatt, G. A., & Gordon, J. R. (Eds.). (1985). *Relapse prevention: Maintenance strategies in the treatment of addictive behaviors.* New York: Guilford Press.

Marlatt, G. A., & Tapert, S. F. (1993). Harm reduction: Reducing the risks of addictive behaviors. In J. S. Baer, G. A. Marlatt, & R. J. McMahon (Eds.), *Addictive behaviors across the life span: Prevention, treatment and policy issues.* Newbury Park, CA: Sage.

McCrady, B. S., & Delaney, S. I. (1995). Self-help groups. In R. K. Hester & W. R. Miller (Eds.), *Handbook of alcoholism treatment approaches: Effective alternatives* (2nd ed.). Needham Heights, MA: Allyn & Bacon.

McLellan, A. T., Childress, A. R., Ehrman, R. N., & O'Brien, C. P. (1986). Extinguishing conditioned responses during treatment for opiate dependence: Turning laboratory findings into clinical procedure. *Journal of Substance Abuse Treatment, 3,* 33–40.

Miller, W. R., & Munoz, R. F. (1982). *How to control your drinking: A practical guide to responsible drinking* (rev. ed.). Albuquerque: University of New Mexico Press.

Monti, P. M., Abrams, D. B., Kadden, R. M., & Cooney, N. L. (1989). *Treating alcohol dependence: A coping skills training guide.* New York: Guilford Press.

Morgenstern, J., & McCrady, B. S. (1992). Curative factors in alcohol and drug treatment: Behavioral and disease model perspectives. *British Journal of Addiction, 87,* 901–912.

Onken, L. S. (1991). Using psychotherapy effectively in drug abuse treatment. In R. W. Pickens, C. G. Leukefeld, & C. R. Schuster (Eds.), *Improving drug abuse treatment.* Washington, DC: U.S. Government Printing Office.

Pavlov, I. P. (1927). *Lectures on conditioned reflexes.* New York: International Publishers.

Prochaska, J. O., DiClemente, C. C., & Norcross, J. C. (1992). In search of how people change: Applications to addictive behaviors. *American Psychologist, 47,* 1102–1114.

Regier, D. A., Farmer, M. E., Rae, D. S., Locke, B. Z., Keith, S. J., Judd, L. L., & Goodwin, F. K. (1990). Comorbidity of mental disorders with alcohol and other drug abuse: Results from the Epidemiologic Catchment Area (ECA) study. *Journal of the American Medical Association, 264,* 2511–2518.

Rimmele, C. T., Miller, W. R., & Dougher, M. J. (1989). Aversion Therapies. In R. K. Hester & W. R. Miller (Eds.), *Handbook of alcoholism treatment approaches: Effective alternatives.* New York: Pergamon Press.

Ross, H. E., Glaser, F. B., & Germanson, T. (1988). The prevalence of psychiatric disorders in patients with alcohol and other drug problems. *Archives of General Psychiatry, 45,* 1023–1031.

Rotgers, F., & Morgenstern, J. (1994). *Processes comprising successful substance abuse treatment: A survey of counselors.* Unpublished manuscript, Rutgers University, Center of Alcohol Studies, Piscataway, NJ.

Sher, K. J. (1987). Stress response dampening. In H. T. Blane & K. E. Leonard (Eds.), *Psychological theories of drinking and alcoholism.* New York: Guilford Press.

Skinner, B. F. (1953). *Science and Human Behavior.* New York: Macmillan.

Sobell, L. C., Sobell, M. B., Toneatto, T., & Leo, G.I. (1993). What triggers the resolution of alcohol problems without treatment? *Alcoholism: Clinical and Experimental Research, 17,* 217–224.

Trimpey, J. (1992). *The small book: A revolutionary alternative for overcoming alcohol and drug dependence* (3rd ed.). New York: Delacorte Press.

Vogel-Sprott, M. (1992). *Alcohol tolerance and social drinking: Learning the consequences.* New York: Guilford Press.

Volpicelli, J. R., Alterman, A. I., Hayashida, M., & O'Brien, C. P. (1992). Naltrexone in treating alcohol dependence. *Archives of General Psychiatry, 49,* 876–880.

Watson, J. B. (1919). *Psychology from the standpoint of a behaviorist.* Philadelphia: Lippincott.

Wikler, A. (1965). Conditioning factors in opiate addiction and relapse. In D. I. Wilner & G. G. Kassenbaum (Eds.), *Narcotics.* New York: McGraw-Hill.

Wikler, A. (1973). Dynamics of drug dependence: Implications of a conditioning theory for research and treatment. *Archives of General Psychiatry, 28,* 611–616.

Wilson, P. H. (1992). Relapse prevention: Conceptual and methodological issues. In P. H. Wilson (Ed.), *Principles and practice of relapse prevention.* New York: Guilford Press.

CHAPTER 8

Behavioral Treatment Techniques for Psychoactive Substance Use Disorders

THOMAS J. MORGAN

BASIC TASKS OF ALL BEHAVIORAL INTERVENTIONS

Whether a clinician is working with substance abuse patients or with a general psychiatric population, there are several essential tasks for the behavioral clinician to accomplish during treatment. These tasks include the following: (1) developing a collaborative, therapeutic relationship, (2) enhancing motivation to make changes, (3) using a functional analysis to make a thorough assessment of the patient's presenting problem, (4) developing and implementing treatment goals, and (5) evaluating treatment progress and terminating the treatment.

Developing a Therapeutic Relationship

The importance of developing a positive therapeutic relationship with patients has been emphasized for many years. Since Rogers (1957) first defined unconditional positive regard, accurate empathy, genuineness, and therapist congruence as necessary therapist characteristics for positive change, the scientific and treatment communities have been interested in the therapeutic relationship and its contribution to successful treatment. In the substance abuse field, Valle (1981) has shown that long-term outcomes for alcoholics could be predicted by the level of a counselor's empathy and general interpersonal skills. Additionally, there is some evidence that alcoholic patients have poorer treatment outcomes when clinicians use a confrontational style in treatment (Lieberman, Yalom, & Miles, 1973; MacDonough, 1976; Miller, Benefield, & Tonigan, 1993).

In developing a positive, collaborative relationship with a patient the clinician should spend some time focusing on several aspects of the therapeutic relationship. One aspect includes defining patient and therapist roles and exploring expectations about treatment. Time is needed to discuss patient experiences with previous treatment and to understand patient expectations about how treatment should proceed. Clinicians should explain to the patient what to expect in the current treatment, such as how long it might last, how sessions are structured, and issues around confidentiality. In defining treatment expectations, patients are told about their responsibilities, such as showing up for appointments, being on time, being sober, and completing homework assignments. For therapists, responsibilities include being on time for appointments, being honest, and giving the patient their "therapeutic all."

Another important aspect of the collaborative relationship is having a sense of empathy for the patient's experiences. McCrady (1993) has suggested some therapist actions to enhance empathy for a substance-abusing patient. Some of these activities include attempting to change an addictive behavior or deeply held habit of his/her own, attending self-help meetings, and listening carefully to the client. Being able to listen to a patient's concerns, experiences, and feelings and having the patient feel heard and accepted are important aspects in developing an empathic relationship. Also, in developing a good therapeutic alliance a clinician can ask questions that reflect an interest in the patient and his/her life outside the substance use. For example, taking some time prior to getting immediately into a substance use history to ask about a patient's family, work, hobbies, or family pet can be an effective way to enhance rapport.

Finally, another essential aspect in developing the therapeutic relationship is helping the patient see that there is hope for change. Assisting patients in identifying small steps taken to change and congratulating them on these accomplishments will help provide them with a sense of hope and increased self-efficacy. Also, facilitating the patient's involvement in self-help groups, such as Alcoholics Anonymous, Narcotics Anonymous, or Rational Recovery, will provide a venue for the patient to see firsthand the extraordinary changes that can be made by those similarly addicted to substances.

Enhancing Motivation to Change

From a traditional disease model perspective, substance-abusing patients were not viewed as terribly motivated to change until they "hit bottom." Personal crises or formal Johnsonian interventions were typical factors that motivated patients to seek treatment (Johnson, 1986). After a patient entered treatment there was less emphasis on maintaining a patient's motivation and relapses; noncompliance or "resistance" was viewed as a patient "in denial." However, viewed from a different perspective, "denial" can be seen as a reflection of differences between the therapist's and patient's definition of the problem. Also, denial can be viewed as the patient's ambivalence about changing his/her addictive behavior as the cost–benefit ratio of making changes will shift over time.

Motivational aspects in substance abuse treatment have more recently become the focus of a great deal of discussion. Miller (1985) has written an excellent article that reviews the concepts of "denial" and motivation in alcoholism treatment. Additionally, Miller and Rollnick (1991) have written a superb text that describes the "how-to" of motivational interviewing with substance abuse clients (e.g., chapters by Allsop & Saunders, 1991; Cox, Klinger, & Blount, 1991; Saunders, Wilkinson, & Allsop, 1991). The main concepts of this type of intervention are that the responsibility for change lies within the patient and the therapist's tasks are to create the type of environment that will facilitate the patient's internal motivation to change. Miller and Rollnick describe the active ingredients of motivational interviewing by using the acronym FRAMES. F is for providing *feedback* about the patient's condition, R includes giving *responsibility* for making the decision to change directly to the patient, A involves giving the patient clear, objective *advice* about making changes in his/her substance use, M provides for giving the patient a *menu* of change options and different strategies for change, E involves the clinician *empathically* providing information and facilitating the discussion of change, and S involves enhancing the patient's sense of hopefulness and *self-efficacy*. The goal in a motivational intervention is to use objective, concrete information about the patient's substance use and its consequences in a fashion that does not elicit resistance from the patient.

Another way to enhance a patient's motivation for change is to adopt a more limited and conservative perspective about defining goals and how they will be accomplished. Prochaska, DiClemente, and Norcross (1992) have described the stages-of-change model, which can be useful in maintaining a patient's motivation. These authors posit five stages of change that individuals pass through on the way to initiating and maintaining changes: (1) precontemplation, in which an individual does not believe that he/she has have a problem that needs changing; (2) contemplation, in which an individual begins to think about the possibility of having a problem but is ambivalent and does not take any action to make changes; (3) preparation, in which an individual now believes that he/she has a problem that needs addressing and begins to consider change options and prepares him/herself to make a change; (4) action, where an individual begins to make specific behavior changes; and (5) maintenance, in which an individual who has made certain changes now makes efforts to maintain these changes. Using this model, a patient who was formerly considered "in denial" is simply viewed as being in a precontemplation or contemplation stage of readiness to change.

Several investigators have written about the importance of enhancing motivation to change through identifying and exploring the conflicts around making a change in behavior (Janis & Mann, 1977; Miller & Rollnick, 1991; Orford, 1985). In addition, Carlson (1991) has developed a comprehensive and practical decisional balance worksheet that is useful in identifying various aspects of a patient's reasons whether or not to use substances. Using these models, the treatment goal is more modest and may simply be for the patient to move from the precontemplation stage to the contemplation stage of change. Working within this model, the goals of treatment are short term and specific. Thus, in working with patients who do not believe they have a substance problem, the goal is not to have them immediately accept being an alcoholic or addict or commit to lifetime abstinence or to teach them how to refuse substances. Rather, the specific and short-term goal would be to work with such patients to see whether they can begin to consider that they might have a problem with substances. This is accomplished by objectively reviewing the consequences associated with substance use as well as reviewing the advantages of using substances.

Making a Thorough Assessment via a Functional Analysis

The hallmark of good behavioral treatment is a thorough understanding of the patient that comes from a comprehensive assessment. In a behavioral assessment, a patient's substance use will be examined by looking at various factors that initiate and maintain the substance use.

One area to assess is the unique precursors or triggers to a patient's substance use. This assessment includes evaluating interpersonal situations, various emotional states, and environmental situations that are associated with a patient's drinking or drug use. For example, one patient may drink heavily in response to feeling angry or anxious. Another patient may drink heavily when in social situations and when there is pressure to drink from peers. Finally, a patient may smoke crack cocaine because the housing project where he/she lives has dealers staking out the entrance to the building. It is important to identify the individualized "triggers" to a patient's substance use as this will be invaluable in the plan to identify and cope with high-risk situations.

The clinician also needs to assess the consequences of the patient's substance use, both from a long- and short-term perspective, as well as defining positive and negative reinforcers associated with the substance use. In identifying consequences, it is important to inquire about many areas of a patient's life. The following are some areas of a person's life that may be affected by substance use:

- *Relationship problems.* Arguments with family and/or friends about substance use; separations, break-ups, or divorce due to alcohol and/or drug use; having family and/or friends become annoyed or criticize patient's alcohol/drug use.
- *Work problems.* Coming in late for work or missing days of work due to intoxication or hangover; being warned at work and/or being fired due to alcohol/drug use; being intoxicated or high while at work.
- *Legal problems.* Being arrested, placed on probation, and/or incarcerated for alcohol- or drug-related offenses such as driving while intoxicated (DWI); being disorderly; possessing controlled dangerous substances (CDS); or possession with intent to distribute.
- *Medical/physical problems.* Having a history of alcohol-related traumas and liver or pancreatic problems, being hospitalized for alcohol- or drug-related illnesses, or having been advised by a physician to quit or cut down on drinking or drug use; having blackouts, hangovers, or withdrawal symptoms such as nausea, shakes, convulsions, or seizures after using substances.
- *Financial problems.* Experiencing heavy debt due to alcohol and/or drug use; not paying bills in order to have money to buy alcohol and/or drugs.
- *Intrapersonal problems.* Having feelings of guilt, shame, and regret about alcohol/drug use; having felt depressed, paranoid, and/or anxious as a result of using alcohol/drugs.

It is important to gather collateral information about the patient's substance use and its effects on other people whenever possible. Gaining a perspective of the patient's substance use from his/her spouse/partner, an employer, a probation officer, and/or a physician can be extremely helpful. Before talking to collaterals it is necessary to discuss the importance of getting collateral information and to obtain the appropriate releases from the patient.

Finally, a clinician should assess a patient's cognitions regarding his/her interpretation of the antecedents or triggers to substance use as well as the patient's expectancies about the effects the substance use will have for him/her. For example, a patient believes that after a particularly long and stressful day at work, "I deserve to have a beer and relax." This cognition highlights the patient's interpretation of personal stress and discomfort as intolerable and his/her sense of entitlement to a stress-free life. Also, it emphasizes the patient's expectation that alcohol will have a soothing, calming effect. (For those readers interested in more detailed accounts of substance abuse assessment, see Hester & Miller, 1989a; Donovan & Marlatt, 1988.)

Developing and Implementing Treatment Goals

Developing individualized treatment plans has been the cornerstone of behavioral treatment. However, within addictions treatment, the traditional disease model has typically prescribed a generic treatment plan for all who have problems with alcohol and drug use. From this traditional perspective, treatment would typically include confrontation of patient denial, education about the disease concept of addiction, and facilitation of the patient into a 12-Step program such as Alcoholics Anonymous or Narcotics Anonymous. Additionally, the goal for all patients would be lifetime abstinence from alcohol and drugs.

From the behavioral perspective, providing different goal options for substance abusers, specifically alcohol abusers, has been consistent with the behavioral tenet of individualized treatment plans. Moderated drinking by alcoholic patients was first reported by Davies (1962) and later suggested by Sobell and Sobell (1976), Miller and Caddy (1977), and Polich, Armor, and Braiker (1981). It was the Sobells' study that received so much attention and controversy from traditional treatment providers. (For a more detailed account of the controlled drinking controversy, see excellent reviews by Nathan & Niaura, 1985; Marlatt, Lanimar, Baer, & Quigley, 1993.) More recently, there has been a consistent and growing literature that supports moderated drinking for some problem drinkers. However, it still is clear that individuals who are alcohol dependent are not appropriate candidates for moderation-based drinking goals. (For an apt review of the literature on controlled drinking, see Rosenberg, 1993.)

From the behavioral perspective it is important that treatment goals are collaboratively determined. Studies have emphasized the importance of the patient's choice of treatment goals. Regardless of goal preferences of treatment providers, studies have shown that patients will ultimately decide on substance use goals that suit them. This includes alcohol-dependent patients who moderate their drinking when treated in an abstinence-based program (McCabe, 1986; Nordstrom & Berglund, 1987; Sanchez-Craig, Annis, Bornet, & MacDonald, 1984; Vaillant & Milkofsky, 1982) as well as patients who abstain from drinking even after they have been treated in a moderation-based program (Miller, Leckman, Delaney, & Tinkcom, 1992; Rychtarik, Foy, Scott, Lokey, & Prue, 1987). Also, having patients self-select their goal is an important factor in the patient's motivation and commitment to treatment (Marlatt et al., 1993; Ogborne, 1987; Sobell, Toneatto, & Sobell, 1992). Finally, goal choice has become more popular as studies have suggested that successful treatment outcomes are more likely if the treatment goals are consistent with the patient's goal preference (Booth, Dale, & Ansari, 1984; Orford & Keddie, 1986).

Evaluating Treatment Progress and Terminating Treatment

As treatment progresses, the therapist needs to continually evaluate the progress of the work or, if there is a lack of progress, to immediately address this issue in treatment. By regularly assessing progress, both therapist and patient can see concrete, positive changes and the patient can be reinforced for making these changes. When progress is not being made toward the treatment goals, both the therapist and patient can identify and discuss any obstacles to reaching treatment goals. It may be that the goals of treatment are unrealistic, the patient has become ambivalent about the original treatment goals, or the assessment of the problems/circumstances in the patient's life are not accurate. When progress is not being made toward achieving treatment goals, the patient and clinician can begin the process of collaboratively redefining treatment goals. It is also extremely helpful to consult with colleagues and supervisors when work with a case becomes "stuck." Ideally, termination of treatment from a behavioral perspective is mutually determined. Treatment ends when goals have been reached or there is an acknowledgment that treatment might follow a different direction and the patient is referred to another practitioner. In terminating treatment, the patient and clinician should accomplish several tasks. One task is to review the treatment and acknowledge and reinforce patient changes. The clinician should highlight the patient's self-efficacy in making changes in treatment and explore other areas of change that might happen outside the therapy. Also during termination there is discussion of "warning signs" that will signal the patient to consider returning to therapy. The clinician can always leave the door open for a future consultation.

Successful treatment can be defined as the degree to which treatment goals have been achieved. Because behavioral treatment values individualized treatment goals, success may be defined quite differently from patient to patient. For one patient it may be a reduction in quantity and frequency of drinking and subsequent reduction or elimination of health, social, and/or emotional problems. For another patient, total abstinence from alcohol and drugs and utilization of a 12-Step program may define success in treatment.

SPECIFIC BEHAVIORAL TREATMENT TECHNIQUES AND INTERVENTIONS

In should be noted that the following description of specific behavioral treatment techniques is relevant for both alcohol- and drug-abusing patients. Due to space constraints I will focus primarily on describing the use of behavioral techniques with alcohol-abusing patients. (For a more comprehensive and detailed description of behavioral treatment with drug abuse populations, see Miller, 1993; Sobell et al., 1992.)

As noted in the previous chapter, classical conditioning assumes that substance users are conditioned to many stimuli in the environment through repeated use of substances in specific settings, with specific people, and according to specific rituals. The cues or "triggers" (conditioned stimuli) for use are quite diverse and unique from individual to individual. In treatment it is assumed that if certain conditioned stimuli are learned to be associated with substance use, then these cues can be unlearned or extinguished. The following section provides a summary of the most well-known treatments for substance abuse disorders following the classical conditioning paradigm.

Aversion Treatments

There are several treatment regimens and specific techniques that are based on the classical conditioning paradigm. One of the first behavioral treatments for substance use disorders, specifically alcohol dependence, was *aversion therapy*. The rationale for this treatment regimen was to pair an aversive experience with the stimuli ("triggers") of drinking so the patient would eventually have a negative reaction to alcohol and thus lose the urge to drink. Over the years, many different types of aversion were used in an attempt to condition an aversive response to alcohol. I discuss here the three most prominent types of aversion therapy.

Electrical Aversion

Early treatment for alcoholism used electrical aversion in which there was a pairing of a painful electrical shock to the site, smell, and taste of a patient's favorite alcoholic beverage. Because of the extremely stressful nature of the treatment, there was need for medical supervision, which made outpatient treatment untenable. Also, not surprisingly, there was a high rate of patient dropout when using electrical aversion therapy. Finally, the use of electrical aversion has been unsuccessful in producing conditioned aversion to alcohol according to Cannon, Baker, and Wehl (1981). In most recent reviews of electrical aversion, the consensus is that this form of treatment is not widely considered a serious treatment for alcohol disorders today (Miller & Hester, 1986; Institute of Medicine, 1990; Lawson & Boudin, 1992; Nathan & Niaura, 1985; O'Leary & Wilson, 1987).

Chemical Aversion

The oldest form of aversion therapy for the treatment of alcoholism is chemical aversion. The idea was that the sight, smell, and taste of alcohol would be paired with nausea (that was chemically induced) in order to set up a negative reaction to drinking and thus reduce the urge to drink. The rationale for using chemical aversion was that the nausea would provide a more realistic aversive association to drinking. It was suspected that electrical aversion was unable to provide a conditioned response to alcohol because a shock was not a realistic, natural consequence of drinking.

In the chemical aversion protocol, patients typically were hospitalized for 10 days and treatment consisted of five treatment sessions. The patient was treated in rooms that were set up to minimize distractions and maximize the visibility of alcohol-related cues such as alcoholic beverages, bottles, and posters with drinking scenes. During the treatment sessions, patients received a nausea-inducing drug (such as an emetine hydrochloride, lithium, or apomorphine) intravenously, which produced nausea within 2 to 8 minutes. Immediately before the first signs of nausea, the patient was given a drink of his/her preferred alcoholic beverage to look at, smell, and eventually drink. More drinks were given to the patient over the next 30 to 60 minutes, as nausea and vomiting continued. At the end of the hospitalization, it was assumed that a conditioned aversive response had been achieved. Booster sessions would be scheduled for reconditioning over the next 6 to 12 months and would be used as either a routine follow-up or an intervention if a patient reexperienced strong urges to drink. Today, chemical aversion treatment techniques are not used as widely as they were in the 1960s–1970s. The questionable ethics of giving alcohol to alcohol-dependent patients (O'Leary & Wilson, 1987), the need for medical supervision and the level of discomfort and stress that chemical aversion provided have made this form of treatment less popular. Studies have shown that chemical aversion can produce an aversion to alcohol, but positive treatment effects are generally lost during longer-term follow-up (6 and 12 months). In recent reviews, it has been suggested that chemical aversion therapy is unwarranted for the treatment of alcoholism (Lawson & Boudin, 1992; Miller & Hester, 1986; Wilson, 1987), although some have been more optimistic about the efficacy of chemical aversion and call for further investigation (Institute of Medicine, 1990).

Covert Sensitization

In covert sensitization, the aversive conditioning to alcohol or drugs occurs through the patients verbal and imaginal modalities. The rationale for using this treatment protocol is that it continues to follow the learning principles of counterconditioning but is not as invasive or painful as electrical and chemical aversion treatments. In addition, medical supervision and special equipment are not needed and covert sensitization procedures can be carried out on an outpatient basis.

In covert sensitization, specific and detailed information is gathered regarding usual antecedents or cues to the patient's alcohol and/or drug use as well as typical negative or feared consequences. These are used in the conditioning scenes. Patients are instructed to relax and imagine as vividly as possible a typical situation in which they are about to use alcohol or drugs. In the imaginal scene, immediately after the patient has used alcohol or drugs he/she is provided a disgusting and specific description of the aversive consequences of the substance use. Such scenarios would include graphic descriptions of nausea, vomiting, hangovers, heart racing, the hurt or frightened look from their children, and other feared natural results of use. These scenes and aversive images are repeatedly paired until the unpleasant images become associated with alcohol and drug use and the urges for substance use have been extinguished.

The imaginal scene may end with the suggestion that the patient will have relief from these symptoms by leaving the situation and avoiding alcohol or drug use in the future. Also, planning and using an imaginal escape route are then utilized in the imaginal scene as soon as the patient begins to feel uncomfortable urges or cravings. The suggestions of relief and positive self-statements are emphasized in this phase.

The data on the efficacy of covert sensitization have been mixed in terms of long-term follow-up (Institute of Medicine, 1990; Lawson & Boudin, 1992; Nathan & Niaura, 1985; O'Leary & Wilson, 1987; Rimmele, Miller, & Dougher, 1989). Rimmele et al. (1989) have noted that the most encouraging results are found in those studies that have specific sensitization procedures and have verified the presence of conditioned aversion. Although the results of covert sensitization's efficacy are mixed, there is general optimism about its viability as a treatment option for substance abuse disorders. Especially when compared to electrical and chemical aversion treatments, it has the advantages of being less intrusive and less physically stressful and can be administered on an outpatient basis. It may not be useful for all patients, especially those who have difficulty with visualizations. (For more specific information about a covert sensitization treatment protocol, see Rimmele et al., 1989.)

Cue Exposure

The intent in cue exposure is to extinguish previously developed conditioned responses, such as craving, heart rate, sweating, shakiness, and ultimately substance use. As one would expect from the classical conditioning paradigm, extinction occurs through repeated exposures of the conditioned stimuli (e.g., stress, sight of cocaine, drug paraphernalia, and smell of beer) without the patient being able to execute the conditioned response (drinking or drug use). Thus, as craving for alcohol and drugs becomes extinguished, the urge and motivation to use these substances are eliminated.

However, it appears clear that exposure alone will not account for significant long-term treatment effects (Monti et al., 1993). Other elements important to address in exposure treatment include self-efficacy expectations, personally relevant cues for substance use, and coping skills training. Empirical support for cue exposure treatments in the areas of phobia and obsessive–compulsive disorders (Foa & Kozak, 1986) and bulimia (Wilson, Rossiter, Kleinfield, & Lindholm, 1986) offer conceptual and theoretical optimism for the use of exposure treatment with substance abuse disorders.

In providing cue exposure treatment, patients are given a rationale about the importance of reducing their craving to use substances and to help them cope with various high-risk triggers. Patients are also given a brief, simple description of the classical conditioning paradigm. In order to individualize treatment, a detailed description and an assessment are needed regarding the patient's preferred drinks and drugs of abuse as well as details regarding specific situations in which the patient uses substances heavily. Treatment typically consists of six to eight sessions, provided in an inpatient facility. Each exposure session begins and ends with an assessment of the patient's subjective and physiological responses to the alcohol cues. Patients receive a series of brief exposures to an alcoholic beverage. Also, patients are exposed to alcohol cues after they have been induced into a negative mood state. (For those readers interested in a more detailed cue exposure protocol, see Monti, Abrams, Kadden, & Cooney, 1989.)

The literature regarding the efficacy of cue exposure treatment is still relatively small. Uncontrolled studies have provided promising results (Institute of Medicine, 1990). Some controlled studies have shown initial positive results in terms of extinguishing craving and withdrawal responses; however, these have not generalized outside the exposure condition (Childress, Ehrman, McLellan, & O'Brien, 1988). In a recent controlled study by Monti et al. (1993), results suggested that alcoholic patients who were given a combination of cue exposure and coping skills training drank significantly less than patients who received only standard treatment. The differences in the drinking outcomes were not seen during the 3-month follow-up but emerged at 6 months.

Behavioral Self-Control Training

According to the Institute of Medicine (1990), since 1980 there have been more treatment outcome studies on behavioral self-control training (BSCT) than on any other treatment modality for alcohol problems. As a treatment modality for alcohol abuse disorders, BSCT has been described as a brief, educationally oriented treatment approach in which patients can achieve a goal of nonproblematic drinking or abstinence. BSCT can be implemented either by a therapist (therapist-directed) or by the patient in the form of a self-help manual (self-directed). There are several advantages for using BSCT over traditional treatment with alcohol-abusing patients. One reason is that some patients refuse to accept an abstinence goal without at least a reasonable attempt at moderated, nonproblematic drinking. A second rationale for using BSCT is that it has the potential to reach a larger, broader population of individuals who are having problems with drinking. Cahalan (1987) has suggested that there are many more problem drinkers than those dependent on alcohol. Additionally, a majority of those with alcohol problems never have any treatment contact with self-help groups or professional services (Institute of Medicine,

1990). Thus, a treatment approach that offers a goal choice may be more attractive for many problem drinkers who do not feel an abstinence goal is necessary and who might otherwise not consider treatment.

The active, effective ingredients of BSCT are believed to be the development of patient self-efficacy and an emphasis on self-control strategies. The patient is given assignments and maintains the primary responsibility for making decisions throughout treatment. BSCT is brief, usually between 6 and 12 sessions with each session being 90 minutes in length. Regular "booster" sessions are typically scheduled in order to solidify gains and to assess patients who may need additional interventions. According to Hester and Miller (1989b), BSCT is made up of specific steps which occur in the following order: (1) setting limits on the number of drinks per day and on peak blood alcohol concentrations (BACs), (2) self-monitoring of drinking behaviors, (3) changing the rate of drinking, (4) practicing assertiveness in refusing drinks, (5) setting up a reward system for achievement of goals, (6) learning which antecedents result in excessive drinking, and (7) learning other coping skills instead of drinking. Homework, role playing, and practice are emphasized in BSCT.

Although a great deal of research has been generated on BSCT over the past 15 years, results have been mixed. Various studies have looked at different treatment populations (DWI offenders, chronic, alcohol-dependent veterans, early-stage problem drinkers), different treatment settings (inpatient, outpatient), different treatment goals (abstinence vs. moderation), and varied treatment delivery (BSCT self-directed vs. BSCT therapist-directed). Many controlled studies suggest that BSCT fares no worse than abstinent-oriented treatments in terms of drinking outcomes and patients have shown significant improvement when compared to control groups. One study (Foy, Nunn, & Rychtarik, 1984) reported that BSCT patients had worse short-term outcomes when compared to an abstinence-oriented treatment, but at long-term follow-up, there were no significant differences in outcomes. Several factors are likely to contribute to the mixed results with BSCT. Treatment packages that are defined as BSCT can vary a good deal in terms of what treatment techniques are used. Also, BSCT has been used with a heterogeneous population and there may be certain types of patients that respond better/worse than others.

Overall, results of controlled empirical studies have suggested that BSCT is generally effective for treating those with alcohol problems. However, in Carey and Maisto's (1985) review of BSCT, the authors concluded that behavioral self-control training appears to provide improvement that is at least comparable to the interventions against which it has been compared. However, more definitive information is needed to determine what are the effective, active ingredients in BSCT and for which specific patients BSCT is most effective.

Broad-Spectrum Treatments

Broad-spectrum treatments are defined as treatment approaches that address not only a patient's substance use but also other problems areas that may be associated with excessive alcohol/drug use. The rationale for this approach is that once individuals have stopped drinking or using drugs, they will be confronted with a variety of problems that will challenge their sobriety due to their lack of effective coping skills. In fact, in analyzing recent relapses among alcohol abusers and opiate addicts, results revealed that most relapses occurred in response to negative emotional states (i.e., anger and frustration) that stem from interpersonal conflict and direct social pressure to resume substance use (Chaney, Roszell, & Cummings, 1982; Marlatt & Gordon, 1985). Broad-spectrum treatments are seen as focusing more on preventing relapse after a patient has gained some stability in his/her early recovery from substance use.

In defining broad-spectrum treatment, there are several specific skills that appear more often in the literature.

Assertiveness Training

Assertiveness training is one of the most widely used examples of this broad-spectrum approach in the treatment of substance abuse. The main focus of assertiveness training is to help patients be more direct and appropriate in expressing their thoughts and feelings. When a patient is more assertive, he/she is better able to resist social pressure to use substances. Additionally, patients are learning how to be assertive in substance-specific situations, but they are also learning how to assert their needs in a variety of settings with different people. It is not uncommon for some patients to be appropriately assertive in some situations but to have difficulty asserting themselves in other situations.

In developing assertiveness skills, specifically for coping with sub-stance use situations, patients are questioned about previous troublesome drinking or drug situations. Patients then role-play with the clinician how they might resist requests to drink or use drugs. Initially, the clinician models appropriate assertiveness skills and takes the role of the person refusing drinks or drugs. Next, the patient takes on the role and practices a variety of drink/drug refusal strategies. These strategies include resisting substance use by (1) requesting others to stop insisting that the patient use, (2) suggesting an alternative activity that is not compatible with drinking or drug use, (3) redirecting the conversation in order to get the topic of discussion off substance use, and (4) maintaining direct eye contact and using gestures, facial expressions, and voice qualities that communicate the patient's resolve not to drink or use.

Stress Management

Stress management is also a popular treatment strategy for substance use disorders. The rationale for including stress management as a treatment component is that stress has been implicated as a significant precursor to substance use and relapse. Oftentimes patients will desire temporary relief from the stressors in their life. Substances such as alcohol, barbiturates, tranquilizers, opiates, and cannabis are often used to escape tension, stress. and anxiety.

Studies that have tested stress management training have included relaxation training, biofeedback relaxation training, and systematic desensitization. Controlled research has shown no positive treatment effects of relaxation training on drinking status (Institute of Medicine, 1990). However, Rosenberg (1979) suggests that relaxation training is related to reduced alcohol consumption, but only for patients who were assessed as having high anxiety. This result is encouraging for those interested in patient–treatment matching.

Social Skills Training

Social skills training offers more general coping skills that can be used in a wide range of problematic situations. The rationale for providing social skills training with substance abusers is the belief that problems in coping are related to the initiation and maintenance of addictive disorders. The emerging coping skills model posits that addictive behavior is a habitual, maladaptive way of coping with stress that can be alleviated through social skills training.

In the standard social skills treatment package, coping skills are taught to deal with negative emotional states, urges to use substances, physical discomfort, the desire to enhance positive emotional states, social pressure, interpersonal conflict, and the desire to enhance positive emotional interactions. As in other behavioral treatment components, it is important to have the patient practice these coping skills *in vivo* in order to enhance self-efficacy and broaden the generalization of the skills.

The controlled literature has shown strong support for the effectiveness of social skills training, especially when used with inpatient alcohol patients in which there are additional treatment components (Chaney, 1989; Institute of Medicine, 1990). (For detailed protocols for social skills training, see Chaney, 1989; Monti et al., 1989; Kadden et al., 1992.)

Contingency Management

It is known that environmental contingencies have an extremely powerful effect on people's behavior. Substance abuse treatment that uses the operant conditioning paradigm emphasizes reinforcing desirable behavior (abstinence) while punishing undesirable behavior (substance use). Many patients enter treatment as part of a implicit contingency contract, such as the spouse who comes to treatment rather than face a divorce, or a person who enters treatment in order to get his/her driver's license back. However, it is interesting that in spite of these strong contingencies, people often continue to use substances. Nathan and Niaura (1985) explain this by noting the unique differences among people and what is rewarding or punishing for one individual is not necessarily rewarding–punishing for another. Additionally, the authors emphasize the need for contingencies to be mutually agreed on, carefully observed, and consistently implemented. The consistent involvement of collaterals and institutions connected with the patient is essential for an effective contingency contract and can often be difficult to obtain. The effectiveness of contingency management programs is mixed depending on the consistency of rewards and punishments being delivered and the type of contingency being used (revocation of professional licenses, increase in methadone dosages, etc.). One of the more successful contingency management programs, the community reinforcement approach, is described next in more detail.

The community reinforcement approach (CRA) is an example of a broad-based, treatment approach that has contingency management as a central theme. Hunt and Azrin (1973) have developed a multidimensional treatment approach in which social, vocational, recreational, and familial reinforcers are contingent upon continuing sobriety. In this broad-spectrum treatment, patients typically receive disulfiram (Antabuse), social skills training, drink refusal skills training, behavioral marital therapy, job training, and social and recreational counseling when appropriate. The treatment focuses on making these various reinforcers (social, familial, vocational, recreational, etc.) contingent upon a patient's continuing sobriety. CRA addresses many lifestyle problem areas related to alcohol abuse, including unemployment, marital problems, isolation, use of leisure time, and social support. The primary goal of CRA is to make the patient's new, sober lifestyle more rewarding than using substances.

The controlled literature on CRA has been impressive. Studies have consistently shown CRA to be effective in reducing alcohol use and in improving patients' general adjustment (Institute of Medicine, 1990; Miller & Hester, 1986). (For a more detailed description of CRA, see Sissin & Azrin, 1989.)

SPECIFIC ISSUES IN IMPLEMENTING SUBSTANCE ABUSE TREATMENT FROM A BEHAVIORAL PERSPECTIVE

Sequencing of Technique Use

Brownell, Marlatt, Lichtenstein, and Wilson (1986) point out that recovery from substance abuse disorders generally can be viewed as following three phases where certain techniques are more appropriate during certain phases.

The first phase of treatment (or any self-change for that matter) is having patients develop a sense of commitment and motivation to making changes in their behavior. This area of treatment has been described in detail earlier in the section "Enhancing Motivation to Change."

The second phase of treatment is initiating early behavior changes. This phase can last from 3 to 6 months during substance abuse treatment. This phase is particularly crucial during the first 3 months when roughly 60% of relapses occur (Hunt, Barnett, & Branch, 1971). During this phase of treatment, there are several tasks and techniques that are most appropriate. First, there is a strong emphasis on actions that facilitate abstinence. These actions include setting up situations that support abstinence through an external focus, such as using residential treatment, prescribing medication (to curb cravings or create an aversion to use), and specifying contingencies with interested parties such as spouses, employers, or the legal system. Also, during this phase the treatment techniques used should be those that assist in initial abstinence. For example, the patient and clinician should focus on identifying high-risk situations for patient use and developing specific plans to use certain coping skills to deal with these situations. Such skills include drink/drug refusal skills, managing urges and cravings, understanding seemingly irrelevant decisions, and managing negative thoughts about substance use. (For more detail about specific coping skills training for early stage recovery, see Monti et al., 1989.)

Finally, there are two activities that are fostered in the patient during this phase of treatment. The first is facilitating patient self-awareness. Patients need to be encouraged and congratulated for efforts to become aware of their urges/craving for substance use, automatic thoughts about substance use, affective reactions, and how all these factors relate to placing the patient in high-risk situations to use substances. Prochaska et al., (1992) have written about the importance of self-awareness (or consciousness raising in their transtheoretical model) for patient's in the early stages of change. The second activity that clinicians need to facilitate in patients is behavioral rehearsal. Patients have often lived through many years of responding to high-risk situations by using substances. Having patients simply listen to lectures on refusing drinks or coping with urges will not be a powerful initiator of behavior change. Patients need to think about these skills during the week when filling out homework exercises and practice these skills during treatment sessions and at home. Bandura's (1986) theory of self-efficacy posits that the most powerful methods of changing self-efficacy (and ultimately behavior) are performance based.

The third phase of treatment is the maintenance of behavior changes. Substance-abusing patients can make changes in their substance use behavior relatively easily. However, it is much more difficult to maintain behavior changes over a length of time. This is where Mark Twain's famous declaration about stopping smoking is relevant. He was quoted as saying, "Quitting smoking is easy . . . I've done it a thousand times." This quote makes the point that the maintenance of change is indeed a difficult task. Clinicians can focus on several areas in order to facilitate the maintenance of change. They can have the patient continue to self-monitor, remain aware of high-risk situations, and regularly weigh the advantages and disadvantages of both sobriety and returning to substance use. This is often difficult for the patient, who has gone a length of time without using substances. The patient's level of confidence is high and the patient does not see the need to be as concerned about recovery issues as he/she did early in treatment. It can be helpful to suggest that patients look at this review process as a preventive exercise, much as their family doctor might do in an annual checkup. The review could be simply completing the decisional balance exercise to get a current view of the pros and cons of their sobriety as well as the pros and cons of a return to substance use.

Another area of focus for maintaining change is to help patients develop and maintain a social support group that is supportive of their sobriety. For many this will include members of a 12-Step program such as Alcoholics Anonymous or Narcotics Anonymous. Other patients who do not utilize 12-Step self-help programs may also develop support networks through their church or synagogue, family members, or other recovery based self-help groups (such as Rational Recovery). The crucial factor in these support groups is that they are supportive of the patient's sobriety and that the support group members are non-substance users (Gordon & Zrull, 1991).

In the maintenance stage there are two general strategies that occur during treatment. One is gradual fading of the external controls that were highlighted in the early recovery stage. Medications are reduced and discontinued, there is less reliance on collaterals, and the locus of control for making changes is emphasized to be the patient. Second, the patient is exposed to progressively more risky and varied drinking/drug situations and encouraged to develop and use alternative coping strategies in these situations. The purpose is to continue to maintain self-efficacy and to enhance the generalizability of the skills.

How Problems Are Addressed and in What Order

When chronic substance abuse patients appear for treatment they often present with a multitude of problems, one of which is their substance use. Often the reason for seeking treatment is a recent crisis and the patient's main concern is resolving the immediate problem, such as an alcohol-dependent husband entering treatment because his wife is talking about getting a divorce. The alcoholic husband may insist that he needs to get into treatment for his "marital problems" and may try to direct the therapy toward focusing on marital communication treatment. Substance abuse patients come into treatment with a variety of concomitant problems, often a consequence of the substance use itself. Extreme stress related to unemployment, financial problems, relationship difficulties, pending legal action, or severe psychiatric symptomology is often found in patients who present for substance abuse treatment. Individuals feel depressed, guilty, and ashamed as they recount the toll their substance use has taken on themselves and others. In addition, some patients have preexisting psychiatric conditions that become prominent as the patient begins abstaining from alcohol and/or drugs. Community studies report between 21% and 39% of individuals who had a substance abuse disorder also met criteria for another diagnosis under the third edition of the *Diagnostic and Statistical Manual of Mental Disorders* (American Psychiatric Association, 1980) (Myers et al., 1984; Regier et al., 1990). In dually diagnosed patients, severe anxiety, depression, or psychotic symptomology may appear and become a significant aspect of treatment.

For the clinician, it is important that the initial focus of treatment is addressing patients' substance use and assisting patients in making changes in their substance use. Without making changes in their substance use, patients cannot begin to make headway in resolving other problems. A slogan from the 12-Step programs is relevant as a patient must remember, "first things first." However, it may be difficult for the clinician to focus on the problem of substance use. There are some patients who come into outpatient sessions each week with a personal crisis that is begging for immediate attention. Other times, patients insist on dealing with relationship problems or feelings of anxiety rather than addressing substance use. It is difficult for a caring clinician not to become engaged with a patient who begins to painfully talk about the abuse/trauma that he/she suffered.

How can a clinician balance the fine line between remaining focused on substance abuse issues and recovery tasks and tending to significant issues that the patient brings into treatment? There are several strategies the clinician can employ:

1. Initially, when briefing patients about what to expect in treatment, make it clear that the first order of business in treatment is to address their substance use. Reminding patients of the association between their substance use and the consequences will be useful in emphasizing the importance of dealing with the substance use first.

2. The clinician can structure the session into "minisessions," where the first third of the session is reserved for patients to talk about their nonsubstance life concerns and the next two thirds of the session are used to focus on initiating and maintaining changes in their substance use. The advantage in this strategy is that patients do have some time to ventilate and vocalize problems that are important to them. Additionally, the clinician may have access to more material that can be used in the substance-focused part of the session. However, a disadvantage of breaking up the session is that the transition between these parts of the session may be incongruous and it relies on the clinician to have good assertiveness skills.

3. Finally, when the clinician finds him/herself in sessions where the treatment is constantly focusing on non-substance-use material this should be a signal to pause and evaluate the treatment. It may be that avoiding discussions and tasks related to the patient's substance use could be part of the patient's ambivalence about changing his/her substance use behavior and reflective of being in a contemplation stage of change. In such cases it is useful then to go back to the tasks in the motivational stage of treatment and work with patients in weighing out the pros and cons of changing their substance use.

How Denial, Resistance, and Lack of Progress Are Addressed

The concept of denial has long been the cornerstone of traditional chemical dependency treatment. Denial has been said to be the "cardinal and integral feature of chemical dependency and the fatal aspect of alcoholism and other drug dependencies" (Hazelden, 1975, p. 9). Additionally, a substance abuser's lack of "motivation" has been used to explain failure to enter, continue in, comply with, and succeed in treatment. Although historically, traditional treatment suggested that confrontation of denial was the essential first step in resolving substance abuse problems, this treatment method has fallen out of favor. Recent literature also suggests that the confrontational approach to treating addictions has not been therapeutic (Lieberman et al., 1973; MacDonough, 1976; Miller et al., 1993).

From a behavioral perspective, "denial" or "resistance" is not seen as a patient trait (Miller, 1985) but rather redefined to reflect a condition in which the patient–therapist definition of the problem is simply not congruent. Once the patient and clinician have differing definitions of the problem, progress in treatment will stall. Thus, rather than defining this problem as some kind of adjective that describes an alleged patient characteristic, it is more accurate to define it as a problem in the therapeutic process (i.e., a "lack of progress"). This description is also more likely to engage the patient to collaborate in resolving the differences in problem definition rather than arguing with the patient to define the problem from the clinician's view.

In traditional treatment, many times there is a struggle to have patients admit their powerlessness over alcohol and to admit to being an alcoholic and/or addict. From the behavioral perspective it is not important for the patient to accept the label or diagnosis of alcoholic/addict. There is still too much stigma associated with these terms (Cunningham, Sobell, & Chow, 1993) and labeling a patient is not seen as particularly helpful in treatment. What behavioral clinicians focus on is the functional role that substance use plays in the patient's life and what problems and/or concerns the patient has experienced due to his/her substance use. By taking this perspective the therapist and patient do not have to struggle over a label and can get to work on agreeing on problem areas for treatment.

In working with patients from the behavioral perspective there are two things to keep in mind regarding patient–clinician agreement on treatment goals. First, it is important to routinely assess patients and their commitment in terms of their original treatment goal. We cannot assume that once a decision is made it is static and etched in stone. It is hoped, in developing the therapeutic relationship and outlining the expectations in treatment, that the clinician has stressed the importance of having patients bring up any thoughts or considerations regarding changes they want to make in their treatment goals. Often patients will not initiate a discussion about changing their treatment goals, especially if they have been having urges or thoughts about returning to drinking. Thus the clinician needs to routinely ask how the patient is feeling about his/her goal choice and whether the patient has entertained any thoughts about returning to controlled drinking. Also, when progress is not forthcoming during treatment, the clinician should pause and reassess the treatment plan. An open, objective discussion about the patient's treatment goals is needed.

How Lapses/Relapses Are Viewed and Used in Treatment

Addiction is characterized by chronic episodes of relapse that Prochaska et al. (1992) describe as being "the rule rather than the exception" (p. 1104). According to Hunt et al. (1971), approximately 60% of patients who completed treatment for smoking, alcohol, and heroin addiction relapsed within the first 90 days. The frequency of relapse has been estimated to be between 70% and 74% within the first year (Hunt et al., 1971; Miller & Hester, 1980). Because relapse is so prevalent, Prochaska et al. (1992) discuss how they have modified their stages-of-change model to include relapse as a stage of change. Their model has become like a spiral where individuals move forward through the stages, have a relapse, and then return to the earlier stages of change, though patients do not start from "square one" but rather have more information and experience than they had in a previous change attempt.

In traditional treatment, there has been a tendency to view relapse as "a dirty word . . . as if the very mention of the word will increase the likelihood of its occurrence" (Chiauzzi, 1991, p. 1). Patients who relapse tend to feel embarrassed, ashamed, and depressed about failing. Counselors' subjective associations to relapse have included descriptions such as "treatment failure," "return to illness," "failure and guilt," and "breakdown" (Marlatt & Gordon, 1985, p. 31).

From a behavioral perspective, clinicians should address the potential of relapse in the early stages of treatment. The clinician should initially discuss with the patient the distinction between a lapse and a relapse. Marlatt and Gordon (1985) define a relapse as a return to a previous state which is characterized by the perception of loss of control. However, a lapse is viewed as an event or situation in which one can take corrective action and not lose control. The cognitive and affective reactions to the first slip or lapse after a period of abstinence exert a significant influence that may determine whether or not the lapse is followed by a complete return to the former level of substance use. The clinician should highlight the differences between a lapse and a relapse and emphasize that a relapse does not need to happen after a lapse. This may be somewhat challenging for patients who have utilized 12-Step programs, where the belief that "one drink, a drunk" (where one drink will inevitably lead to a return of out-of-control drinking) has been emphasized as a characterization of the disease of addiction. To suggest that one can control that one drink (or drinking/drug use episode) and return to recovery may be interpreted by the patient as, "Hey look, I can control my drinking/drug use." It becomes less of a departure from traditional 12-Step philosophy to bridge these seemingly disparate views by emphasizing the commonalities. If one experiences a slip, 12-Step supporters would emphasize, "don't drink and go to meetings," where individuals would be able to talk about their slip and learn from it. Similarly, from the behavioral perspective, though taking a more empowering perspective (one drink is *not* equated to an immediate return to old substance use patterns), patients are encouraged to stop, look at the lapse, and use it to learn how to improve their sobriety.

The clinician should advise the patient that lapses or "slips" are part of the recovery process for many individuals and if one were to occur, the patient should have an "emergency plan" ready to implement that would keep the lapse from becoming a full-blown relapse. The clinician should convey to the patient that the lapse can be used as a learning experience by reviewing what happened, identifying where the patient may have been caught off guard, and reexamining the patient's decision to change.

The advantage of this open discussion of lapses and relapses is that it provides an honest appraisal of what the patient might expect. Patients can expect that if they slip, all is not lost and they can come into treatment and use the slip as a way of learning more about themselves and the plans they have to stay sober. Historically, relapse has been viewed as a "dirty" word and both patients and clinicians colluded in not talking about it. When lapses/relapses are not talked about in the early stages of treatment, they come across as forbidden material. Thus, if a patient slips, the internal sense of disappointment in him/herself as well as his/her embarrassment and shame make it extremely difficult to come into treatment and use the slip effectively.

How to Integrate Other Treatment Supports
Such as Self-Help Groups and Medication

Utilization of other treatment supports can be a valuable adjunct to a behaviorally oriented substance abuse treatment. Self-help groups as another form of support in treatment are valuable tools to add to the patient's recovery armamentarium. Although there has been little empirical support for the efficacy of self-help groups, clinically we know that participation in self-help groups can be extremely helpful for many patients. Research in the area of social support and recovery also suggests that individuals who are involved with a nonusing support network have better treatment outcomes (Gordon & Zrull, 1991).

Self-help groups have been a prominent part of the substance abuse treatment field for many years. Twelve-Step groups such as Alcoholics Anonymous and Narcotics Anonymous have been the cornerstone of traditional treatment and are well-known to most counselors in the substance abuse treatment field. The development of alternative self-help groups has grown a great deal in the recent past. The emergence of Rational Recovery in the past decade offers a self-help alternative that is theoretically more compatible with the behavioral/social learning model. (For a more detailed description of Rational Recovery, see Trimpey, 1989; Tate, 1993. See also McCrady & Delaney, in press, for an excellent, comprehensive chapter reviewing self-help groups in substance abuse treatment.)

The use of medication in substance abuse treatment has often been a part of the treatment for patients with a concurrent psychiatric disorder. As noted earlier, there is a large overlap between psychiatric disorders and psychoactive substance use disorders. The use of psychotropic medications will be appropriate in many cases in order to effectively treat the psychiatric disorder. Because symptoms resulting from the chronic use of substances often mimic psychiatric symptoms (such as depression, anxiety, and paranoia) it is important to conduct a thorough assessment of the patient's psychiatric history and allow a long enough period of abstinence to determine whether the psychiatric symptoms resolve as a function of the patient's sobriety. There will be instances when patients have a preexisting psychiatric condition that has been exacerbated by their substance use, and it will likely remain even in recovery. Referral to a psychiatrist who has experience treating patients with addictions would be ideal. Those patients who also participate in 12-Step recovery meetings may feel uncomfortable in taking medication as they might believe they are not totally drug-free. However, today most 12-Step groups accept the need for some individuals to be taking medications for psychiatric conditions. In fact, Alcoholics Anonymous World Services has published a pamphlet specifically regarding the use of medications and recovery (Alcoholic Anonymous, 1984).

SUMMARY

Of the many treatment approaches reviewed, those that have the most empirical support are behaviorally based (Miller & Hester, 1986). The behavioral model with emphasis on assessment, evaluation, and treatment matching lends itself well to studies of effectiveness. Given the current health care atmosphere, these elements are quite important. The behavioral approach offers patients more options and flexibility in treatment. However, in treating substance use disorders from a behavioral perspective, one of its strengths is also one of its biggest drawbacks. By individualizing treatment, it is difficult to study "treatment" because the "package" will vary from individual to individual. In the future, there needs to be continued efforts to focus research attention on the active elements in successful behavioral treatment, particularly taking into account matching patient and treatment variables. There is a need to foster translation, dissemination, and training in implementation of behavioral approaches to front-line substance abuse counselors. Finally, the future of behavioral treatment is likely to include more focus on harm reduction (Marlatt et al., 1993) and providing brief interventions with populations of people that have less severe substance use problems.

CASE ILLUSTRATION

The following is a case example using cognitive-behavioral treatment techniques in the treatment of alcohol dependence. Certain information and aspects of the case were altered in order to protect the privacy of the patient and to highlight various aspects of the treatment.

Background and History

Jim is a 35-year-old married white male who was referred to outpatient treatment at the recommendation of his attorney after an arrest for his second DWI. Jim lives with his wife Sharon in a rented apartment. He and Sharon have been married for 8 years and have two daughters, 6 and 4 years of age. Jim is a high school graduate and is employed full time as a project manager for a local construction company.

Assessment Procedure

In addition to the clinical interview, Jim completed the Inventory of Drinking Situations–100 (Annis, 1982) and the University of Rhode Island Change Assessment Scale (DiClemente & Hughes, 1990). The Inventory of Drinking Situations (IDS) is a 100-item questionnaire that asks about the likelihood that a patient will drink heavily in a variety of situations. Scores are provided for eight subscales and include the following: drinking as a response to unpleasant emotions, physical discomfort, pleasant emotions, testing personal control, urges to drink, conflict with others, social pressure to drink, and pleasant times with others. The University of Rhode Island Change Assessment Scale (URICA) is a 32-item questionnaire that asks patients about their intentions to make changes regarding a problem behavior. A patient's scores are converted to a change profile that shows an individual's score on each of the stages of change according to Prochaska and DiClemente's model. The stages include precontemplation, contemplation, action, and maintenance.

Past Alcohol and Drug Use History

When Jim was 8 years old he first tasted alcohol after his father gave him a sip of wine during a family gathering. At age 16, during his junior year in high school, Jim began to drink regularly. He reported drinking three to five times per month, usually after school sporting events or social activities. He described drinking "just beer" and would typically have three or four cans. He first became intoxicated, at age 16, when he drank four beers and "many" shots of whiskey before getting sick and passing out. Since graduating from high school, Jim has been drinking consistently to the present. Over the past 12 years, Jim stated that he has been drinking daily, typically having four beers after work. During the weekends, Jim described drinking 6 to 10 beers and "shots" of whiskey when he would go to the bar with friends. During the last 2 years, Jim stated that he has "cut down" on his drinking, typically having four beers per day and drinking to excess (six beers and two shots of whiskey) roughly once a month. The longest period Jim reported being abstinent from alcohol was for 1 month after his first arrest for DWI at age 25.

Jim reported a history of marijuana and cocaine use. During his senior year of high school, Jim tried marijuana while at a party and shared a joint with a friend. He used marijuana episodically during the remainder of high school, but only when someone provided it at a party. Since high school, Jim smoked marijuana irregularly and the last time he used was a year before his marriage to Sharon. He strongly insisted that he has never had a problem with marijuana and rather proudly reported that he never purchased any for himself.

Jim first used cocaine when he was a senior in high school. He was at a party where someone brought out cocaine and he snorted part of a "line." Jim described the experience as generally "uncomfortable" and the cocaine not really "doing anything for me." He has not used cocaine since that time.

Initial Phase of Treatment

During these sessions, the primary focus of treatment was to develop a therapeutic relationship, conduct a thorough assessment of Jim's substance use, and enhance his motivation to change.

Developing a Therapeutic Relationship

Jim expected to be told to stop drinking and seemed surprised when I discussed the expectations for the current treatment. I advised him that we would spend a good deal of time looking at his drinking from many different perspectives. My goal for our working together was to have open discussions about his drinking, and I emphasized that the ultimate decision about his drinking would be left up to him. We would work together to look at all facets of his drinking critically so that he could make an informed choice about making any changes.

Functional Analysis

Initially, Jim seemed guarded and vague about his alcohol use and subsequent problems. However, he responded favorably to a nonjudgmental stance about his drinking and the emphasis that I was interested in helping him. As the early sessions progressed, Jim provided more detailed information about his substance use and resulting consequences. Over the course of the first four sessions, using both the IDS and URICA and clinical interviews, Jim reported the following consequences or concerns about his drinking:

- Recent loss of driver's license due to second DWI occurring 2 months prior to his entry into treatment.
- First DWI arrest occurred when he was 25 years old.
- Relationship problems due to his alcohol use. He noted that the current stressors with his wife and children are related to his drinking. Jim also conceded that the break-up with his girlfriend, 9 years ago, was also partially due to his use of alcohol.
- Physical concerns regarding his drinking, which included hangovers, nausea, increased tolerance, and unclear thinking.
- Concerns about the financial impact of his drinking, notably the legal costs for his DWI, missing work, and the actual cost of buying alcohol.
- Personal concerns about having blackouts, changes in his "personality," and periodic loss-of-control drinking and ultimately feeling guilty and ashamed of himself.

Commitment and Motivation to Change

In listening to Jim's perception of his drinking and noting his responses on the URICA, it appeared that Jim was in the contemplation stage of change. He strongly agreed with the following URICA statements regarding his drinking "problem": I may be part of the problem, but I don't really think I am. I have worries but so does the next guy. Why spend time thinking about them? Maybe this place will be able to help me. I've been thinking that I might want to change something about myself. Jim's endorsement of these items reflect his ambivalence about viewing his drinking as a problem that needs changing.

At this point in treatment, we worked together on completing a decisional balance worksheet using a modified version of the Carlson model. The goal of this exercise was to identify the advantages and disadvantages of changing his drinking habits as well as the pros and cons of not changing. Jim's decisional balance worksheet is provided in Figure 8.1.

In completing the decisional balance worksheet, I emphasized that in order to make an informed choice about his drinking, it was important to look at all facets of the decision critically. Also, I spent some time getting an idea from Jim about his current life goals and having him describe his view of himself as a person. This information would be used in highlighting discrepancies between the characteristics he used in defining an ideal self and the characteristics defining himself as a drinker. Jim reported that he had some interest in going back to school and developing a closer relationship with his wife and children. He described himself as "hard working, caring, and fun-loving" and was proud of his abilities in working with his hands.

As noted in Figure 8.1, Jim reported a number of disadvantages in continuing to drink. In reviewing this list of drawbacks to drinking, Jim reported that he was most concerned about the impact his drinking was having upon his daughters, the financial burdens he was experiencing, and the fact that his health had been affected.

In going over the advantages of his drinking, Jim had some difficulty acknowledging any "good" things about his drinking. In fact, he quickly responded, "what, do you think I'm nuts, there is nothing good about my drinking." However, with some prompting, Jim reported the following advantages of drinking: He enjoyed the camaraderie with friends and coworkers, he felt relaxed and entitled to have a "couple beers," a few drinks helped him fall asleep after a stressful day, and drinking served to help Jim "forget about it all" when having problems at home or work.

Figure 8.1 also has Jim's list of advantages and disadvantages of sobriety. Jim stated that an advantage of sobriety would be that he would

PROS AND CONS OF ABSTINENCE AND EARLY RECOVERY

Pros of abstinence	Cons of abstinence	Coping with the difficulties of abstinence and early recovery
1. Feel better physically 2. Improved relationship with Sharon 3. Improved relationship with daughters 4. Having more money 5. Being less nervous, fearful, and guilty 6. Improve self—e.g., going back to school	1. Nervous and uncomfortable in social situations 2. Coworkers giving me a hard time 3. Loss of friends 4. Life is mundane, unrewarding 5. Face reality (stress, insomnia, arguments, anger) 6. Change is work	1. Stress management, relaxation exercises 2. Assertiveness training, drink refusal skills 3. Participation in self-help groups 4. Cognitive restructuring, pleasant activities schedule 5. Assertiveness, stress management, communication skills training 6. Cognitive restructuring

PROS AND CONS OF CONTINUED ALCOHOL AND/OR DRUG USE

Disadvantages of using alcohol/drugs	Advantages of using alcohol/drugs	Achieving the same benefits without using alcohol/drugs
1. Financial burden and legal problems 2. Problems with wife—risk divorce 3. Health and physical problems 4. Alienating daughters 5. Feeling lousy about self 6. Stuck in a "rut" regarding work	1. Comaraderie with coworkers 2. Relaxed and comfortable in social situations 3. Celebrating a job well done 4. Avoid uncomfortable feelings like anger, hurt 5. Help fall asleep when stressed	1. Development of social network of nondrinking people 2. Stress management, relaxation training, drink refusal skills 3. Cognitive restructuring, rewarding nondrinking activities 4. Cognitive restructuring, Communication skills training 5. Relaxation training

FIGURE 8.1. Jim's decisional balance worksheet.

feel better physically, not risk further legal or health problems, and consequently, would feel less nervous, fearful and guilty. Also, Jim saw that by not drinking he would save money, his family life would improve significantly, and they would be "one big happy family."

Jim reported that a disadvantage of sobriety would be his initial discomfort at work by not drinking with his coworkers, as he expected certain individuals would give him a hard time about not drinking. Jim also feared he would lose friends and his life would become mundane and boring if he stopped drinking. Further, he expected significant discomfort if he were not able to drink to help himself with stress and insomnia. Finally, Jim saw that not drinking was going to be a fair amount of work and would require that he spend time and energy on making many changes in his life.

Jim reported that going over the decisional balance exercise was a sobering (he initially did not realize the pun) experience. At this time, he indicated that his intention was to stop drinking for an extended period, but he was not sure whether he would pursue a goal of lifelong abstinence.

Initial Behavior Change

The next phase of treatment included making initial behavior changes to support Jim's goal of abstinence. We needed to determine what situations would be "high risk" for Jim to return to drinking. In addition to the decisional balance worksheet, Jim's responses to the IDS were helpful in determining his unique high-risk situations. Jim's IDS profile is provided in Figure 8.2. After going over the IDS and clarifying several situations, it was determined that Jim tended to drink more heavily in situations that reflected social pressure to drink, in response to feelings of pleasant emotions, and in response to conflicts with others.

During the bulk of the sessions in this phase of treatment, Jim and I focused on developing coping skills that would assist Jim in abstaining from drinking. On the decisional balance worksheet, in the portion dealing with the advantages of drinking, we completed a section that identified specific strategies to achieve the same benefit but without drinking. Additionally, we recognized that the disadvantages of sobriety were relevant and focused on developing strategies to cope with these drawbacks as well. These portions of the decisional balance worksheet are also included Figure 8.1.

Use of Specific Skills to Cope with High-Risk Situations

Due to space limits, I will describe the strategies developed for one of Jim's three high-risk situations: social pressure to drink.

Jim reported drinking heavily when friends or coworkers asked him to join them for drinks after work. Because Jim was working every day, it was important to first develop strategies for him to use at work. Jim described a typical working day and how he would get invited to have a few drinks with coworkers at the end of the day. We discussed the possible reactions his coworkers might have if he were to decline having a drink with them. We also discussed the possibility of Jim's socializing with his coworkers after work but drinking soda instead of alcohol, as well as the option of Jim's going home right after work and not staying with his coworkers. Jim decided that it would be too tempting to stay after work and drink soda while others were drinking beer. We role-played different ways he would refuse a coworker's request to stay after work and drink. Initially, Jim felt he could not tell his coworkers that he was no longer drinking because he had an alcohol problem. He wanted to tell his coworkers that he was not staying after work because he had errands to run. We discussed how it was not ideal for Jim to make excuses about not drinking because he would continue to get invitations to drink from his coworkers as they would not know he was no longer drinking. However, because Jim would be immediately facing the invitations to drink, it was decided to "use whatever works" initially and work on developing the skills to become more direct with his coworkers about his intention to

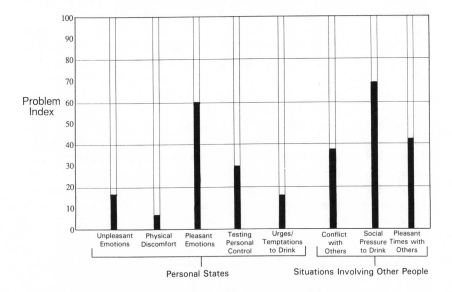

FIGURE 8.2. Jim's IDS profile.

abstain from drinking. Over the course of several sessions, Jim was successful in avoiding invitations to remain after work to drink. We began to discuss various ways he could tell his coworkers about his decision not to drink and role-played several of the most promising. Jim was able to come up with the strategy to tell a couple of his coworkers (who were better friends) that he was no longer drinking. He decided to tell these friends that he really felt drinking was getting in the way of his plans for the future and that he was feeling great physically since he stopped drinking. He also planned to ask for his friends' support if other coworkers started to give him a hard time about not drinking. In fact, Jim reported that there was another coworker who did not drink and we discussed how Jim might begin to spend time after work with this man in pursuing nondrinking, pleasurable activities. In addition to specific drink refusal skills, I had Jim identify and monitor any urges or cravings for drinking after work. Once Jim began to recognize these urges, he learned how to interrupt these urges by distracting himself, leaving the situation, or simply waiting it out. Jim was quite successful in developing alternative, nondrinking activities to fulfill his need for social contact and relief from a hard day at work.

The preceding description of the treatment with Jim represented roughly 14 sessions and occurred over approximately 5 months. Jim utilized this phase of treatment effectively. He was consistent in his attendance, he generally completed homework assignments, and he was an active participant in the sessions. Jim had less success with expanding his social support network and particularly becoming involved in self-help meetings. He tried one Rational Recovery meeting but said that it was too difficult to get to the meeting as it was some distance from his home. Jim also attended two or three Alcoholics Anonymous meetings but had difficulty with identifying himself as an "alcoholic." He said that it sounded like such a condescending and judgmental term.

Coping with a Lapse

Over a 2-month period, approximately 5 months into treatment, Jim called to cancel three or four treatment sessions due to illness and overtime at work. In a phone conversation with Jim attempting to reschedule the latest canceled appointment, I asked Jim how he was doing and if he was having any difficulties remaining sober. Jim's response was vague, but he eventually indicated that he had been drinking over the last 2 weeks. He said that drinking was not as much fun as he expected and predictably Sharon was extremely angry with him. Further, Jim described that he felt guilty and ashamed with himself.

In discussing Jim's lapse, it became apparent that he became extremely busy and focused on work, which he described as "burning the candle at both ends." Sharon was generally happy with his sobriety, but they continued to have periodic arguments that Jim described as "shit from the past." Often, when Jim would work late Sharon would question him relentlessly about what he was doing and who he was with. Jim felt he was doing well by not hanging around with his coworkers, but he spoke of feeling "lonely and alone." When Sharon questioned Jim or was suspicious of his late hours, he became angry and resentful. His automatic thoughts were quite "hot" and included self-statements such as: "What's her problem, why doesn't she trust me?" "All this work I've done to get sober and she can't appreciate my efforts," and "I might as well be drinking for all the support I get from someone so ungrateful." Shortly after an intense augment, Jim said he went to a local bar and ended up getting drunk.

In response to Jim's relapse, Jim and I developed a treatment plan that included the following: (1) periodic couple sessions with Sharon to focus more directly on communication skills and being able to talk about expectations and anger from the past, (2) renewing Jim's commitment to an abstinence goal and focusing on daily self-monitoring of automatic thoughts around expectations for himself and Sharon, and (3) suggesting more directly that Jim begin to develop a support group of recovering peers, through either Rational Recovery or Alcoholics Anonymous.

Maintenance and Termination Phase

The final stage of treatment with Jim focused on reestablishing his sobriety and maintaining general lifestyle changes and new social supports. Jim was able to become consistently involved in Alcoholics Anonymous meetings, although we spent a number of sessions challenging his cognitions about the label "alcoholic." Once Jim was able to become involved in Alcoholics Anonymous he developed several friendships that he was able to rely on during challenging times. Another important aspect of this phase was Jim and Sharon's work toward openly communicating with one another. We continued to have periodic couple sessions that focused on giving Jim and Sharon long-term assignments around rebuilding trust and expressing anger. Approximately 4 months after his lapse, Jim asked about how treatment would end. He indicated that he felt he had benefited a good deal from treatment but was ready to "strike out on his own." I suggested that we plan to meet another three or four times over a 3-month period to focus on reviewing our treatment and solidifying a long-term recovery plan. Jim agreed to this plan; however, after our first session of the termination period, he canceled the next appointment. Jim eventually ended treatment over the phone and during that interaction I congratulated him for his progress and reinforced his plans for long-term recovery. Jim told me he still thinks about our first sessions when we completed the decisional balance worksheet and what a powerful impact it had on him. Jim said he planned to continue to keep his worksheet in his wallet so that he could refer to it regularly and have it as a reminder.

In summary, Jim worked hard in his treatment and was quite involved in completing assignments and participating in role-play situations. Jim responded well to the collaborative nature of the treatment relationship and the practically oriented focus of the behavioral treatment model. Treatment with Jim was typical in several ways. During treatment, often an individual will experience a lapse or relapse as Jim did. This should not be seen as a "failure" but as an opportunity to learn and develop more effective skills for remaining sober. Also, the manner which Jim ended treatment was not unusual. A planned, final session to review treatment and terminate is often the exception rather than the rule. Clinicians need to be flexible in ending with patients in a variety of mediums, such as termination by phone or mail.

REFERENCES

Alcoholics Anonymous (1984). *The A.A. member: Medications and other drugs.* New York: Alcoholics Anonymous World Services.

Allsop, S., & Saunders, B. (1991). Reinforcing robust resolutions: Motivation in relapse prevention with severely dependent problem drinkers. In W. R. Miller & S. Rollnick, *Motivational interviewing: Preparing people to change addictive behavior* (pp. 236–247). New York: Guilford Press.

American Psychiatric Association. (1980). *Diagnostic and statistical manual of mental disorders* (3rd ed.). Washington, DC: Author.

Annis, H. M. (1982). *Inventory of Drinking Situations.* Toronto: Addiction Research Foundation of Ontario.

Bandura, A. (1986). *Social foundations of thought and action: A social cognitive theory.* Englewoood Cliffs, NJ: Prentice Hall.

Booth, P. G., Dale, B., & Ansari, J. (1984). Problem drinkers' goal choice and treatment outcome: A preliminary report. *Addictive Behaviors, 9,* 357–364.

Brownell, K. D., Marlatt, G. A., Lichtenstein, E., & Wilson, G. T. (1986). Understanding and preventing relapse. *American Psychologist, 41,* 765–782.

Cahalan, D. (1987). *Understanding America's drinking problem: How to combat the hazards of alcohol.* San Francisco: Jossey-Bass.

Cannon, D. S., Baker, T. B., & Wehl, C. K. (1981). Emetic and electric shock alcohol aversion therapy: Assessment of conditioning. *Journal of Consulting and Clinical Psychology, 49,* 360–368.

Carey, K. B., & Maisto, S. A. (1985). A review of the use of self-control techniques in the treatment of alcohol abuse. *Cognitive Therapy and Research, 9,* 235–251.

Carlson, V. B. (1991). Testing a decisional balance worksheet for substance abusers: Factors related to intentions regarding treatment and abstinence (Doctoral dissertation, Rutgers University, 1991). *Dissertation Abstracts International,* 5526B.

Chaney, E. F. (1989). Social skills training. In R. K. Hester & W. R. Miller (Eds.), *Handbook of alcoholism treatment approaches: Effective alternatives* (pp. 206–221). Elmsford, New York: Pergamon Press.

Chaney, E. F., Roszell, D. K., & Cummings, C. (1982). Relapse in opiate addicts: A behavioral analysis. *Addictive Behaviors, 7,* 291–297.

Chiauzzi, E. J. (1991). *Preventing relapse in the addictions: A biopsychosocial approach.* New York: Pergamon Press.

Childress, A., Ehrman, R., McLellan, A. T., & O'Brien, C. (1987). Conditioned craving and arousal in cocaine addiction: A preliminary report. In L. S. Harris (Ed.), *Problems of drug dependence 1987: Proceedings of the 49th annual scientific meeting, committee on problems of drug dependence* (NIDA Monograph 81). Rockville, MD: National Institute on Drug Abuse.

Cox, W. M., Klinger, E., & Blount, J. P. (1991). Alcohol use and goal hierarchie: Systematic motivational counseling for alcoholics. In W. R. Miller & S. Rollnick, *Motivational interviewing: Preparing people to change addictive behavior* (pp. 260–271). New York: Guilford Press.

Cunningham, J. A., Sobell, L. C., & Chow, M. C. (1993). What's in a label? The effects of substance types and labels on treatment considerations and stigma. *Journal of Studies on Alcohol, 54,* 693–699.

Davies, D. L. (1962). Normal drinking by recovered alcoholics. *Quarterly Journal of Studies on Alcohol, 23,* 94–104.

DiClemente, C. C., & Hughes, S. O. (1990). Stages of change profiles in outpatient alcoholism treatment. *Journal of Substance Abuse, 2,* 217–235.

Donovan, D. M., & Marlatt, G. A. (Eds.). (1988). *Assessment of addictive behaviors.* New York: Guilford Press.

Foa, E. B., & Kozak, M. S. (1986). Emotional processing of fear: Exposure to corrective information. *Psychological Bulletin, 99,* 20–35.

Foy, D. W., Nunn, B. L., & Rychtarik, R. G. (1984). Broad-spectrum behavioral treatment for chronic alcoholics: Effects of training in controlled drinking skills. *Journal of Consulting and Clinical Psychology, 52,* 218–230.

Gordon, A. J., & Zrull, M. (1991). Social networks and recovery: One year after inpatient treatment. *Journal of Substance Abuse Treatment, 8,* 143–152.

Hazelden. (1975). *Dealing with denial.* Center City, MN: Hazelden Caring Community Services.

Hester, R. K., & Miller, W. R. (Eds.). (1989a). *Handbook of alcoholism treatment approaches: Effective alternatives.* Elmsford, NY: Pergamon Press.

Hester, R. K., & Miller, W. R. (1989b). Self-control training. In R. K. Hester & W. R. Miller (Eds.), *Handbook of alcoholism treatment approaches: Effective alternatives* (pp. 141–149). Elmsford, NY: Pergamon Press.

Hunt, G. L., & Azrin, N. H. (1973). A community-reinforcement approach to alcoholism. *Behaviour Research and Therapy, 11,* 91–104.

Hunt, W. A., Barnett, L. W., & Branch, L. G. (1971). Relapse rates in addictions programs. *Journal of Clinical Psychology, 27,* 455–456.

Institute of Medicine. (1990). *Broadening the base of treatment for alcohol problems.* Washington, DC: National Academy Press.

Janis, I. L., & Mann, L. (1977). *Decision-making: A psychological analysis of conflict, choice, and commitment.* New York: Free Press.

Johnson, V. E. (1986). *Intervention: How to help someone who doesn't want help.* Minneapolis, MN: Johnson Institute.

Kadden, R., Carroll, K., Donovan, D., Cooney, N., Monti, P., Abrams, D., Litt, M., & Hester, R. (1992). *Cognitive-behavioral coping skills therapy manual: A clinical research guide for therapists treating individuals with alcohol abuse and dependence.* (NIAAA Project MATCH Monograph series, Vol. 3, DHHS Publication No. ADM 92–1895). Rockville, MD: National Institute on Alcohol Abuse and Alcoholism.

Lawson, D. M., & Boudin, H. M. (1992). Alcohol and drug abuse. In M. Hersen & A. S. Bellack (Eds.), *Handbook of clinical behavior therapy with adults* (pp. 293–318). New York: Plenum Press.

Lieberman, M. A., Yalom, I. D., & Miles, M. B. (1973). *Encounter groups: First facts.* New York: Basic Books.

MacDonough, T. S. (1976). Evaluation of the effectiveness of intensive confrontation in changing the behavior of alcohol and drug abusers. *Behavior Therapy, 7,* 408–409.

Marlatt, G. A., & Gordon, J. R. (Eds.). (1985). *Relapse prevention: Maintenance strategies in the treatment of addictive behaviors.* New York: Guilford Press.

Marlatt, G. A., Larimar, M. E., Baer, J. S., & Quigley, L. A. (1993). Harm reduction for alcohol problems: Moving beyond the controlled drinking controversy. *Behavior Therapy, 24,* 461–504.

McCabe, R. J. R. (1986). Alcohol-dependent individuals sixteen years on. *Alcohol and Alcoholism, 21,* 85–91.

McCrady, B. S. (1993). Alcoholism. In D. H. Barlow (Ed.), *Clinical handbook of psychological disorders: A step-by-step treatment manual* (2nd ed., pp. 362–395). New York: Guilford Press.

McCrady, B. S., & Delaney, S. (in press). Self-help groups. In R. K. Hester & W. R. Miller (Eds.), *Handbook of alcoholism treatment approaches: Effective alternatives* (pp.160–175). Elmsford, NY: Pergamon Press.

Miller, W. R., & Hester, R. K. (1980). Treating the problem drinker: Modern approaches. In W. R. Miller (Ed.), *The addictive behaviors: Treatment of alcoholism, drug abuse, smoking, and obesity* (pp. 11–141). Elmsford, NY: Pergamon Press.

Miller, W. R., & Hester, R. K. (1986). The effectiveness of alcoholism treatment: What research reveals. In W. R. Miller & N. Heather (Eds.), *Treating* addictive behaviors: Processes of change (pp. 121–174). New York: Plenum Press.

Miller, W. R. (1985). Motivation for treatment: A review with special emphasis on alcoholism. *Psychological Bulletin, 98,* 84–107.

Miller, W. R. (1993). Behavioral treatments for drug problems: Where do we go from here? In L. S. Onken, J. D. Blaine, & J. J. Boren (Eds.), *Behavioral treatment for drug abuse and dependence* (NIDA Research Monograph 137, NIH Publication No. 93–3684, pp. 303–321). Washington, DC: U.S. Government Printing Office.

Miller, W. R., Benefield, R. G., & Tonigan, J. S. (1993). Enhancing motivation for change in problem drinking: A controlled comparision of two therapist styles. *Journal of Consulting and Clinical Psychology, 61,* 455–461.

Miller, W. R., & Caddy, G. R. (1977). Abstinence and controlled drinking in the treatment of problem drinkers. *Journal of Studies on Alcohol, 38,* 896–1003.

Miller, W. R., Leckman, A. L., Delaney, H. D., & Tinkcom, M. (1992). Long-term follow-up of behavioral self-control training. *Journal of Studies on Alcohol, 53,* 249–261.

Miller, W. R., & Rollnick, S. (1991). *Motivational interviewing: Preparing people to change addictive behavior.* New York: Guilford Press.

Monti, P. M., Abrams, D. B., Kadden, R. M., & Cooney, N. L. (1989). *Treating alcohol dependence: A coping skills training guide.* New York: Guilford Press.

Monti, P. M., Rohsenow, D. J., Rubonis, A. V., Niaura, R. S., Sirota, A. D., Colby, S. M., Goddard, R., & Abrams, D. B. (1993). Cue exposure with coping skills treatment for male alcoholics: A preliminary investigation. *Journal of Consulting and Clinical Psychology, 61,* 1011–1019.

Myers, J. K., Weissman, M. M., Tischler, G. L., Holzer, C. E., Leaf, P. J., Orvaschel, H., Anthony, J. C., Boyd, J. H., Burke, J. D., Kramer, M., & Stoltzman, R. (1984). Six-month prevalence of psychiatric disorders in three communities. *Archives of General Psychiatry, 41,* 959–967.

Nathan, P. E., & Niaura, R. S. (1985). Behavioral assessment and treatment of alcoholism. In J. H. Mendelson & N. K. Mello (Eds.), *The diagnosis and treatment of alcoholism* (pp. 391–45). New York: McGraw-Hill.

Nordstrom, G., & Berglund, M. (1987). A prospective study of successful long-term adjustment in alcoholic dependence: Social drinking versus abstinence. *Journal of Studies on Alcohol, 48,* 95–103.

Ogborne, A. C. (1987). A note on the characteristics of alcohol abusers with controlled drinking aspirations. *Drug and Alcohol Dependence, 19,* 159–164.

O'Leary, K. D., & Wilson, G. T. (1987). Alcoholism and cigarette smoking. In K. D. O'Leary & G. T. Wilson (Eds.), *Behavior therapy: Application and outcome* (pp. 293–319). Englewood Cliffs, NJ: Prentice Hall.

Orford, J. (1985). *Excessive appetites: A psychological view of addictions.* New York: Wiley.

Orford, J., & Keddie, A. (1986). Abstinence or controlled drinking in clinical practice: A test of the dependence and persuasion hypothesis. *British Journal of Addictions, 81,* 495–504.

Polich, J. M., Armor, D. J., & Braiker, H. B. (1981). *The course of alcoholism: Four years after treatment* (National Institute on Alcohol Abuse and Alcoholism). Santa Monica, CA: Rand Corporation.

Prochaska, J. O., DiClemente, C. C., & Norcross, J. C. (1992). In search of how people change: Applications to addictive behaviors. *American Psychologist, 47,* 1102–1114.

Regier, D. A., Farmer, M. E., Rae, D. S., Locke, B. Z., Keith, S. J., Judd, L. L., & Goodwin, F. K. (1990). Comorbidity of mental disorders with alcohol and other drug abuse. *Journal of the American Medical Association, 264,* 2511–2518.

Rimmele, C. T., Miller, W. R., & Dougher, M. J. (1989). Aversion therapies. In R. K. Hester & W. R. Miller (Eds.), *Handbook of alcoholism treatment approaches: Effective alternatives* (pp. 128–140). Elmsford, NY: Pergamon Press.

Rogers, C. R. (1957). The necessary and sufficient conditions for therapeutic personality change. *Journal of Consulting Psychology, 21,* 95–103.

Rosenberg, H. (1993). Prediction of controlled drinking by alcoholics and problem drinkers. *Psychological Bulletin, 113,* 129–139.

Rosenberg, S. D. (1979). *Relaxation training and a differential assessment of alcoholism.* Unpublished doctoral dissertation (University Microfilms No. 8004362), California School of Professional Psychology, San Diego.

Rychtarik, R. G., Foy, D. W., Scott, T., Lokey, L., & Prue, D. M. (1987). Five–six-year follow-up of broad-spectrum behavioral treatment for alcoholism: Effects of training controlled drinking skills. *Journal of Consulting and Clinical Psychology, 55,* 106–108.

Sanchez-Craig, M., Annis, H. M., Bornet, A. R., & MacDonald, K. R. (1984). Random assignment to abstinent and controlled drinking: Evaluation of a cognitive-behavioral program for problem drinkers. *Journal of Consulting and Clinical Psychology, 52,* 390–403.

Saunders, B., Wilkenson, C., & Allsop, S. (1991). Motivational intervention with heroin users attending a methadone clinic. In W. R. Miller & S. Rollnick (Eds.), *Motivational interviewing: Preparing people to change addictive behavior* (pp. 279–292). New York: Guilford Press.

Sissin, R. W., & Azrin, N. H. (1989). The community reinforcement approach. In R. K. Hester & W. R. Miller (Eds.), *Handbook of alcoholism treatment approaches: Effective alternatives* (pp. 242–258). Elmsford, NY: Pergamon Press.

Sobell, M. B., & Sobell, L. C. (1976). Second-year treatment outcome of alcoholics treated by individualized behavior therapy: Results. *Behaviour Research and Therapy, 14,* 195–215.

Sobell, L. C., Toneatto, A., & Sobell, M. B. (1992). Behavior therapy. In R. B. Millman & J. G. Langrod (Eds.), *Substance abuse: A comprehensive textbook* (pp. 479–505). Baltimore: Williams & Wilkins.

Tate, P. (1993). *Alcohol: How to give it up and be glad you did, a sensible approach.* Altamonte, FL: Rational Self-Help Press.

Trimpey, J. (1989). *A revolutionary alternative for overcoming alcohol and other drug dependencies: The small book.* New York: Delacorte Press.

Vaillant, G. E., & Milkofsky, E. S. (1982). Natural history of male alcoholism: IV. Paths to recovery. *Archives of General Psychiatry, 39,* 127–133.

Valle, S. K. (1981). Interpersonal functioning of alcoholism counselors and treatment outcome. *Journal of Studies on Alcohol, 42,* 783–790.

Wilson, G. T. (1987). Chemical aversion conditioning as a treatment for alcoholism: A re-analysis. *Behaviour Research and Therapy, 25,* 503–516.

Wilson, G. T., Rossiter, E., Kleinfield, E., & Lindholm, L. (1986). Cognitive-behavioral treatment of bulimia nervosa: A controlled evaluation. *Behaviour Research and Therapy, 24,* 277–288.

CHAPTER 9

Motivation and Addictive Behaviors: Theoretical Perspectives

BILL SAUNDERS
CELIA WILKINSON
TANIA TOWERS

Motivation has long been viewed as a matter of importance in the addictions field (see, e.g., Lemere, O'Hollaren, & Maxwell, 1958; Mindlin, 1959; Sterne & Pittman, 1965). Indeed, Sterne and Pittman (1965) noted that "Probably in no other condition is so much verbal concern manifested for the patient's motivation to recover as in alcoholism" (p. 41). They further reported from interviews with some 200 "alcoholism" counselors that the overwhelming majority considered that the client's motivation was either "very important" or "essential" for successful treatment.

However, whereas motivation may generally be deemed to be of considerable importance, there is much less agreement as to the actual nature of motivation. As anecdotal support of this statement at a recent addictions counselling course run by one of the authors (B. Saunders) the 50 or so participants were asked to rate motivation in terms of its importance and its influence on the counselling of problem drug users. As with the Sterne and Pittman finding, the consensus was that motivation was "very" or "extremely" important. However, when participants were asked to define motivation, the troublesome nature of the concept became all too apparent. They could not reach agreement. Definitions included "powerful inner drives"; "an individual's acknowledgement that there were problems"; "recognition by the individual of the need for change"; and reference to deep-seated, but nebulous, "unconscious forces."

However, our participants are not alone in being unsure as to the true meaning of the term "motivation." Any reference to standard psychological textbooks will reveal a variety of broad definitions, most of which refer to inner drive states, the operation of incentives, decision-making processes, or some form of intervening process that impels the individual into action. Not surprisingly, Reber (1985) noted that the term "motivation" was "extremely important but definitionally elusive" (p. 454).

Given the elusiveness of the concept of motivation, it is useful to review succinctly the major psychological theories of motivation and then compare and contrast them with the pertinent thinking in the addictions field.

THE PSYCHOLOGY OF MOTIVATION

Drives as Motivation

Historically, motivation has been linked to the notion of drive states. Essentially, motivation is deemed as being akin to physiological needs such as hunger, thirst, or sex. The organism is driven by unsatisfied "within the skin" needs. A definition of motivation based on this conceptualization is that motivation is "an intervening process or an internal state of an organism that impels or drives it to action. In this sense motivation is an energizer of behavior" (Reber, 1987, p. 454).

In terms of addiction behavior, drive theory is clearly consistent with relief drinking and, presumably, the other psychobiological elements of the alcohol dependence syndrome (Edwards & Gross, 1976). Another good example of drive theory is the "genetic predisposition" argument, especially that proposed by Noble (1993) in which a dopamine allele (a gene variant) is suspected of being associated with the development of alcohol dependence. Noble has written:

> It may be hypothesized that individuals carrying the A1 allele, having fewer D2 dopamine receptors in brain reward areas, inherit a deficit in central reward mechanisms. Alcohol (as well as other drugs) by releasing dopamine in the brain activates the fewer receptors of A1 allelic subjects, thus producing a more enhanced euphoria and reward when compared to A2 allelic individuals. The experience of these marked pleasurable feelings in A1 allelic subjects may induce them to further use, and with the development of tolerance increased use of alcohol until dependence on this drug occurs. (1993, pp. 287–288)

Although not everyone is as persuaded as Noble of the reliability and the validity of the "alcoholism is genetic" argument or the role of the D2 allele (e.g., see Goldman 1992; or Saunders & Phillips, 1993), Noble's position is a good example of drive theory.

One key criticism of the drive model is that it centers the locus for behavior almost beyond the will of the individual. Drug use is driven by within-the-skin factors rather than the individual electing consciously to engage in any specific behavior. Historically, drive models were initially challenged by, and then incorporated with, behaviorist or learning models of motivation.

Learning as Motivation

It is indisputable that much of our behavior is based on learning. We learn what we like to do by behaving in certain ways and then experiencing the consequences of our actions. Positive and negative reinforcement (the removal of a noxious stimulus) as well as punishment shape our behaviors, and this includes drug use. Also, as Siegel (1983) has interestingly articulated, drug use, and even dependence and tolerance, can be classically conditioned. As noted earlier, drive theories have usually been seen as complementary to the behavioral perspective in that whereas drives may initiate behavior, it is the consequences of the action that reinforce or repress the occurrence of the behavior in the future.

From the perspective of the addictions arena, the use of aversion techniques in the late 1950s and the advent of behavioral techniques to inculcate controlled drinking behaviors (most particularly the severe electrical techniques adopted by Lovibond & Caddy, 1970) are classic examples of a behaviorist paradigm in operation. However, as time has passed strict aversive and punishment regimens have fallen into disuse. The reasons for this relate to general difficulties with a straight behaviorist view of the world—most particularly the veto on cognition. Humans "think" and as Ellis (1982) has adroitly remarked, what people think about their behaviors, before and after doing them, strongly influences the way they behave. The emergence of cognitive-behavioral approaches to the management of maladaptive human behaviors has been primarily due to the acknowledgment that humans are more purposeful than stimulus and response psychology would allow.

Decision Making as Motivation

West (1989) noted that "the most prevalent common sense view of motivation is that people do things because they perceive them as being better in some way than not doing them" (p. 71).

It is possible from this elegantly simple position to introduce the notion of motivation as a decision-making process. A number of decision-making models exist. In essence, all are connected by the idea that decision making involves the evaluation of alternative courses of actions by assessing the potential positive and negative attributes of each choice (Keeney, 1982).

A classic decision making model is that of subjective expected utility (SEU) (Edwards, 1954). Basically, it is the "what's in it for me" approach to life in that the anticipated personal (subjective) usefulness (utility) of any future course of action is deemed to be of importance in determining an individual's eventual behavior. In the theory, it is postulated that people anticipate both positive and negative consequences of a behavior. The central hypothesis is that when individuals are confronted with two or more options, they will select the one that, relative to the other options, will provide the most benefit and is the least aversive (i.e., has the greatest personal value). The SEU model is an "as if" model. This means that it is assumed that people do not consciously weigh up all the pros and cons related to a decision, but they act "as if" they have.

Based on this model, Sutton (1987) developed an instrument to investigate whether an SEU model could adequately explain individuals' attempts to cease smoking. He surveyed some 960 smokers in the UK and had them complete a comprehensive questionnaire. Incorporated in this questionnaire was a list of 32 potential consequences of ceasing or continuing to smoke on which subjects were required to report their "confidence and intentions, their subjective probabilities and utilities." At 6-month follow-up Sutton (1987) found that the instrument had good predictive validity in that it was able to differentiate between the successful and unsuccessful quitters.

Other investigators have not been able to replicate Sutton's finding. For example, Hopkins (1989) investigated the relationship between SEU and successful outcome with a sample of clinic-attending problem drinkers and found that subjects' SEU ratings for abstinence at intake were not predictive of either eventual success or failure. In fact, she found a simple 4-point Likert scale requiring drinkers to indicate their degree of confidence in modifying their drinking a better predictor of successful outcome.

In attempting to explain her findings, Hopkins (1989) stated: "The concept of motivation as measured by utility theory may be too narrow in its focus to account for maintenance of a commitment to change drinking behavior, even in the short term" (p. 64). In conclusion, she cited Mann (1989) and suggested that there was a need to use more sophisticated instruments that took into account the cognitive and emotional processes that influence individuals' decision making.

West (1989) has also raised this issue. He said that a problem with SEU and indeed many other decision-making models is that they assume that the individual cognitively weighs the pros and cons in a rational, unemotive manner. Indeed, the SEU model has been disarmingly criticized by Schoemaker (1982), who noted that it was "an extreme but tenable attitude to view the SEU model as an interesting theoretical construction which is useless for real-world decision-making" (p. 556).

In effect, individuals do not possess the cognitive ability required to process the extensive amount of information often involved in making a rational calculated decision. Simon (1976) coined the term "bounded-rationalists" to describe human decision makers. Due to individuals" limited "information-processing capacity" the best they can expect to achieve is to make decisions they perceive as "good enough."

There are also other difficulties with the notion of humans as rational actors. As Tversky and Kahneman (1981) have noted, if individuals made decisions in a rational manner, we would expect some "consistency" and "coherence" in their decision outcomes. However, Tversky and Kahneman (1981) reported many instances in which individuals demonstrate neither consistency nor coherence. They noted that in making a decision, all individuals progress through the same process—they are confronted with a number of options from which they can choose and any particular decision will bring about particular results. Tversky and Kahneman (1981) showed, however, that it is possible to "frame" a decisional question in different ways and that the nature of the framing of the decisional question affects the eventual decision. They demonstrated that when two scenarios with identical possible outcomes were presented to subjects, the respondents differed in their stated choices depending on whether the question was framed in terms of possible gains or losses. This difference in the framing of the decisional question caused a significant decisional shift from "risk-aversive" to "risk-taking" styles of decision making, despite the fact that "rationally" the problem was the same.

Given the above considerations, the idea that the perceived value of options drives behavior looks unlikely and suggests that successful applications of utility models may be aberrant. However, with regard to the work of Sutton (1987) it is necessary to acknowledge that he utilized a modified form of SEU, one that also incorporated assessment of respondents' belief in their ability to succeed in quitting. This is known as a value-expectancy paradigm in that it was deemed that both the value of the perceived behavior *and* the individuals' belief in their ability to achieve the goal determine the eventual outcome. Confidence in one's ability to master tasks, or self-efficacy to cite its psychological label, has been demonstrated to be an important psychological component in successful task completion (Bandura, 1977). The proposal, that in order to attempt a task individuals have to value the outcome and expect they can do it, appears quite reasonable.

However, Klar, Nadler, and Malloy (1992) have recently challenged this view. They have argued, from analyses of students' attempts to change various aspects, or "domains," of behavior (e.g., to be more punctual, to stop smoking, to be more sociable, or to be more independent), that it is the desirability of the outcome that drives behavior more than the perceived likelihood of success. They concluded from the reports of some 200 students over 25 domains of behavioral change that individuals "are ready to invest costly resources even when their expectancy to obtain that outcome is meager, or, when their past record with change is poor" (p. 77).

Klar et al. (1992) also cited Cantor and Langston (1989), who wrote:

In many cases, individuals give relatively little independent weight to their chance of success and base their decisions and actions on value related information—primarily, how much they would desire a given outcome. The strength of the cosmetic and fashion industry seems to depend on the fact that people cannot or will not realistically estimate their probability of achieving the sought after goal, but instead base their actions on how much they want the desired outcome. (pp. 217–218)

Similarly, Fitzgibbon and Kischenbaum (1992) have noted that despite relatively modest results, the weight-loss industry continues to prosper. In effect, irrespective of high failure rates, the desirability of weight loss has increased to the point that more and more people are engaging in attempts to diet. This is an interesting argument, and if Klar et al. (1992) are correct, the critical implication for addiction counselors is to consider how they can enhance the desirability or value of abstinence or reduced intake in what may be considered increasingly drug consumerist societies.

Also of potential interest is another of Klar et al.'s (1992) findings: Whereas measures of the desirability of change were related to actual attempts at change, two other psychological variables were also of importance. These were low feelings of self-worth and high levels of personal dissatisfaction with present life. The more emotionally "distressed" individuals were, the more they were likely to engage in action. Emotion as a driving force for behavior is often acknowledged, but coming to grips with the role of emotion in human behavior is less well articulated.

Emotion as Motivation

Clearly, decision making is not an absolutely rational process and in one recent text on the decision sciences (Kleindorfer, Kunreuther, & Schoemaker, 1993) the following is noted:

> The view we adopt in this book . . . is that humans have many limitations and biases and that these provide the key to understanding what they will do in choice situations. To put it simply people do not have immense memory, perceptual abilities or information- processing abilities. . . . Human emotions are also important in understanding decision making. Consider problem acceptance for example. It is a widely held view that a major reason that many choice situations are resolved in favor of doing nothing (the celebrated status quo solution) is fear. Accepting a problem implies accepting responsibility for resolving the resulting choice dilemma. This can be a very threatening experience, especially if the results of the decision-making activity are publicly announced. Other emotional factors, such as love, hate, regret, and disappointment, may also be seen as very important to understanding choice processes in many problem contexts. (p. 11)

So far so good, but in the remaining 400 pages of the book, "emotion" received just one mention and even that was in passing. This is not in any way to demean the text but to highlight that the contribution of emotion to decisional models of motivation is poorly articulated. As an aside, it is probably useful to stress that some cognizance of the "celebrated status quo" solution is of relevance to the addictions field in that the common predilection of clients to persist with drug use despite contraindications is not atypical human behavior. Most of us, when in doubt, dither and continue with the old ways.

One model that has acknowledged an emotive component to decision making is Janis and Mann's (1977) "conflict theory." Mann (1989) stated: "Cognitive processes may predominate in the typical hypothetical choice problem studied in the laboratory, but strong emotions and motives exert a powerful influence on the major life choices faced in the home, the workplace, the clinic" (p. 144).

Janis and Mann (1977) proposed the Decisional Balance Sheet of Incentives as a schema for understanding the cognitive, emotional, and motivational aspects of decision making. Within the decisional balance schema the gains of undertaking a behavior are contrasted with the perceived costs of that action *and* the costs and benefits of not undertaking the behavior. Thus, it is not the total number of gains and losses the decision maker perceives that influences his/her decision but the number of gains and losses in comparison to each other. It is a comparative as opposed to an absolute (e.g., SEU) model and one that Janis and Mann contend is closer to what we do when we make decisions.

Janis and Mann (1977) classified the gains and losses that accrue from any particular decision as being of one of four types:

1. *Utilitarian gains and losses for self.* This encompasses the anticipated instrumental consequences of the decision in relation to personal utilitarian goals.
2. *Utilitarian gains and losses for significant others.* This takes into account the anticipated instrumental consequences of the decision in relation to the goals of other individuals or groups to which the decision maker is linked (e.g., family and friends).
3. *Self approval and disapproval.* This includes such nontangible aspects as moral standards, ego ideals, and components of self-image and are related to the decision maker's self-esteem.
4. *Approval or disapproval by significant others.* The anticipated approval or disapproval in relation to the decision from individuals and groups with whom the decision maker is associated.

According to Janis and Mann (1977), all four considerations should be taken into account when significant decisions are made. However, they believed that there are four defective styles of coping behavior that affect the quality of an individual's decision. These are:

1. *Unconflicted inertia.* Individuals continue to respond as they are currently doing because they have not systematically evaluated other alternatives.
2. *Unconflicted change.* Individuals may perceive an alternative option as being more favorable than their current action and respond to the alternative option without considering all factors related to the change.
3. *Defense avoidance.* Individuals adopt a particular course of action which may be inappropriate and damaging because they do not perceive the alternative options as being more favorable.
4. *Hypervigilance.* An individual believes he/she must respond immediately. Consequently, the decision is made without considering the consequences of this option or other alternatives that may be more appropriate.

In employing one of more of these defective coping styles, individuals are considered likely to produce a defective balance sheet and consequently make inept decisions. This may be of little consequence to an individual when minor day-to-day decisions are being made, but the use of these styles may have far-reaching, negative implications on major decisions, such as the decision to continue or curtail drug use.

Janis and Mann (1977) have argued that to avoid such difficulties a vigilant decision-making style is more appropriate. Vigilance involves reviewing all the possible options and considering the likely consequences of each one. The final decision will be made only after the individual has examined the information gathered and, thereby, can make an informed, "rational" decision.

Janis and Mann (1977) have investigated the usefulness of applying a balance sheet format for making important decisions and, on balance, the results favor the adoption of vigilant procedures in that subjects who used such strategies were much less likely to report "postdecisional distress," irrespective of the eventual outcome of the decision. In essence, having made a careful and considered choice, people are, come what may, more content with the decision they made.

Colten and Janis (1982) examined the impact that completing a decisional balance sheet had on participation at a weight-loss clinic. Eighty women who attended a weight-loss clinic were randomly assigned to one of four possible treatment conditions. Initially, they participated in either a low or high self-disclosure interview. They then explored the pros and cons of the alternative options to following a 1,200-calorie diet or, alternatively, were involved in a general discussion about the 1,200-calorie diet. The investigators reported that after tracking the women's performance over a 1-month period the treatment condition combining high self-disclosure with the balance sheet procedure resulted in superior outcomes, with subjects being more successful in their weight loss and in conforming to the clinic program.

Balance sheet procedures were also incorporated into a successful relapse prevention program (Saunders & Allsop, 1991) in which severely alcohol-dependent clients were randomly allocated to conventional care, a relapse discussion group, or a relapse prevention skills group. The last group remained sober for significantly longer, and even if members relapsed, they relapsed less severely. Thus, utilizing a conflict–decisional framework may be of value in responding to addiction behavior.

Interestingly, work recently reported by McMahon, Jones, and O'Donnell (1994) found that social drinkers mediate their drinking decisions by reference to both positive and negative alcohol expectancies, whereas with problem drinkers negative expectancy was more closely associated with drinking decisions than with positive expectancies. This study suggests that emphasizing the clients' perceived negative expectancies may be useful in tipping the balance toward change.

Finally, it is relevant to cite the work of Apter (1982), who outlined a psychological model of human behavior called reversal theory. The theory is complex in terms of both the model itself and the words used to describe aspects of the model (e.g., "paratelic," "telic," and "metamotivational"). Recently, the model has been utilized in relation to addictive behaviors such as gambling (Brown, 1989) and to the field in general (Miller, 1985a). In brief, Apter has suggested that behavior is driven by the interaction of a number of states that are "bistable." A bistable variable is one that operates in one of two mutually exclusive positions, (e.g., a light switch that is either on or off. Other bistable states include the gearing on motor boats, which allows the vessel to go either backwards or forwards, and the literary example, suggested by Miller (1985a), of Dr. Jekyll and Mr. Hyde. The movement from one aspect of the state to the other is known as a reversal. Apter has suggested that one of the bistable states of human behavior is the telic–paratelic state. Basically, when in telic mode the individual is goal oriented and behaving in a way that is useful for survival. Alternatively, when in the paratelic state the individual has switched from work to play in that paratelic behaviors are not necessary for human survival but are undertaken for their pleasurable, perhaps even harmful, aspects. Paretelic state behavior includes things such as partaking in sport, engaging in artistic pursuits, and, presumably, drug use.

Apter (1982) argued that reversals occur because the individual has become satiated or frustrated with the state he/she is in or because of external contingencies. An important assumption of reversal theory is that human behavior is inconsistent and to some degree unpredictable. Kerr (1993) has proposed in relation to sporting performance, that the use of cognitive techniques may be of value in focusing players in an appropriate state, yet it has to be noted that there is little evidence to date that interventions can be deployed to 'lock' people into appropriate states. As Miller (1985a) noted, perhaps Apter's (1982) greatest contribution is that his model allows a different perspective through which to view and appreciate some of the vagaries of human behavior.

The Psychology of Motivation Summarized

It is always difficult to distill the essential wisdoms from reviews such as the above. The language of psychological science tends to cloak, and even at times obscure, what is the essence of the matter. However, we would like to propose, using the language of everyday life, that there are some common and valuable themes to be gleaned from an appreciation of the psychology of motivation. The first, and not surprising, is that human beings are not rational actors. To quote Shakespeare, individuals "are but poor players who strut and fret their hour upon the stage." But we are not totally irrational actors either. We are not absolute flotsam and jetsam at the whim of the winds and waves of our existence. Shakespeare knew that the human condition is one that involves making choices, and often difficult choices at that. We make decisions, we try to weigh, however inconsistently and inaccurately, the options that are presented to us. We try to be purposeful, but in weighing our options, our judgments are often distorted and disturbed by our emotional state. Yet, paradoxically, our emotions may just be the prime movers of our behavior. What we do often has to do with what we desire. Our desires may change and our behaviors may look inconsistent to the casual observer. When presented with difficult choices, especially those that are perceived as involving losses whichever way we leap, we procrastinate and dither. The old way is chosen despite some internal doubts as to the wisdom of its selection. Then having made a decision to change our ways we are confronted with new circumstances and new choices. Shall we stick with our resolution or revert back to the old way?

Finally, we contend that all behavior is motivated. There is no such thing as "unmotivated" behavior. The key question to determine is: What is the direction of that motivation? Which way will our imperfect, apprehensive, and perplexed decision maker decide is the best bet?

MOTIVATION AND THE ADDICTIONS FIELD

So how well do the above considerations fit with the ideas on motivation that pertain in the addictions field? It is necessary to note that confusion over what is generally meant by motivation is exacerbated in the addictions field by differences of opinion as to the very nature of addiction itself. That old, and somewhat tedious, debate as to whether addiction is best perceived as a disease-like state or as a learned behavior affects the ideas of motivation that are used. As with other areas within the addictions arena, it is possible to identify distinct differences in orientation between the traditional (disease) and the cognitive-behavioral schools of thought.

The understanding of motivation that pertains within the traditional school is well reflected in the following viewpoints. Mindlin (1959) operationally defined motivation as the clients' willingness to become actively involved in treatment; determination to change in addition to not drinking and their preparedness to make sacrifices for therapy. Similarly, Stunkard (1961) equated motivation to patients' recognition of their disability, realization of the need for therapy, and appreciation that such help would ameliorate their condition. Nir and Cutler (1978) concluded that motivation is multidetermined and reflects a wide variety of defensive constellations (e.g., denial, lack of insight, lack of awareness, ego syntonicity, and fear of change) while Davis (1987) suggested that motivation should be determined by clients' readiness to acknowledge a problem, request treatment, cooperate with treatment, or all three.

After reviewing the literature, Miller (1985b) not surprisingly concluded that "motivation is often used as an antonym for terms such as denial and resistance and a synonym for constructs such as acceptance and surrender" (p. 86).

Additional aspects of what may be deemed the traditional model of addiction behavior come from the work of Davies (1979, pp. 454, 456), a medical sociologist, who observed Scottish psychiatrists interviewing people with alcohol-related problems. Two quotes from his work are useful exemplars.

> *Psychiatrist* (after seeing a patient with alcohol dependence): "What a dreadful person. Aaaah! Just awful. I can't decide whether he's an inadequate personality or an inadequate psychopath. He's certainly terribly immature. He's no motivation whatsoever. When he left us last time he did nothing to help himself. Quite honestly we can do nothing for the likes of him. I'd like to just throw him out of the door."

> *Another psychiatrist* (after seeing another alcohol-dependent person): "Och, we were short of time. He was going to tell me lies anyway. He was going to tell me that he's just been drinking a bit excessively. You know, he says that he just knocks back the drink to spite his wife. It's all a pack of lies. . . . They all tell lies. I bear no malice saying that. I just find it's best to work on the assumption that they are lying."

The above statements from Davies's observational study illustrate several themes that in any appraisal of motivation need to be addressed. The first is the idea of "no motivation," that people who choose not to change are not motivated at all or are exhibiting an "unmotivated syndrome paradigm" (DiCicco, Unterberger, & Mack, 1978). Sterne and Pittman (1965) found that many alcoholism counselors' supported the notion that alcoholics can be divided into two classes, those who have motivation and those who do not.

A second facet of the above quotations is that without motivation there is nothing the counselor can do for the client. It is implied that clients must enter treatment motivated and already inclined to change themselves. If they are not so prepared, the therapist may quite legitimately "throw them out of the door." Sterne and Pittman (1965) found that this view was common. The majority of counselors they interviewed considered there was little they could do to manipulate motivation and many felt that it was not their business to do so. For example, "there is not much need, with the shortage of manpower, to solicit business with someone who you think isn't motivated to benefit" (p. 48). This perspective is further illustrated by reference to Lemere et al. (1958) who wrote "a genuine desire on the part of the patient to stop drinking is the *sine qua non* of any treatment of alcoholism" (p. 598). Similarly, Moore and Murphy (1969) reported that "when the patient willingly admits his problem and is sincerely motivated to change, the battle is largely won, irrespective of the treatment technique" (p. 599).

A third and vital issue reflected in the above quotations is the notion that drug users are incapable of telling the truth. An apposite example of this perspective was reported in DiCicco et al. (1978). An employee who "denied" he had a drinking problem was told by the worksite medical director: "Shut up and listen. . . . Alcoholics are liars, so we don't want to hear what you have to say" (p. 599).

This view of the untruthfulness of problem drug users has been succinctly encapsulated in catch-phrases such as "alcoholism is a disease of denial." For example, Wilson (1985) noted that "the alcoholic patient often cannot recognize his [*sic*] disorder and accept the need for treatment because of his own profound denial," and Gitlow (1980) described alcoholism as "the only disease that tells people they don't have it" (p. 94).

A final issue is that motivation is frequently assessed by reference to the individual's eventual behavior—"after he left us . . . he did nothing to help himself." In this case motivation is an after-the-event attribution, which is determined by whether or not people do well. Those who succeed are deemed to have had motivation, while those who do badly have had little or none. This perspective meant that there was little need to evaluate treatment practices. If treatment resulted in poor outcome, it was not the treatment or the clinician who was at fault but rather "the unmotivated client" (Sterne & Pittman, 1965).

Fortunately, for problem drug users at least, this traditional view has been challenged, and in some cases superseded, by the cognitive-behavioral model of motivation applied to addictive behavior. When this happens a number of key distinctions become apparent.

The Idea of "No Motivation"

The first contrast, as Davies (1984) has adroitly noted, is that the damning epithet—the client has "no motivation"is no longer available. The decision to carry on drinking when there are contraindications is motivated behavior, even though it may irk and irritate others. As Davies (1984) stressed, all problem drug users are motivated (many of them powerfully so) but usually in the direction of continuing to use.

Therapeutic Intervention and Motivational Direction

Second, as noted above, the traditional view is that clients need to come to clinics committed to change. Within the cognitive-behavioral paradigm this is not the case. This change in perspective is in part due to the important contribution of Prochaska and DiClemente (1986, 1992). Working predominantly with nicotine users, Prochaska and DiClemente outlined what has become known as the stages-of-change model. They established that drug users can be identified as being in different stages in the behavioral change process. Those drug users who are unwilling, at present, to change their drug use are in the first stage. These "precontemplators," in Prochaska and DiClemente's terms, have been classified by DiClemente (1991) as falling into one of four types—the reluctant, the rebellious, the resigned, and the rationalizer. Reluctant precontemplators appear to lack insight or are passive in respect to acknowledging that there may be a problem with their behavior. Rebellious precontemplators have a big "investment" in the problem behavior and want to maintain control in making decisions about changing their behavior. The resigned precontemplators perceive change as being too difficult and believe they do not have the energy, or ability, to successfully make changes. Rationalizing precontemplators believe they have successfully examined the positive and negative aspects of the behavior and, on balance, have decided the behavior is not a problem for them personally.

As a caveat to DiClemente's view of the nature of precontemplators, we must remember that Prochaska and DiClemente have worked, almost exclusively, with nicotine users, the majority of whom (perhaps as high as 95%) are dependent on nicotine. This is clearly not the case with alcohol consumption, where the prevalence of alcohol dependence in the community may be somewhere in the order of 6% (Stockwell, Sitharthan, McGrath, & Lang, 1994). Thus, it is possible to speculate that many alcohol users (or for that matter cannabis, cocaine, LSD, Ecstasy, or heroin users) while being precontemplators are not rationalizing, resistant, reluctant, or resigned but are in fact "revelers." They enjoy their drug use and perceive it as being beneficial. For example, Towers (1994), using a decisional balance measure, found that social drinkers who could be classified as precontemplators reported more benefits than costs to their alcohol use. In effect, they deemed themselves to be "happy users."

However, as time passes negative consequences may begin to accumulate, and happy users (and presumably even the resigned, rebellious, reluctant, and rationalizing precontemplators) may begin to consider, "Is my drug use really worth it?" This group—the "contemplators" is interesting because research with both smokers (Velicer, DiClemente, Prochaska, & Brandenburg, 1985) and alcohol users (Towers, 1994) indicates that for them, the good and the bad things of drug use are finely balanced. Additionally, as individuals begin to perceive that the costs are rising respective to the benefits, they enter the third stage of being "ready for action" which has also been called determination (Prochaska, DiClenente, & Norcross, 1992).

When this ambivalence becomes sufficiently strong a decision is made that change has to happen. This is the "action" phase. Presumably, it is this group that was traditionally viewed as being motivated, because they attend clinics espousing the view that they need, perhaps even want, to change their behavior. Also, it is possible to surmise that those persons who traditionally have been labelled "unmotivated" were in fact contemplators, or "reveling" precontemplators.

To return, however, to consideration of the stage-of-change model, from action emerges the fifth and final stage, which is maintenance. Individuals in this category have taken effective action and have achieved sustained (in excess of 6 months) change.

The importance of this model is, as Prochaska and DiClemente (1986) argued, that different therapeutic strategies need to be deployed at different stages in the change process. They also note that ideas as to what constitutes effective counselling could include the nudging of a precontemplator into contemplation or the contemplator into being a "ready for action-er." Furthermore, as Tober (1991) has well stated, it is the drug counselors responsibility to engage effectively with people across the spectrum of change, including precontemplators, and tailor the counselling style to where "the client is at" in the change process. She has argued quite forcefully that a client's being unwilling to quit does not relieve the counselor of the responsibility to engage with the client effectively. Such involvement may include giving advice, which limits the damage from continued use.

A Matter of Denial

Reference to the work of Tober (1991) is appropriate because it introduces the third identified aspect of the traditional school of thought—that of denial and the untruthful nature of clients with addiction problems. Tober noted that working with precontemplators can be a frustrating business for counselors and that these frustrations in turn result in the cultivation of negative attitudes, where pre-contemplators are described as people who "lie about their drinking," "deny they have a problem," or are "unmotivated to change." In an attempt to keep the counselor's own attribution system intact, individuals in precontemplation are blamed for their refusal to comply with treatment and ultimately [are] excluded from it or written off as a "treatment" failure. But there is another way at looking at it. The frustrations experienced by specialist and primary counselors alike are the product of continually setting inappropriate goals. (p. 37)

By amplifying Tober's perspective it is possible to argue that many of the traits deemed in the traditional school to be the hallmark characteristics of problem drug users (e.g., denial, untruthfulness, and lack of motivation) are but a reflection of inappropriate intervention. Clients often resist and are recalcitrant because the addiction counselor is locked into strategies (e.g., "how to stop") that are inconsistent with the client's position in the change process. If a client is still making up his/her mind about the need to curtail or cease drug use, admonition or instruction on how to achieve abstinence is unlikely to be well received. In a similar vein, Miller (1983) argued that denial is a product of the nature of the interaction between therapist and client and that, rather than being a characteristic of the client, denial is in fact the result of poor and inappropriate counselling.

"Denial" as Cognitive Conflict

Nonetheless, even the most skilled cognitive-behaviorist counselor will encounter clients who are reluctant to discuss fully the nature of their difficulties. While it may be tempting to label this "denial," an alternative perspective is to consider a reluctance to disclose self-damning evidence as a psychological defense induced by cognitive conflict. In order to examine this idea, it is useful to refer to a number of studies that have investigated giving up addiction behavior.

For example, Stimson and Oppenheimer (1982), in their 10-year follow-up of some 130 heroin users attending drug dependence clinics in London, noted about heroin users giving up that "at anytime there are some advantages in continuing as an addict and some in ceasing. The conflict between reasons for continuing and reasons for stopping is a source of tension. In retrospectively assessing their lives, many [addicts] saw a shift in the balance between advantages and disadvantages as having led them to make a decision to stop using drugs" (p. 160). This quotation merits serious consideration. Stimson and Oppenheimer are suggesting that many drug users, rather than being unaware of the adverse consequences of their actions (i.e., being in denial) are in fact involved in an internal battle between what may be described as the pleasure and the pain of drug use. Orford (1985), in his authoritative review of "excessive appetites" or addictions, has similarly written that "motivation for change derives from an accumulation of 'losses,' 'costs' or harm resulting from behavior—these exceed 'gains,' 'benefits' or pleasurable outcomes to such a degree that the conflict between desire to continue and other needs require a decision to be made with regard to the behavior" (p. 210). What is being proposed here is that rather than drug users being unable to see the consequences of their actions, they are aware of the costs and this awareness prompts action. However, what of the recalcitrant, apparently nonadmitting client?

Although there are many theories of addiction behavior, a comprehensive psychological model proposed by Orford (1985) may help answer this question. In essence, Orford has argued that what might be considered the hallmark features of addiction behavior—the ambivalence, the broken promises, the unreliability, the binges, the rationalizations, and even the denial—are in fact the consequences of an individual being considerably conflicted about a behavior. Orford has written that "what characterizes an 'ism' or a mania, or a strong and troublesome appetite, as distinct from relatively trouble-free, restrained, moderate or normal appetitive behavior, is the upgrading of a state of balance into one of conflict" (p. 233). According to Orford it is this cognitive conflict, or internal battle between "I want to do this very much, but I know that I really shouldn't," that lies at the heart of compulsive, excessive behavior. If Orford is right, any "addict" is constantly having to choose between very strong desires to use and acute apprehensions as to the nasty consequences. As we have long recognized, such conflict is the antithesis to sound decision making. Indeed, Abelson (1963) coined the delightful phrase "hot cognitions" to describe decision making when under emotional duress. As noted earlier, the difficulty with decisions made under such circumstances, as opposed to those reached via "cool cognition," is that they are inherently fallible.

Herein then lies a possible explanation for the apparent vacillations of problem drug users. Promises to abstain are all too frequently replaced by decisions to use "just once more." Whilst such relapses may look like a lack of motivation, according to Orford they in fact reflect that the user is acutely troubled by what he/she is doing. Orford has written that when "subject to opposing motives of great strength it is difficult to know one's own mind, let alone behave with any consistency" (p. 239).

The significance of Orford's cognitive-conflict model of addictive behavior for the understanding of motivation is that there is a paradox to be grasped and understood. A drug user may exhibit all the behavioral features traditionally presumed as being indicative of no motivation, and even denial, at the very time he/she is most acutely conscious of all the dangers and deficits inherent in drug use. The very worst excesses may actually occur when the drug user is most troubled and most conflicted by what he/she is doing. One client recently described her excessive behavior as being "stupid". When asked how it felt to be doing something stupid, she noted that the very stupidity of it made her feel so wretched that she did it even more. There was, she said, no point in doing a stupid thing a little. It were to be done it had to be done excessively. When further asked as to what she thought about as she engaged in the behavior she noted: "I don't look at the costs, I just do it."

Engaging in behavior that one knows to be wrong or self-defeating is likely to induce a sense of not wishing to look at the possible consequences of the behavior. Any reflection on the potential of disaster is too detrimental, too intrusive, to the moment of pleasure. It is also too psychologically discomforting and unsettling.

To conclude this perspective on denial, we must note that denial may occur not because individuals are incapable of seeing what they are doing to themselves but because they choose not to look. If they look, they may have to tell themselves to quit and, in the stages of change prior to taking action, that is too dreadful a decision to consider.

Contrasting Counseling Styles and Perspectives

Obviously, adoption of such a paradigm has implications for the management of addictive behavior. This is the subject of the accompanying chapter by Bell and Rollnick (Chapter 10, this volume); however, it is relevant to encapsulate what may be viewed as the essential theoretical differences between the traditional and emerging schools of thought and how these are reflected in the rationale and style of counseling. Table 9.1 is a modified version outlined by Miller (1989) and Stockwell, Gregson, Osbourne, and Bolt (1989).

Clearly, if Table 9.1 is accepted as an accurate portrayal of the differences between the two schools of thought within the addictions field, marked differences as to how motivation is perceived, and how it is therefore addressed, exist. One model of motivation and addictive behavior, which is based on incorporation of cognitive-behavioral perspectives, is outlined by Cox and Klinger (1988). They have written: "Our model of alcohol use depicts people as deciding to drink or not to drink on the basis of whether the positive affective consequences that they expect to derive from drinking outweigh those that they expect to derive from not drinking" (p. 53). As we can appreciate, this is a standard "value" model of behavior. The interest of the Cox and Klinger model is that it also includes the individual as a social actor with past learning, expectancies, and emotional processes. The model incorporates historical factors (e.g., sociocultural experience, personality characteristics, and past reinforcement from drinking), current factors (e.g., positive and negative incentives and severity of alcohol dependence), and expected factors (e.g., outcome expectancies for drug use or abstinence). In many ways this is the most comprehensive motivational model yet outlined specifically for the addictions field.

Motivation and Giving Up Addictive Behaviors

It is relevant to conclude this chapter with reference to the literature on giving up addictions, particularly that drawn from the accounts of people who achieved change without formal treatment. Such literature is replete

TABLE 9.1. Perspectives on Motivation and Addiction Behavior

Perspective on	Disease model	Emerging model
Concept of client	Someone who will not face up to the reality of his/her drug use. Confrontation and education required.	Someone who can acknowledge that drug use causes some problems but is also aware that drug use provides very real benefits.
Focus of clinical sessions	To make clients aware of the nature and severity of their drug use.	To elicit and assess the concerns clients may have about drug use and other current problems.
Aim of session	To have clients acknowledge their addiction, admit that they cannot control their drug use, and commit themselves to abstinence.	Have clients consider the advantages and disadvantages of continuing, and of stopping, their current drug use and assist them to decide one way or the other.
Style of session	Therapist controlled and directed.	Therapist led but client centered.
Therapist's role	To educate, instruct, advise, confront, and direct clients about the nature of their addiction behavior and tell them how to solve their difficulties	To assist clients in making decisions about their future drug use (to continue, to curtail, or to cease) and provide supportive, goal-directed counseling.

with mystery and ambiguity, but we believe it is consistent with the psychology of motivation.

The first reference is to Stewart (1987) who in her autobiographical account of heroin use wrote:

> Hunting for a reason to stop that outweighs the drive to stay hooked is the major problem. During one soul-searching session I neatly listed advantages and disadvantages of taking smack. Potential consequences of using heroin including being charged with an offense, starring in a scandal, losing home, job, health, wealth, friends, and credibility of every kind. Advantages were impossible to find. The following statements appeared on the list of reasons not to stop: "It [heroin] makes life easy"; "I'm scared to stop" and "I don't feel like it." A moment's thought contradicted the first two and left me confronted by the third. I did not "feel like it." I did not stop, but logic had not assisted the choice. (p. 152)

As we have suggested, perhaps straight-forward rationality is insufficient. However, what is sufficient to prompt change is elusive as evidenced by Knupfer's (1972) report on how problem drinkers resolved their problems without entering treatment. She noted:

> In explaining why they quit respondents often gave strangely trivial reasons. One man after seventeen years of drinking a fifth of whiskey daily said "I seen it wasn't doing me no good, so I quit."
>
> Another began going with a woman (his future wife) and was ashamed for her to see him drunk. Another walked into his favorite bar one day and the bartender began telling him about the fancy car he had just purchased. The respondent thought to himself indignantly "he's buying that car with my money, goddamn it and what have I got?" Then and there he decided to quit. (p. 272)

The researcher or clinician interested in understanding the motivational process whereby people give up their addictions is challenged by a core difficulty inherent in the above quotations. Stewart suggested that logic does not help but Knupfer emphasized the curiousness of the giving-up process. Is giving up addiction, and thereby the motivation for so doing, something that will, at the end of the day, always remain slightly beyond comprehension?

It may be, for as John F. Kennedy is cited as saying: "The essence of ultimate decisions remains impenetrable to the observer—often, indeed to the decider himself. . . . There will always be the dark and tangled stretches in the decision making process—mysterious even to those who may be most intimately involved" (from Sorensen, 1963, p. 67).

It is just possible that the decision to give up well-established but maladaptive behaviors is an idiosyncratic and emotional process that pertains to values within the individual: some intrinsic sense of what they are about, the meaning of their life, what they perceive to be their allotted and proper roles. For many the decision to quit is a difficult and dubious decision driven more by the recognition of the need to make changes than the desire to do so. As one client recently noted, her decision to give up drinking was generated by the realization that eventually the pain of change was less than the pain of staying the same.

In this chapter we have deliberately focussed on the "front end" of the change process. The acute task for the counselor is to assist the client in coming to a robust resolution to change. It is a nudging, catalytic, psychological interaction. Once the decision to change has been made, action strategies come into play that will, we hope, sustain the initial resolution. However, as is all too apparent, the decision to quit is often shortlived and the human foible of changing one's mind often results in relapse. It is absolutely vital to stress that social factors, the quality of one's existence—family, friends, relationships, job—and the experience that change is a good bet are the things that sustain and reinforce the initial decision to quit. Motivation is then an ongoing process. However, it is a process in which the desire and energy for any specific goal will ebb and flow. All of us feel, on some days, more motivated to achieve or change than on others.

Most "addicts" do give up their addictive behaviors. Tam Stewart, who was not persuaded by logic, did eventually quit. The tale of her recovery is the conclusion of this chapter. It is our contention that her description reflects much of what we have contended is important in motivation and addictive behavior. It is, we believe, a salutary tale. She reports it thus:

> I have been in and around the heroin scene in Liverpool for many years. Last summer I kicked my heroin habit. I did not really decide to stop. The decision was forced upon me. Things had been hotting up for a while: the bank was on my back; I had nothing left to sell; there was no direction, no creativity, no hope. Sanity was being sucked up the tube. I became marginally paranoid. People were following me. Trips to score caused panic, paranoia, actually something close to terror. I ditched my car for someone else's. They would not know the number. They would not be able to get me. At night I slept with "It" a hand's reach away—but would I wake in time? Every dawn the door was kicked in by a phantom drug squad and I held my breath listening for their footsteps. I slept with the curtains parted so I would wake at first light to pre-empt their beastly plans.
>
> In this month July, I rowed and raged, I fell out with people. I cried a

lot. And I slumbered on, blissful much of the time, in rash, brittle, oblivion, numbed and Lethe-lulled on a pillow of never, never, never. Relationships became erratic, but Bobby and I united in mutual need. We got a system going. We were never without. And we were scared, very scared, we might have to be. The money was always found. Food went by the board. We went nowhere except to score. Or to visit other devotees on similar errands. I lost weight. One particular Sunday the paranoia peaked.

We went down around lunchtime to our usual place. The weather was hot. Very hot. There was a party spirit on the streets. Loud music wailed. Rastas hung out of windows in Warwick Street, bare-chested and celebratory, but the scorched grass at the roadside reeked of dog shit and discontent buzzed through the ghetto with the flies. I waited. He was out. Come back in three-quarters of an hour. We did. Sorry. Come at 3 o'clock. Try later. By now there was a queue. A rag-taggle bunch of desperate people who did not care who saw them or who knew what they wanted—so long as they got it. And got it fast. They argued about who would be first when something turned up. The lunacy continued. In car, in taxis, on motor bikes they set off in convoy to another part of the city. I waited. They had no luck. The madness went on. I went home. I gave up. I would just get sick.

Bobby turned up at teatime. Everything was all right again. Our eyes and noses were dry once more. We had spent six hours of the day and a lot of anxiety just for that. To say nothing of the £60. Self-disgust was swelling like an over-ripe boil. I had almost had enough. I resolved to get the hell out while I was still sane. I resolved to stop. There were no more mountains to climb this side of September; no job, no tasks, nothing. I phoned a friend in London. I could stay there.

Tuesday was the last of it. At the station I panicked. £20 had been dispatched at the last moment. But Bobby did not make it back with the supplies and I left on the train, beside myself, nearly stepping off to wait, after all, for as long as it took. In the toilet, before we even passed Edge Hill, I whacked off the last of what I had. The journey passed in seconds, the few when I had my eyes open. Getting my bags to the taxi was quite hard.

I came off in London. It was not easy. I spent August in Wales, looking to the green countryside for a sense of renewal and well-being. In the autumn I began this book. (Stewart, 1987, pp. 1–2)

REFERENCES

Abelson, R. (1963). Computer simulation of "hot" cognition. In S. Tomkins & S. Messick (Eds.), *Computer simulation of personality*. New York: Wiley.

Apter, M. (1982). *The experience of motivation: The theory of psychological reversals*. London: Academic Press.

Bandura, A. (1977). Self-efficacy: Toward a unifying theory of behavioral change. *Psychological Review, 84*, 191–215.

Brown, I. (1989). Relapses from a gambling perspective. In M. Gossop (Ed.), *Relapse and addictive behavior.* London: Tavistock/Routledge.

Cantor, N., & Langston, C. (1989). Ups and downs of life tasks in a life transition. In L. Pervin (Ed.), *Goal concepts in personality and social psychology.* Hillsdale, NJ: Erlbaum.

Colten, M., & Janis, I. (1982). Effects of self-disclosure and the decisional balance sheet procedure in a weight reduction clinic. In I. Janis (Ed.), *Counseling on personal decisions: Theory and field research on helping relationships.* New Haven, CT: Yale University Press.

Cox, M. W., & Klinger, E. (1988). A motivational model of alcohol. *Journal of Abnormal Psychology, 97,* 168–180.

Davies, P. (1979). Motivation, responsibility and sickness in the psychiatric treatment of alcoholism. *British Journal of Psychiatry, 134,* 449–458.

Davies, J. (1984). A psychological look at willpower and motivation. *Salud.* The Alcohol Studies Centre, Paisley College of Technology, Scotland.

Davis, D. (1987). *Alcoholism treatment: An integrative family and individual approach.* New York: Gardner Press.

DiCicco, L., Unterberger, H., & Mack, J. (1978). Confronting denial: An alcoholism intervention strategy. *Psychiatric Annals, 8,* 596–606.

DiClemente, C. (1991). Motivational interviewing and the stages of change. In W. R. Miller & S. Rollnick, *Motivational interviewing: Preparing people to change addictive behavior.* New York: Guilford Press.

Edwards, G., & Gross, M. (1976). Alcohol dependence: Provisional description of a clinical syndrome. *British Meidcal Journal, 1,* 1058–1061.

Ellis, A. (1982). *Rational–emotive therapy and cognitive behavior therapy.* New York: Springer.

Fitzgibbon, M., & Kirschenbaum, D. (1992). Who succeeds in losing weight? In Y. Klar, J. Fisher, J. Chinsky, & A. Nadler (Eds.), *Self change: Social, psychological and clinical perspectives.* New York: Springer-Verlag.

Gitlow, W. (1980). An overview. In S. Gitlow & H. Peyser (Eds.), *Alcoholism: A practical treatment guide.* New York: Grune & Stratton.

Goldman, D. (1992). Commentary. *Annual Review of Addictions Research and Treatment, 2,* 217–221.

Hopkins, C. (1989). *Drinkers' motivation to change their drinking behavior: An application of subjective expected utility.* Unpublished M. App. Sc. (Psych.) dissertation, Curtin University of Technology, Perth, Western Australia.

Janis, I., & Mann, L. (1977). *Decision making: A psychological analysis of conflict, choice and commitment.* New York: Collier Macmillan.

Klar, Y., Nadler, A., & Malloy, T. (1992). Opting to change: Students' informal self-change endeavours. In Y. Klar, J. Fisher, J. Chinsky, & A. Nadler (Eds.), *Self change: Social, psychological and clinical perspectives.* New York: Springer-Verlag.

Kleindorfer, P., Kunreuther, H., & Schoemaker, P. (1993). *Decision sciences: An integrative perspective.* Cambridge, England: Cambridge University Press.

Knupfer, G. (1972). Ex-problem drinkers. *Life history research in psychopathology, 2,* 256–280.

Lemere, F., O'Hollaren, P., & Maxwell, T. (1958). Motivation in the treatment of alcoholism. *Quarterly Journal of Studies on Alcohol, 19,* 428–431.

Lovibond, S., & Caddy, G. (1970). Discriminative aversive control in the moderation of alcoholics' drinking behavior. *Behavior Therapy, 1,* 437–444.

McMahon, J., Jones, B., & O'Donnell, P. (1994). Comparing positive and negative alcohol expectancies in male and female social drinkers. *Addiction Research, 4,* 349–365.

Mann, L. (1989). Becoming a better decision maker. *Australian Psychologist, 24,* 141–155.

Miller, W. R. (1983). Motivational interviewing for problem drinkers. *Behavioural Psychotherapy, 11,* 147–182.

Miller, W. R. (1985a). Addictive behaviour and the theory of psychological reversals. *Addictive Behavior, 10,* 177–180.

Miller, W. R. (1985b). Motivation for treatment: A review with special emphasis on alcoholism. *Psychological Bulletin, 98,* 84–107.

Miller, W. R. (1989). Increasing motivation for change. In R. K. Hester & W. R. Miller (Eds.), *Handbook of alcoholism treatment approaches: Effective alternatives.* Elmsford, NY: Pergamon Press.

Mindlin, D. (1959). The characteristics of alcoholics as related to prediction of therapeutic outcome. *Quarterly Journal of Studies on Alcohol, 20,* 604–619.

Moore, R., & Murphy, T. (1969). Denial of alcoholism as an obstacle to recovery. *Quarterly Journal of Studies on Alcohol, 22,* 597–609.

Nir, Y., & Cutler, R. (1978). The unmotivated patient syndrome: Survey of therapeutic interventions. *American Journal of Psychiatry, 135,* 442–447.

Noble, E. (1993). The genetic transmission of alcoholism: Implications for prevention. *Drug and Alcohol Review, 12,* 283–290.

Orford, J. (1985). *Excessive appetites: A psychological view of addiction.* Chichester, England: Wiley.

Prochaska, J. O., & DiClemente, C. C. (1986). Towards a comprehensive model of change. In W. R. Miller & N. Heather (Eds.), *Treating addictive behaviors: Processes of change.* New York: Plenum Press.

Prochaska, J. O., & DiClemente, C. C. (1992). Stages of change in the modification of problem behaviors. In M. Hersen, R. M. Eisler, & P. M. Miller (Eds.), *Progress in behavior modification.* Newbury Park, CA: Sage.

Prochaska, J. O., & DiClemente, C. C., & Norcross, J. C. (1992). In search of how people change: Applications to addictive behaviors. *American Psychologist, 47,* 1102–1114.

Reber, A. (1985). *Dictionary of psychology.* London: Penguin.

Saunders, B., & Allsop, S. (1991). Alcohol problems and relapse: Can the clinic combat the community? *Journal of Community and Applied Social Psychology, 1,* 213–221.

Saunders, B., & Phillips, M. (1993). Is alcoholism genetically transmitted? And are there any implications for prevention? *Drug and Alcohol Review, 12,* 291–298.

Schoemaker, P. (1982). The expected utility model: Its variants, purposes, evidence and limitations. *Journal of Economic Literature, 20,* 529–558.

Siegel, S. (1983). Classical conditioning, drug tolerance and drug dependence. In Y. Israel, F. Glaser, H. Kalant, R. Popham, W. Schmidt, & R. Smart (Eds.), *Research advances in alcohol and drug problems* (Vol. 7). New York: Plenum Press.

Simon, H. (1976). *Administrative behavior: A study of decision making processes in administrative organizations.* New York: Free Press.

Sorensen, T. (1963). *Decision making in the White House: The olive branch and the arrows.* New York: Bantam.

Sterne, M., & Pittman, D. (1965). The concept of motivation: A source of institutional and professional blockage in the treatment of alcoholics. *Quarterly Journal of Studies on Alcohol, 26,* 41–57.

Stewart, T. (1987). *The heroin users.* London: Pandora.

Stimson, G., & Oppenheimer, E. (1982). *Heroin addiction: Treatment and control in Britain.* London: Tavistock.

Stockwell, T., Gregson, A., Osbourne, J., & Bolt, J. (1989, July). *Motivational interviewing with problem drinkers: A controlled trial of a method for reducing client dropout.* Paper presented at the Winter School in the Sun Conference, The Alcohol and Drug Foundation, Brisbane.

Stockwell, T., Sitharthan, T., McGrath, D., & Lang, E. (1994). The measurement of alcohol dependence and impaired control in community samples. *Addiction, 89,* 167–174.

Stunkard, A. (1961). Motivation for treatment. *Comprehensive Psychiatry, 2,* 140–147.

Sutton, S. (1987). Social–psychological approaches to understanding addictive behaviours: Attitude-behaviour and decision making models. *British Journal of Addiction, 82,* 355–370.

Towers, T. (1994). *The development of a decisional balance scale to change drinking behaviour.* Unpublished M. Psych. dissertation, Curtin University of Technology, Perth, Western Australia.

Tober, G. (1991). Helping with pre-contemplator. In R. Davidson, S. Rollnick, & I. McEwan (Eds.), *Counseling problem drinkers.* London: Tavistock/Routledge.

Tversky, A., & Kahneman, D. (1981). The framing of decisions and the psychology of choice. *Science, 211,* 453–458.

Vaillant, G. (1983). *The natural history of alcoholism: Causes, patterns, and paths to recovery.* Cambridge, MA: Harvard University Press.

Velicer, W., DiClemente, C., Prochaska, J., & Brandenburg, N. (1985). Decisional balance measure for assessing and predicting smoking status. *Journal of Personality and Social Psychology, 48,* 1279–1289.

West, R. (1989). The psychological basis of addiction. *International Review of Psychiatry, 1,* 71–80.

Wilson, G. (1985). Intervention by the clinician to motivate the alcoholic. *Australian Alcohol and Drug Review, 4,* 94–100.

CHAPTER 10

Motivational Interviewing in Practice: A Structured Approach

ALISON BELL
STEPHEN ROLLNICK

Motivational interviewing has attracted increasing attention over the past 10 years, particularly in the treatment of people experiencing problems with substance use. When questioning their initial interest in motivational interviewing, a common response from trainees is that they want to know "what motivates people to change" or to learn "how to motivate the unmotivated." On calling for definitions of motivation from workshop participants, most responses center around change, with motivation involving a movement in a positive direction toward changing the undesirable behavior. Motivational interviewing begins, however, with the premise that people are in fact *quite* motivated (but perhaps not always in the direction we in the business of change would want them to be).

Motivational interviewing arose in response to a trend in the treatment of people experiencing alcohol and other drug problems, an approach involving the use of direct confrontation and persuasion. The confrontational approach was based on the premise that alcoholics and addicts possess extraordinary levels of defense mechanisms such as denial, projection, and rationalization, characteristics seen as inherent personality traits that constitute a unique lack of motivation for change. William Miller (1983, 1985) proposed that motivation or, more to the point, seeming lack of motivation, is *not* an inherent, static personality trait or problem but more a reflection of a state of readiness to change, which fluctuates from one time or situation to another and is affected by a variety of both internal and external factors.

The style of the therapist is considered to be an important factor in the client–counselor interaction. In fact, the approach taken by the therapist can be a powerful determinant of client resistance or change. "Motivation for change does not simply reside within the skin of the client, but involves an interpersonal context" (Miller & Rollnick, 1991, p. 35). Carl Rogers (1961) examined a number of studies of interactions within helping relationships and concluded that the helping person was an integral factor in determining whether the relationship was "growth-promoting or growth-inhibiting" (p. 41). Rogers also noted that clients found it unhelpful when therapists gave direct and specific advice regarding decisions. More recently, a number of studies (Patterson & Forgatch, 1985; Miller & Sovereign, 1989, cited in Miller & Rollnick, 1991; Miller, Benefield, & Tonigan, 1993) demonstrated that the level of client resistance was directly related to the level of confrontation from the therapist. The style of the counselor was also a predictor of client outcome, with the greater the level of confrontation, the more likely the client was drinking 1 year later (Miller & Sovereign, 1989; Miller et al., 1993).

Paradoxically, however, motivational interventions are both confrontational and nonconfrontational. "Confrontation is a goal of all counseling and psychotherapy and is a prerequisite for intentional change" (Miller & Rollnick, 1991, p. 13). Confrontation of perceived client denial is avoided; rather, the aim is for the client to reach a state of self-confrontation and cognitive reappraisal through awareness and self-examination. Confrontation in this sense is a *goal* rather than a *style* of counseling. To see one's situation clearly is a first step toward change. Thus, confrontation by one's self, rather than by the therapist or some other source, is seen as essential for change.

The client's own perception of his/her situation is essential to the therapeutic process. Brissett (1988) claims that "those individuals who deny the judgement that they are alcoholic (or addict) are not necessarily wrong, do not necessarily suffer from some illness. . . . What comes to be labelled as denial may be little more than a declaration of personal independence" (p. 394). The need for an individual to accept a label "alcoholic," for example, can be a source of resistance between the client and counselor and is not necessary to the change process. What is considered more important is to assist the client through the decision-making process and to strengthen commitment for change. The aim of motivational interventions is, therefore, to elicit from the client any concerns related to the behavior, and personal reasons for change.

TWO KEY CONCEPTS

The practice of motivational interviewing requires an understanding of two central concepts: (1) people are at different stages of readiness for change, and (2) the experience of ambivalence is normal and understandable (Rollnick, Heather, & Bell, 1992). Both are essential factors in the decision-making process and will have an impact on the client's perception of any intervention and the outcome.

Readiness for Change

Originally developed by Prochaska and DiClemente (1986), the stages-of-change model (Figure 10.1) is important to the practice of motivational interviewing as it proposes that change is a process rather than a discrete event. (See Saunders, Wilkinson, & Towers, Chapter 9, this volume, for a more detailed explanation of the stages.)

   Motivation is understood in terms of the client's stage of change, with differing therapist tasks at different stages of change (Miller & Rollnick, 1991). The precontemplator, classified as "the happy user," is not likely

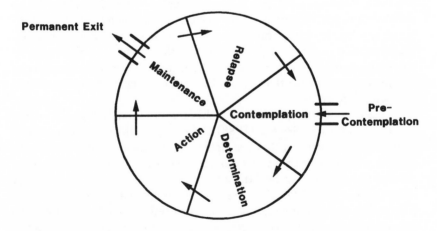

FIGURE 10.1. Prochaska and DiClemente's six stages of change. From Miller and Rollnick (1991). Copyright 1991 by The Guilford Press. Reprinted by permission.

to be seen within the treatment setting unless coerced into therapy by a concerned party. People in a state of precontemplation are therefore, most likely to be labeled as being in denial and to appear resistant to treatment (DiClemente, 1991). With the precontemplator, the aim is to raise some doubt within the client and to increase the perception of risks associated with current substance use by providing information and feedback.

The contemplator is typified by a state of ambivalence about the drug-using behavior: "I want to and I don't want to" (Miller & Rollnick, 1991). Contemplators are often caught in a state of conflict between the benefits and costs of continued use. A confrontational approach with someone in a state of contemplation may push the client toward defending the benefits of continued use, which is likely to result in seeming denial of any problem or concern raised by the therapist (Rollnick, Kinnersley, & Stott, 1993). The recommended approach with the contemplative client is to explore the two sides of the drug-using behavior and to tip the balance toward change.

The stage between contemplation and action is one of determination, a process of preparation for change before any action is taken (DiClemente et al., 1991). Preparation is important to the change process because the reasons for attempting change, as well as the strength of the original resolution will effect the quality of outcome, such as the likelihood of relapse occurring (Allsop & Saunders, 1991). The client's sense of self-efficacy, or belief in his/her ability to carry out and succeed with a chosen task, is likely to influence the movement from determination into action. There is also a likelihood of heightened ambivalence as the client moves toward a point of choice. Thus, the task of the therapist when working with a client in the determination stage is to strengthen the commitment for change by helping the client to determine the best course of action to take (Miller & Rollnick, 1991).

In the action stage, any plans for change are implemented. It is important that the client chooses his/her own action plan and perceives that change is desirable. It is also important at this stage to acknowledge that the client is likely to experience an ongoing sense of ambivalence or a continued weighing of the costs and benefits of change. Clients at this stage require a sense of reward for any success achieved. The maintenance of change involves a continued vigilance of the change process and the achievement of personal goals. Relapse prevention strategies, which include a review of the original resolution for change, are important to the maintenance of change. Relapse, although perhaps not desirable, is seen as a normal and almost inevitable part of the change process. The aim of motivational interventions at this stage is to minimize any problems associated with a lapse or relapse by assisting the client to renew the original commitment for change and thus recommence the process of contemplation and determination for action.

The stages-of-change model provides an alternative to thinking about motivation as a personality trait; client behavior is viewed in terms of the total process or cycle of change. The practice of motivational interviewing focuses on the importance of matching the client's stage of readiness to change with the treatment. Rather than focusing solely on the action and maintenance phases of the change process, the aim is first to assist the individual to work through the contemplation and decision-making stages, by acknowledging that ambivalence and indecision are normal and important processes in the cycle of change. It can also be a more rewarding way of working with clients as it measures change in small steps, thus decreasing the likelihood of therapeutic nihilism, which can be problematic when working with substance abuse clients.

Ambivalence

Ambivalence about substance use is a common and normal experience, with fluctuations between the desire for continued use and change being the source of conflict. In relation to continued use, the heroin user, for example, may find that while heroin provides a state of euphoria and relaxation, at the same time heroin use costs a lot of money and is affecting his/her relationships with other people. On the side of changing the behavior, the heroin user may feel that although stopping the use of heroin may decrease the risk of problems with the law, the loss of a certain lifestyle or the possibility of discomfort in withdrawal is undesirable. These may be strong opposing forces, caught between a state of "I really want to use heroin very much" versus "I know I really shouldn't use it" (Saunders, Wilkinson, & Allsop, 1991, p. 280). Although the process of decisional conflict may not be conscious, it can be a powerful force within the client–counselor interaction. Ambivalence can be a factor even for people voluntarily seeking, and it can continue into the action and maintenance stages. "In many cases, working with ambivalence is working with the heart of the problem" (Miller & Rollnick, 1991, p. 38).

Attempting to persuade someone who is ambivalent is likely to lead to resistance and seeming denial. Arguments related to the costs of use or benefits of change from the therapist will lead clients to defend the other side of their position (i.e., the benefits of continued use and the costs of change). Thus, ambivalence is often misconstrued as a sign of resistance or denial (Miller, 1983). It is important to the therapeutic relationship that the client's conflict is recognized as an essential part of the change process. Acknowledgment and exploration of the two sides of the conflict, with the aim of encouraging the client to consider the cost–benefit equation, can be the key to change.

THE STRUCTURE
OF MOTIVATIONAL INTERVIEWING

The practice of motivational interviewing has developed over the past 10 years, owing to the variety of clinical applications and differing interpretations of the theory. The method described in the following sections is based on a series of strategies we developed within the course of a research project. The hospital-based intervention study was aimed at motivating non-help-seeking excessive drinkers to reduce their alcohol consumption. Our approach formed the basis of brief motivational interviewing (see Rollnick et al., 1992). The use of key strategies is based firmly on the principles of motivational interviewing but is more structured than the method described by Miller and Rollnick (1991). It has also proved to be a useful teaching method for both specialist alcohol and drug counselors and more generalist health workers. (See Figure 10.2.)

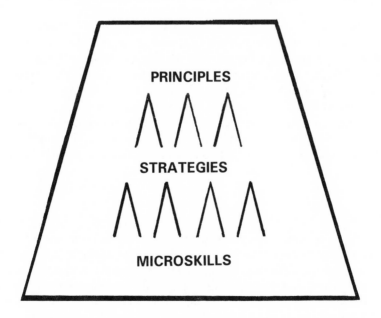

FIGURE 10.2. A model of structured motivational interviewing.

The manner in which the strategies interconnect with the principles of motivational interviewing and the core counseling skills, essential to the client-centered approach, are demonstrated in the case scenario that follows the description of each level.

Principles

There are five key principles underlying the practice of motivational interviewing (Miller & Rollnick, 1991).

Express Empathy

Rogers (cited in Miller, 1983) claimed that an essential ingredient in the counseling process is one of "accurate empathy." This does not imply the need for total identification with the client but, rather, an expression of understanding and acceptance of the client's position. Any ambivalence is accepted as normal and understandable, thus decreasing the level of resistance between the client and the counselor.

Develop Discrepancy

Essentially, the counselor must create and amplify in the client's mind a discrepancy between the current behavior and personal goals or beliefs about oneself (e.g., the person who smokes yet values his/her physical health). The principle works on the assumption that change is prompted when a divergence between present behavior and personal goals becomes uncomfortable. In practice, this discomfort derives from eliciting and clarifying important goals with the client and exploring the consequences of the present behavior that conflicts with those goals. The aim is for the client to achieve a state of self-confrontation and to present reasons for change.

Avoid Argument

Arguments are counterproductive and serve only to increase the level of client resistance and counselor frustration. Arguments with clients can take a number of forms (e.g., direct confrontation or attempts to persuade the person with logic or evidence of physical damage). Labeling can also be a source of conflict between the therapist and the client. The acceptance of a label, in the form of "alcoholic" or "problem," for example, is not viewed as a prerequisite for treatment.

Roll with Resistance

The essential ingredients of motivational interventions aim to decrease client resistance. However, clients may express hostility or opposition to treatment for any number of reasons, for example, because they were coerced into therapy or due to past counseling experiences. Rather than meeting resistance with confrontation or argument, it is met with reflection or reframing. The energy of client resistance is seen as a positive sign and something that requires exploration rather than something that needs to be broken down by confrontation. Resistance is also recognized as a possible indication of the mismatch between the client's stage of change and the focus of the therapy.

Support Self-Efficacy

The client's perception of his/her ability to carrying out a course of action and achieve certain goals will affect the likelihood of change being attempted. As the client is ultimately responsible for choosing and carrying out personal change, this perception is essential to the change process. An analogy that illustrates the movement from determination into action involves the parachutist who, before jumping from an airplane at great height, believes that the parachute will open and that the landing will be achieved safely. To help the person anticipating change to drinking or drug-using behavior, we must instill a sense of confidence in the individual's own plan of action and the achievement of the desired outcome.

Strategies

The strategies provide the structure for the practice of motivational interviewing. There are a number of different strategies that can be used to enhance client motivation within the therapeutic interaction (Rollnick et al., 1992). The four key strategies that are discussed provide part of a menu of possible strategies from which to choose. The choice of strategy will depend on the level of rapport between the client and counselor, the client's stage of change, and the therapist's perception of the level of concern.

"Exploring a Typical Day or Session"

The essence of this strategy is to obtain a "snapshot" of the client's situation in relation to the use of a particular substance. As an opening strategy, an exploration of a recent and specific "day in the life of" the client will provide for an assessment of substance use in the context of the client's reality, as well as an indication of the level of client concern. Asking the client to go through a specific day in some detail will also build rapport, as the counselor expresses an interest in understanding the client's situation.

"Good Things and Less Good Things of Substance Use"

An exploration of the two sides of the client's substance use serves a number of purposes. The first is to express empathy for the client's position. In addition, by eliciting from the client the benefits and costs of his/her alcohol or drug use, the strategy is also a useful way of assessing the stage of change and the degree of ambivalence within the client. It is important, however, that the therapist does not presume that the costs or "less good things" related to substance use are a source of concern to the client, and that the therapist avoid the use of terms such as "problem" or "concern." Rather, the strategy creates and amplifies a sense of decisional balancing within the client, with the aim of facilitating client reflection and sources of possible concern.

"Providing Information"

The provision of information, feedback, or advice can be an important focus within counseling. However, the manner in which information is provided can make the difference between a confrontation–resistance struggle and a therapeutic interaction. One of the traps that many helpers fall into when delivering advice is the "expert–problem solver" trap, which leaves the client in either a passive or a defensive position. Before information is given, it is important to assess whether the client actually wants any information or advice. It also important to assess what the client already knows in relation to the effects of substance use, for example, in order to avoid duplicating client knowledge. Such an assessment also increases client self-efficacy by acknowledging that the client is likely to be informed to some extent on the issue of substance use. When providing advice or feedback, it is important to allow time for the client to discuss the personal implications of the information given. Finally, it is left up to the client as to what he/she does with the information.

"Exploring Concerns"

The exploration of concerns begins with an assumption that the client has some concerns or problems related to substance use. Asking someone in precontemplation, for example, about his/her concerns is likely to be met with confusion or resistance. The purpose of this strategy is to move the client toward the goal of motivational interviewing, by eliciting reasons for concern in detail. Following an exploration of each concern, time is allowed for the client to contemplate his/her position. The therapist is then in a position to assist the client through the decision-making process.

Microskills

The third but essential level in the practice of motivational interviewing involves the use of client-centered counseling skills. The skills of *open questioning, reflective listening, affirmation,* and *summary* are the essential ingredients in motivational interviewing, as they provide an opportunity for the client to explore his/her own situation. Without the use of these core skills, motivational interventions are not possible, as client-centered techniques form the foundation stone on which practice is built.

A second paradox exists, however, within motivational interviewing. Although the practice relies on nondirective counseling skills, the use of key strategies provides a structure for direction as does the use of selective reflection and questions. Thus, the therapist is in a position to subtly steer the client toward change.

Putting It All Together

The interplay between the principles, strategies, and microskills forms the practice of motivational interviewing. One further essential ingredient is the style of the therapist. As stated earlier, the therapist's style is a powerful determinant of client resistance and change (Miller & Rollnick, 1991). An attitude of acceptance and understanding for the client's situation, and a sense of trust in the client's judgment and decisions, is crucial to the process.

CASE ILLUSTRATION

It is a difficult task to convey through a single, written scenario the full essence of motivational interviewing in practice (as it would be with any counseling approach). It is also obvious but important to note that each case will be different in practice; as Miller and Rollnick (1991) state: "No particular case can demonstrate the rich variety of situations and problems you will face, nor the range of ways in which these challenges can be met"

(p. 139). However, the purpose of the case illustration is to demonstrate in particular, the interplay among the principles, microskills, and selected strategies.

Although motivational interviewing can be used in a variety of situations, with different client groups, the scenario that follows demonstrates the use of motivational interviewing within a general hospital setting. The therapist involved is a clinical nurse. A case such as this shows that motivational interviewing can be particularly useful as a form of brief intervention in opportunistic settings such as hospitals or in general practice (Rollnick et al., 1993). It is our contention that alcohol and other drug problems should not be viewed simply as a "specialist" problem, as the majority of people experiencing potential or real problems will never be seen by an alcohol or other drug counselor or present to specialist services (Rollnick & Bell, 1991) An Australian Quality Assurance Project report on the management of alcohol problems (Mattick & Jarvis, 1993) concludes that brief interventions in primary health care settings are highly recommended, as these are the situations in which people experiencing alcohol or other drug problems are most likely to be detected.

Motivational interviewing is also considered an effective form of intervention in the broader health care setting as the majority of clients encountered are most likely to be in earlier stages of change, such as precontemplation or contemplation (Rollnick et al., 1992). Because of the opportunistic nature of the interaction (i.e., the client is not asking for help), there is also great potential for resistance to arise, particularly if the client senses that he/she is being labeled or being told what to do. Consequently, motivational interviewing is a recommended approach for health care workers faced with the task of addressing the issue of substance use.

Janis Mann is a 35-year-old woman who has been admitted to a hospital medical ward following referral by her general practitioner. Janis has a history of hypertension, and due to recent complaints of epigastric pain, it is also suspected that she suffers from a peptic ulcer. On admission to hospital, routine medical assessment was carried out, which included an estimate of alcohol and other drug use as well as a number of laboratory tests. Janis indicated that she drank wine on most days, up to one bottle, and occasionally took one or two temazepam to help her to sleep. The laboratory tests revealed abnormal liver function (elevated gamma GT) and high blood lipids. Janis's blood pressure on admission was 140/100. Because of the clinical picture, there was a need for further assessment of the client's alcohol intake and its possible contribution to her current health problems. However, the manner in which the issue of alcohol use was broached is important; the temptation to use the information from Janis's history and pathology results as evidence needs to be avoided.

It is also important to consider timing in this situation. It is better to choose a time when the client is feeling more comfortable and not in any physical distress. The way in which the alcohol or other substance use is raised can be a crucial first step. Rapport building is essential, which is one good reason for the client's primary nurse to address the issue, rather than bringing in a specialist alcohol and other drug counselor. The session begins with rapport building, through a discussion of general health and lifestyle issues, before the subject of alcohol use is raised.

NURSE: Good morning, Janis. How are you feeling today?

JANIS: A lot better, thanks. My stomach pains seem to be going. Although, I find it really hard to sleep in this bed. Sleeping's not easy at the best of times. I'll be glad to go home to the comfort of my own pillow. Hopefully, I'll be able to go home in the next couple of days.

NURSE: I'm sorry to hear you're not comfortable. I'll try to find you a better pillow. It sounds like you're looking forward to leaving the hospital.

JANIS: Yes. Actually, I'm really missing work, surprisingly enough!

NURSE: Tell me a bit about your work. What sort of work do you do?

JANIS: I'm an accountant with a large company. It's really busy, particularly at the moment as it's the end of the financial year. We've all been working really long hours lately to try to catch up with all the work.

NURSE: It sounds like your work is pretty stressful.

JANIS: Yes. It sure is! Sometimes I think about doing something else, perhaps even going solo. But most of the time I enjoy it and the people I work with. I don't really know what I'd do with myself if I stopped working.

NURSE: So even though work's stressful, you find it rewarding.

JANIS: Hmm . . . well, most of the time. Sometimes I find it too stressful. I find it really hard to unwind after working all day which leaves me too tired to enjoy the rest of my life.

NURSE: You find it difficult to relax at the end of the day. What sorts of things do you do to help you to relax?

JANIS: I like to go swimming or for a walk. I find exercise helps me to unwind, to forget about everything. But I haven't done much exercise lately. I just don't seem to have the time or the energy at the moment.

NURSE: So, exercise is a way of relaxing for you. What else do you do to help you to relax?

JANIS: I like to go out with friends. I have a couple of close friends I like to go out with; we have a few drinks and a few laughs. Most of them are as busy as I am though, so I haven't seen much of them lately. I tend to spend a lot of time at home alone recovering from the day's events.

NURSE: It sounds like you have very little time for pleasure and relaxation at the moment. What do you do when you're at home?

JANIS: Oh, I usually feel exhausted at the end of the day. I haven't been bothered cooking much lately. I usually buy something to eat on the way home. Sometimes I buy a bottle of wine; I find a couple of drinks help me to relax. I suppose my eating habits haven't helped my health very much.

[Commentary: Summary is a useful way to acknowledge what the client has said and to then raise the issue of alcohol use.]

NURSE: Janis, you have mentioned a number of things about your current lifestyle, such as the long hours you work and the stress you feel under. You spoke about having very little time or energy for relaxation or to enjoy times with your friends. You also mentioned your diet and your use of alcohol. I'd like to spend some more time discussing with you a number of things about your health and lifestyle, such as stress and diet. One of the things I'd also like to talk to you about is your use of alcohol.

JANIS: Oh? I know I've probably been drinking too much lately, but it's not really a problem. I only drink to help me to relax and I only ever drink wine.

[Commentary: One of the times when resistance is most likely to arise is when the subject of substance use is raised. Spending time building rapport will help to decrease the level of resistance between the client and the counselor. The next step is to "roll with resistance" and to choose a strategy that expresses a sense of empathy with the client, rather than getting stuck on the "problem" label. At this stage, it is possible to assume that the client is at a stage of either precontemplation or early contemplation. By choosing the strategy "Good Things and Less Good Things" to explore the two sides of drinking, the nurse will be able to further assess the client's readiness for change and decrease the level of resistance that comes up. It is important that the nurse does not draw on the "evidence" of the client's level of alcohol consumption from the admission records at this stage.]

NURSE: The purpose of our discussion is certainly not to label you with a problem; that's really not my concern. I'm more interested in your health and lifestyle and where your use of alcohol fits in.

JANIS: Well, as I said, I sometimes have a few glasses of wine to help me to relax after work. I don't get drunk at all, and I never drink anything except wine.

NURSE: Janis, you mentioned that one of the good things about having a drink is that it helps you to relax after work. What other things do you enjoy about having a drink?

JANIS: Drinking is a part of socializing and having a good time. As I said, I like to have a few drinks and a laugh with a couple of friends. We all do. I don't drink like I used to at parties or at the bar when I was at university. That's when I used to really drink.

NURSE: So you like to have a drink with friends, and you used to drink at the bar in your student days. Would you say you drink less now than when you were at university?

JANIS: Hmm . . . that's a difficult question. I probably drink more regularly now than in those days. We didn't have a lot of money to drink all the time at university. We used to have a big night out about once a fortnight. No . . . as I said I drink more regularly now, but I don't drink as much in one night, and I don't really get drunk any more, not like we all used to.

NURSE: Drinking is a part of your social times and you drink more regularly now than you did at university, as part of relaxing at home after work. What other good things are there about having a drink for you?

JANIS: Well, it helps me to sleep. I haven't been sleeping very well lately with work and other worries. I don't like to take sleeping tablets as I've heard that you can become dependent on them. I find I sleep better after a couple of glasses of wine.

NURSE: So wine helps you to sleep and wake up more rested.

JANIS: It certainly helps me to sleep but I don't always wake up rested. I'm not very good in the mornings; I usually take a while to get started. I've always been slow in the mornings.

NURSE: It sounds like, even though you have a good sleep after having a few drinks, you wake up feeling tired. You're not sure if the alcohol has anything to do with being slow to get started.

JANIS: Hmm . . . well there are some mornings when I feel worse, sometimes if I've been out late with friends. But I never miss work. This stay in hospital is the first time I've missed work for years.

[Commentary: Now that the client has raised a possible concern, a summary of the good things about alcohol use will help to direct the discussion toward the other side of alcohol use.]

NURSE: Janis, you have mentioned a number of good things about drinking, such as how it helps you to relax and unwind, and that alcohol sometimes helps you to sleep. You also mentioned sometimes you wake up feeling unrested, particularly if you have been out with friends. What other less good things are there about drinking for you? What are the things you don't quite like as much about alcohol?

JANIS: Well . . . I don't really like drinking too much if I'm out. I hate feeling out of control; not that I ever get really drunk these days. But sometimes I drink too much when I'm feeling nervous.

NURSE: So drinking helps you to feel comfortable when you feel nervous, but sometimes it can make you feel uncomfortable, out of control.

[Commentary: Deploying discrepancy.]

JANIS: Hmm . . . sounds silly really.

NURSE: What else don't you like about drinking?

JANIS: To tell you the truth, I'm pretty worried about my health, especially because I have ended up in the hospital. I've been waking up with pains, and as you know, the doctors seem to think I have an ulcer.

NURSE: You have some health concerns at the moment. The ulcer and the raised blood pressure may be due to the stress you are currently under and your diet.

[Commentary: Paradox is sometimes a useful strategy to elicit from clients their own arguments for change.]

JANIS: Yes. It probably is. But I can't help but wonder about my drinking. I know I feel less like eating after I've had a couple of glasses of wine.

NURSE: So, Janis, even though there are a number of good things about drinking, such as how it helps you to relax, on the other hand, you are wondering whether alcohol may be contributing to your current health problems.

JANIS: Hmmm . . .

NURSE: I wonder, would you like to spend some time talking about some of the health effects of alcohol?

JANIS: I have got some idea myself from what I've read in magazines and newspapers. I've heard alcohol's pretty bad for the liver. I also remember reading that women shouldn't have more than two drinks a day or something. But I always wondered where they got that figure from. Most of the people I know drink more than the recommended levels and they all seem OK to me.

NURSE: The suggested two drinks a day is a surprise to you.

JANIS: Well yes. I've had more than that for years and I haven't felt any effects. . . . Maybe not up until now . . . but I don't know whether I'm sick because of drinking. Do you think my drinking has caused me to be in hospital?

NURSE: Well, there is a possibility that alcohol, along with the other lifestyle factors you have mentioned such as stress and diet, may have contributed to you currently being unwell. The health literature does suggest that conditions such as high blood pressure and peptic ulcers can be related to alcohol consumption. You also mentioned the effects of alcohol on the liver, and sometimes this can show up on blood tests.

JANIS: What about my blood tests—What do they show?

NURSE: Your liver function tests do show some abnormalities.

JANIS: (*Silence*)

NURSE: Janis, you seem a bit surprised by the information I have given you. What do you make of it all?

JANIS: I suppose I have been hitting it pretty hard lately. It's not like I'm an alcoholic though. I stopped drinking altogether for three months last year.

NURSE: So you had a time alcohol free. Why was that?

JANIS: I suppose I was trying to live a healthier lifestyle. I took up swimming every day and ate better as well. But as work got busier, I just got back into the routine of missing meals and drinking again.

NURSE: It sounds like drinking tends to fit into a cycle, when your work gets busy.

JANIS: Hmm . . . but I can't see life getting any easier, not unless I stop working, and I can't see that happening for quite a few years yet. But I can't afford to get sick either. I don't know what to do.

NURSE: What do you think you would like to do?

[Commentary: The "expert–problem solver" trap was avoided. Although providing information and advice can be a useful next step, it can be premature.]

JANIS: Well . . . as I said, I enjoy drinking and I know I can stop if I want to. But I am worried how I might have affected my health. Should I stop drinking altogether? I don't know whether I want to do that.

[Commentary: Although the client appears to be moving toward the stage of determination or preparation for change, a state of heightened ambivalence is likely to be experienced by the client, particularly as she has reached a point of choice. It is therefore important not to push for a decision but to allow some time for the client to consider the information and possibilities.]

NURSE: Janis, we have talked quite a lot this morning about your health and lifestyle and where your use of alcohol fits in. It sounds like even though there are a few positive things about drinking, you can see that alcohol may be contributing to your health concerns. You also sound uncertain as to what you want to do. I can give you some literature to read about the effects of alcohol on health, as well as some further information about the recommended alcohol consumption that you mentioned. But it's really up to you what you do with that information. Perhaps we can spend some time later talking about the possibilities for you.

JANIS: OK. Thanks. You have given me a lot to think about.

NURSE: In the meantime, I'll see if I can find you a more comfortable pillow!

The case of Janis Mann is illustrative of the interaction between the principles, strategies, and microskills of motivational interviewing. An important factor in change in relation to health related problems is that the individual needs to be aware of his/her feelings about the health threat (Sutton, 1987). Allowing the client time to contemplate the information given and the factors that arose in the discussion is important at this stage.

CLIENT CHOICE IN GOAL SETTING

The next step in the process would involve strengthening any decision for change and negotiating possible treatment goals. In helping the client to take the next step, it is important not to fall into the trap of becoming too directive or overprescriptive, as this may push the client back into a state of contemplation. In essence, the process of deciding on plans for action involves eliciting from the client his/her own ideas and choices, with the therapist acting as a resource person. "The client is expected to make the final decision, rather than simply to agree with a decision already reached by the counselor" (Miller, 1983, p. 154). Studies have shown that a superior outcome is likely at 1 year after treatment if a client chooses his/her own options for change (Miller & Hester, 1986). The reality is that clients are in a position to know what best suits them and are ultimately responsible for carrying out any plans of action. An attitude of trust in the client's decision and abilities is essential to the change process. "It is important not to confuse what we hope or plan for clients (therapist goals), their hopes for themselves (client goals) and what they actually achieve (client outcomes)" (Miller, 1987, p. 134).

CONCLUSION

Motivational interviewing is a directive, client-centered counseling style for helping people resolve ambivalence about behavioral change. Although the ideas central to motivational interviewing have been developed within the context of working with people experiencing problems related to alcohol or other drug use, the model can be applicable to any situation involving the negotiation of behavioral change (Rollnick et al., 1993). Motivational interviewing, however, is not just about motivating change; it is about utilizing the client's own motivation.

Motivational interviewing is not a panacea. It is an approach that works with some people, some of the time, in some situations. It is proposed as an approach that is particularly useful for working with clients experiencing ambivalence or conflict about the behavior and the possibility of change. Motivational interviewing can be integrated within a broad range of strategies and can also be used to prepare a motivational foundation for other approaches (Miller & Rollnick, 1991). If the client is highly motivated to change, motivational interviewing might not be necessary, but the therapist may find it useful to reinforce the client's motivation by exploring what the client hopes to achieve by changing (Mattick & Jarvis, 1993).

Motivational interventions require a shift in counselor focus. It is about learning to take the passenger seat and trusting the client to take control of the steering wheel.

REFERENCES

Allsop, S., & Saunders, B. (1991). Reinforcing robust resolutions: Motivation in relapse prevention with severely dependent problem drinkers. In W. R. Miller & S. Rollnick, *Motivational interviewing: Preparing people to change addictive behavior.* New York: Guilford Press.

Brissett, D. (1988). Denial in alcoholism: A sociological interpretation. *Journal of Drug Issues, 18,* 385–402.

DiClemente, C. C. (1991). Motivational interviewing and the stages of change. In W. R. Miller & S. Rollnick, *Motivational interviewing: Preparing people to change addictive behavior.* New York: Guilford Press.

DiClemente, C. C., Prochaska, J. O., Fairhurst, S. K., Velicer, W., Velasquez, M., & Rossi, J. S. (1991). The process of smoking cessation: An analysis of the precontemplation, contemplation, and preparation stages of change. *Journal of Consulting and Clinical Psychology, 59,* 295–304.

Mattick, R. P., & Jarvis, T. (Eds.). (1993). *An outline for the management of alcohol problems: Quality assurance project.* Canberra: Australian Government Publishing Service.

Miller, W. R. (1983). Motivational interviewing with problem drinkers. *Behavioral Psychotherapy, 11,* 147–172.

Miller, W. R. (1985). Motivation for treatment: A review with special emphasis on alcoholism. *Psychological Bulletin, 98,* 84–107.

Miller, W. R. (1987). Motivation and treatment goals. *Drugs and Society, 1,* 133–151.

Miller, W. R., Benefield, R., & Tonigan, S. (1993). Enhancing motivation for change in problem drinking: A controlled comparison of two therapist styles. *Journal of Consulting and Clinical Psychology, 61,* 455–461.

Miller, W. R., & Hester, R. K. (1986). Matching problem drinkers with optimal treatments. In W. R. Miller & N. Heather (Eds.), *Treating addictive behaviors: Processes of change.* New York: Plenum Press.

Miller, W. R., & Rollnick, S. (1991). *Motivational interviewing: Preparing people to change addictive behavior.* New York: Guilford Press.

Miller, W. R., & Sovereign, R. C. (1989). The check-up: A model for early intervention in addictive behaviors. In T. Loberg, W. R. Miller, P. E. Nathan, & G. A. Marlatt (Eds.), *Addictive behaviors: Prevention and early intervention* (pp. 219–231). Amsterdam: Swets-Zeitlinger.

Patterson, G. R., & Forgatch, M. S. (1985). Therapist behavior as a determinant for client noncompliance: A paradox for the behavior modifier. *Journal of Consulting and Clinical Psychology, 53,* 846–851.

Prochaska, J. O., & DiClemente, C. C. (1986). Toward a comprehensive model of change. In W. R. Miller & N. Heather (Eds.), *Treating addictive behaviors: Processes of change.* New York: Plenum Press.

Rogers, C. R. (1961). *On becoming a person.* London: Constable.

Rollnick, S., & Bell, A. (1991). Brief motivational interviewing for use by the nonspecialist. In W. R. Miller & S. Rollnick, *Motivational interviewing: Preparing people to change addictive behavior.* New York: Guilford Press.

Rollnick, S., Heather, N., & Bell, A. (1992). Negotiating behavior change in medical settings: The development of brief motivational interviewing. *Journal of Mental Health, 1,* 25–37.

Rollnick, S., Kinnersley, P., & Stott, N. (1993). Methods of helping patients with behavior change. *British Medical Journal, 307,* 188–190.

Saunders, B., Wilkinson, C., & Allsop, S. (1991). Motivational intervention with heroin users attending a methadone clinic. In W. R. Miller & S. Rollnick, *Motivational interviewing: Preparing people to change addictive behavior.* New York: Guilford Press.

Sutton, S. (1987). Social-psychological approaches to understanding addictive behaviors: attitude–behavior and decision-making models. *British Journal of Addiction, 82,* 355–370.

CHAPTER 11

Integrating Psychotherapy and Pharmacotherapy in Substance Abuse Treatment

KATHLEEN M. CARROLL

Although this book focuses on the theory and technique of psychotherapeutic approaches commonly used in the treatment of substance abuse, medications also play a vital role in the treatment system. This chapter reviews (1) the differences in the roles and functions of psychotherapy and pharmacotherapy in the treatment system, (2) the potential advantages of the two forms of treatment alone and in combination, and (3) concentrating on the treatment of alcohol, opioid, and cocaine use (the forms of substance abuse for which pharmacotherapies have been developed and play a prominent role in the treatment system), the major pharmacologic approaches, with emphasis on studies evaluating how outcomes from pharmacologic treatments can be enhanced and extended by combining them with psychotherapy.[1]

THE ROLE OF PSYCHOTHERAPY

There are over 300 "brand names" of psychotherapy (Beutler, 1991), many of which have been applied to substance abusers. Most types of psychotherapy for substance abuse (including the ones described in the preceding chapters in this volume) address several common issues and tasks, despite often wide differences in theory, technique, strategies, and providers. Although different approaches and theories vary in the degree to which emphasis is placed on these common tasks, some attention to these issues is likely in any successful treatment (Rounsaville & Carroll, 1992). Moreover, it should be noted that most of these areas are specific to psychosocial treatments; that is, currently available pharmacotherapies would be expected to have little or no effect in the following areas.

Setting the Resolve to Stop

Rare is the substance abuser who seeks treatment without some degree of ambivalence regarding cessation of drug use. Even at the time of seeking treatment, which usually occurs only after drug-related problems have become severe, drug abusers usually can identify many ways in which they want or feel the need for drugs and have difficulty developing a clear picture of what life without drugs might be like (Rounsaville & Carroll, 1992). Moreover, given the substantial external pressures that may precipitate application for treatment, many patients are highly ambivalent about treatment itself. Ambivalence must be addressed if patients are to experience themselves as active participants in treatment; if the patient perceives treatment as wholly imposed upon him/her by external forces and does not have a clear sense of personal goals for treatment, it is likely that any form of treatment will be of limited usefulness. Motivationally based treatments, such as those described in this volume (Bell & Rollnick, Chapter 10) and elsewhere (Miller & Rollnick, 1991; Miller, Zweben, DiClemente, & Rychtarik, 1992), concentrate almost exclusively on strategies intended to bolster the patient's own motivational resources. However, review of the preceding chapters in this volume reveals that most approaches include, typically as part of assessment and preparation for treatment, some evaluation of what the patient stands to lose or gain through continued substance use as a means to enhance motivation for treatment and abstinence.

Teaching Coping Skills

Social learning theory posits that substance abuse may represent a means of coping with difficult situations, positive and negative affects, invitations by peers to use substances, and so on. By the time substance use is severe enough for treatment, it may represent the individual's single, overgeneralized means of coping with a variety of situations, settings, and states. If stable abstinence is to be achieved, treatment must help patients recognize the high-risk situations in which they are most likely to use substances and develop other, more effective means of coping with them. Although cognitive-behavioral approaches concentrate almost exclusively on skills training as a means of preventing relapse to substance use (e.g., Carroll, Rounsaville, & Keller, 1991; Kadden et al., 1992; Marlatt & Gordon, 1985; Monti, Abrams, Kadden, & Cooney, 1989), most treatment approaches touch on the relationship between high-risk situations and substance use to some extent.

Changing Reinforcement Contingencies

By the time they seek treatment, many substance abusers are spending the preponderance of their time on acquiring and using substances and recovering from their substance use, to the exclusion of other endeavors and rewards. The abuser may be estranged from friends and family and have few social contacts who do not use drugs. If the abuser is still working, employment often becomes only a means of acquiring money to buy drugs, and the fulfilling or challenging aspects of work have faded. Few other activities, such as hobbies, athletics, and involvement with community or church groups, can stand up to the demands of substance dependence. Typically, rewards available in daily life are narrowed progressively to those derived from drug use, and other diversions may be neither available nor perceived as enjoyable. When drug use is brought to a halt, its absence may leave the patient with the need to fill the time that was spent using drugs and to find rewards that can substitute for those derived from drug use. Thus, most psychosocial treatments encourage patients to identify and develop fulfilling alternatives to substance use, as exemplified by the community reinforcement approach (CRA) (Azrin, 1976), which stresses the development of alternate reinforcers and vocational rehabilitation.

Fostering Management of Painful Affects

The most commonly cited reasons for relapse are powerful negative affects (Marlatt & Gordon, 1985), and many psychodynamic clinicians (Khantzian, 1975; Wurmser, 1978) have suggested that failure of affect regulation is a central dynamic underlying the development of compulsive drug use. Moreover, the difficulty many substance abusers have in recognizing and articulating their affect states has been noted in several populations (Keller, Carroll, Nich, & Rounsaville, in press; Taylor, Parker, & Bagby, 1990). Thus, an important common task in substance abuse treatment is to help develop ways of coping with powerful dysphoric affects and to learn to recognize and identify the probable cause of these feelings. To foster the development of mastery over dysphoric affects, most psychotherapies include techniques for eliciting strong affects within a structured or protected therapeutic setting and then enhancing the patients' ability to identify, tolerate, and respond appropriately to them (Rounsaville & Carroll, 1992). Again, whereas psychodynamic treatments emphasize the role of affect in the treatment of cocaine abuse (Keller, Chapter 4, and Leeds & Morgenstern, Chapter 3, this volume), many forms of psychotherapy for substance abuse include a variety of techniques for coping with strong affect.

Improving Interpersonal Functioning and Enhancing Social Supports

A consistent finding in the literature on relapse to drug abuse is the protective influence of an adequate network of social supports (Longabaugh, Beattie, Noel, Stout, & Malloy, 1993; Marlatt & Gordon, 1985). Typical issues presented by drug abusers are loss of or damage to valued relationships occurring when using drugs was the principal priority, failure to achieve satisfactory relationships even prior to having initiated drug use, and inability to identify friends or intimates who are not themselves drug users (Rounsaville & Carroll, 1992). Many forms of treatment, including family therapy (McCrady & Epstein, Chapter 5, and McKay, Chapter 6, this volume), 12-Step facilitation (Wallace, Chapter 1, and Nowinski, Chapter 2, this volume), interpersonal therapy (Rounsaville, Gawin, & Kleber, 1985), and network therapy (Galanter, 1993), make building and maintaining a network of social supports for abstinence a central focus of therapy.

THE ROLE OF PHARMACOTHERAPY

Pharmacotherapies play a variety of roles in the treatment of substance abuse, which differ from those of psychotherapy in their course of action, time to effect, target symptoms, and durability of benefits (Elkin, Pilkonis, Docherty, & Sotsky, 1988a, 1988b). Typically, pharmacotherapies have a much more narrow application than do psychotherapies for substance abuse. That is, most psychotherapies are applicable in many types of treatment settings (e.g, inpatient, outpatient, and residential) and modalities (e.g., group, individual and family) and to a wide variety of populations. For example, a 12-Step, behavioral, psychodynamic, or motivational approach can be used regardless of whether the patient is an opiate, alcohol, cocaine, marijuana, or barbiturate user. On the other hand, most pharmacotherapies are applicable only to a single class of substance use and exert their effects over a comparatively narrow band of target symptoms. For example, methadone produces cross-tolerance for opioids but would not be expected to have a direct effect on cocaine use; disulfiram produces nausea after alcohol ingestion but not after ingestion of other substances. Roles and indications for pharmacotherapy in the treatment of substance dependence disorders include the following:

Detoxification

For those classes of substance that produce substantial withdrawal syndromes (e.g., alcohol, opioids, and sedative–hypnotics), medications are frequently needed to reduce or control often dangerous symptoms associated with withdrawal. Agents such as methadone, clonidine, naltrexone (Charney et al., 1986), and, more recently, buprenorphine (Kosten & Kleber, 1986), are typically used for the management of opioid withdrawal. Alcohol withdrawal is treated with barbiturates or long-acting benzodiazepines when appropriate. Withdrawal from barbiturates and sedative–hypnotics usually involves closely monitored, gradual reductions of the substance or the substitution of a cross-tolerant, longer-acting drug, often phenobarbitol (Alling, 1992). Because some of these agents, particularly the barbiturates, are likely to be misused by some patients, detoxification is usually done in an inpatient or closely controlled setting. Furthermore, the role of psychotherapy during acute detoxification is typically extremely limited due to the level of discomfort, agitation, and confusion the patient may experience. Therefore, the integration of psychotherapy and detoxification agents are not discussed in this chapter.

Stabilization and Maintenance

An example of the use of a medication for long-term stabilization of drug users is methadone maintenance for opioid addicts, a treatment strategy that involves the daily administration of a long-acting opioid (methadone) as a substitute for the illicit use of short-acting opioids (typically heroin). Methadone maintenance permits the patient to function normally without experiencing withdrawal symptoms, craving, or side effects, as a daily dose of methadone in a stabilized patient prevents withdrawal symptoms for 24 to 36 hours. Although methadone maintenance remains a somewhat controversial approach, the large body of research on methadone maintenance indicates that it fosters treatment retention, provides the opportunity to evaluate and treat other problems and disorders that often coexist with opioid dependence (e.g., medical, legal, and occupational problems), may reduce the risk of HIV (human immunodeficiency virus) infection through reducing intravenous drug use, and provides a level of stabilization that permits the inception of psychotherapy and other aspects of treatment (Lowinson, Marion, Joseph, & Dole, 1992).

Antagonist and Other Behaviorally Oriented Pharmacotherapies

Another pharmacologic strategy is the use of antagonist treatment, that is, the use of medications that block the effects of specific drugs. An example of this type of approach is naltrexone, an effective, long-acting opioid antagonist. Naltrexone is nonaddicting, does not have the reinforcing properties of opioids, has few side effects, and, most important, effectively blocks the effects of opioids. Therefore, naltrexone treatment represents a potent behavioral strategy: As opioid ingestion will not be reinforced while the patient is taking naltrexone, unreinforced opioid use allows extinction of relationships between conditioned drug cues and drug use. For example, a naltrexone-maintained patient, anticipating that opioid use will not result in desired drug effects, may be more likely to learn to live in a world full of drug cues and high-risk situations without resorting to drug use. A related, but quite different, behaviorally oriented pharmacologic approach is the use of antidipsotropics, the most commonly used agent being disulfiram, where anticipation of the unpleasant alcohol–disulfiram reaction represents a significant deterrent to alcohol use.

Treatment of Coexisting Disorders

An important role of medications in the treatment of substance use is as treatment for coexisting psychiatric disorders which may precede or play a role in the maintenance of drug dependence. The frequent co-occurrence of psychiatric disorders, particularly affective and anxiety disorders, with substance use disorders is well documented in a variety of populations and settings (Anthony & Helzer, 1990; Meyer, 1986; Regier et al., 1990; Rounsaville et al., 1991; Rounsaville, Weissman, Kleber, & Wilber, 1982). Given that psychiatric disorders often precede development of substance use disorders, several researchers and clinicians have hypothesized that individuals with primary psychiatric disorders may be attempting to self-medicate their psychiatric symptoms with drugs and alcohol (Khantzian, 1975; Wurmser, 1978). Thus, effective pharmacologic treatment of the underlying psychiatric disorder may improve not only the psychiatric disorder but also the perceived need for and therefore the use of illicit drugs and alcohol. Examples of this type of approach include the use of antidepressant treatment for depressed alcohol (Shaw, Donley, Morgan, & Robinson, 1975), opioid (Kleber, Weissman, Rounsaville, Prusoff, & Wilber, 1983; Nunes, Quitkin, Brady, & Stewart, 1991), and cocaine-dependent (Gawin & Kleber, 1986b; Ziedonis & Kosten, 1991) individuals, and methylphenidate treatment of cocaine abusers with residual symptoms of attention deficit hyperactivity disorder (Khantzian, Gawin, Kleber, & Riordan, 1984).

MODELS OF PSYCHOTHERAPY
AND PHARMACOTHERAPY, ALONE
AND IN COMBINATION

Psychotherapy as Sole Treatment

Some form of psychosocial treatment, be it psychotherapy, behavioral therapy, or counseling, is available in the vast majority of substance abuse treatment centers (Onken & Blaine, 1990) and is the backbone of substance abuse treatment. With the exception of opiate addiction, where the modal form of treatment is methadone maintenance, psychotherapy is likely to be the sole form of treatment received by substance-abusing patients. Research findings suggest that psychotherapy is sufficient and effective treatment for many cocaine (Carroll, Rounsaville, & Gawin, 1991; Rawson, Obert, McCann, & Mann, 1986) and alcohol (Holder, Longabaugh, Miller, & Rubonis, 1991; Miller & Hester, 1986) users; however, treatment of opioid dependence with a purely psychotherapeutic approach has typically had disappointing results (Rounsaville & Kleber, 1985).

Despite the ubiquity of psychotherapeutic treatments for substance abusers, there are several drawbacks of purely psychotherapeutic approaches. First, across different types of psychotherapeutic approaches, rates of dropout during treatment and relapse after treatment are high. Thus, there is ample opportunity for the adjunctive use of other forms of treatment, such as pharmacotherapy, to enhance treatment retention and outcome. Second, despite consistent findings pointing to the effectiveness of psychotherapy, no treatment has emerged from well-controlled clinical trials as superior to other psychotherapies (Luborsky, Singer, & Luborsky,

1975; Smith, Glass, & Miller, 1980). One interpretation of these findings is that different types of patients may respond differently to different treatments, and by aggregating outcome data across different types of patient characteristics, differential treatment outcomes may be obscured (Finney & Moos, 1986). Instead, by "matching" substance abusers to the particular type of treatment, or combination of treatment approaches, that best meets their needs and problems, outcome for treatment may be greatly enhanced.

Pharmacotherapy as Sole Treatment

Pharmacotherapeutic treatments for substance abusers delivered alone, without psychotherapeutic support, are usually seen as insufficient as a means of promoting stable abstinence in drug abusers. As described earlier, most pharmacotherapies are comparatively specific and narrow in their actions and may help to detoxify, stabilize, or treat coexisting disorders but are rarely considered 'complete treatments' in and of themselves. Furthermore, because few patients will persist or comply with a purely pharmacotherapeutic approach, pharmacotherapies delivered alone, without any supportive or relationship elements, are usually not considered feasible (Elkin et al., 1988b; Karasu, 1990).

Even when pharmacotherapy is seen as the primary treatment, as in the case of methadone maintenance, some form of psychosocial treatment is used to provide at least a minimal supportive structure within which pharmacotherapeutic treatment can be conducted effectively. Furthermore, it is widely recognized that drug effects can be enhanced or diminished with respect to the context in which treatment is delivered. That is, a drug administered in the context of a supportive clinician–patient relationship, with clear expectations of possible drug benefits and side effects, close monitoring of drug compliance, and encouragement for abstinence, is more likely to "warm up the drug" and enhance its effectiveness than a drug delivered without such elements (Klerman, 1963). Thus, even for primarily pharmacotherapeutic treatments, a psychotherapeutic component is almost always included to foster patients' retention in treatment and compliance with pharmacotherapy (Docherty, Marder, Van Kammen, & Siris, 1977; Elkin et al., 1988a).

Psychotherapy Combined with Pharmacotherapy

In this model, psychotherapy and pharmacotherapy are conceived of as having specific and unique therapeutic properties that, when combined, may interact in many ways. Uhlenhuth, Lipman, and Covi (1969) described four models for such effects: additive (in which the effect of combined treatment equals the sum of their individual effects), potentiation (in which the effect of the combined treatment is greater than the sum of the two individual treatment effects), inhibition (where the combined treatment is less than the sum of their individual effects), and reciprocation (where the effect of the combined treatments equals the individual effect of the more potent intervention). In general, research evidence suggests best outcomes for combined psychotherapy and pharmacotherapy, (i.e., additive or reciprocal effects) and has not supported inhibition of effects. There are several possible reasons for the benefits of combinations of psychotherapy and pharmacotherapy.

Improvement over a Broader Range of Symptoms

Extein and Bowers (1979) differentiate between state disorders, described as time-limited, autonomous, and unresponsive to psychotherapeutic intervention (such as acute psychoses or delirium), and trait disorders, defined as "dysfunctional qualities which individuals tend to develop and carry throughout life and which become manifest as predictable patterns for interaction and response to stress. Such patterns tend not to be responsive to medication but respond better to psychosocial treatment" (Extein & Bowers, 1979, pp. 690–691). State and trait disorders are conceived of as independent, but one or both may be present in any one individual.

Substance abuse can be conceived of as having attributes of both state and trait disorders in varying degrees among different abusers: Pharmacotherapy or other forms of medical intervention are generally essential when state disorders are present (e.g., withdrawal symptoms associated with physical dependence, drug intoxication, and drug-induced psychoses) that would not be expected to respond to psychotherapy. Similarly, psychotherapy may be indicated for those trait aspects of substance abuse upon which pharmacotherapy would be expected to have little impact (e.g., fostering motivation to reduce substance use, restricting availability of drugs and alcohol, avoiding situations associated with use, developing non-substance-using social supports) (Carroll, 1993).

Psychotherapy and pharmacotherapy work through different mechanisms and target different symptoms areas or problems. By increasing the number of symptom areas potentially improved through combining psychotherapy and pharmacotherapy, one may dramatically improve the "hit rate" among substance abusers, who typically present with heterogeneity of symptoms and problems (Carroll, 1993). Combining different forms of treatment that are likely to work on different sets of symptoms may be an effective strategy for treating the broad and variable range of symptoms and problems substance abusers face.

Patient–Treatment Matching

Even for the most effective forms of psychotherapy and pharma-cotherapy, treatment response is incomplete. That is, not all patients respond equally well to treatment and no single form of treatment is sufficient for all substance abusers. This is to be expected, as substance abusers are heterogeneous and may present at a variety of different levels of severity, psychopathology, psychosocial functioning, and social supports and stability. Combining psychotherapy and pharmacotherapy to meet the needs of a diverse patient population is thus an important strategy for enhancing the effectiveness of substance abuse treatment. For example, a substance abuser with a coexisting depressive disorder may be greatly helped by receiving antidepressant treatment for depressive symptoms combined with a psychotherapeutic approach that addressed substance use. Similarly, as pharmacologic treatment is usually indicated for more severe substance dependence, the addition of pharmacotherapy may increase treatment effectiveness for more severe, poor-prognosis patients. Thus, by combining psychotherapy and pharmacotherapy to "match" treatment to the needs of specific patients, treatment is more likely to be effective by meeting the needs of a diverse patient population.

Offsetting Drawbacks of the Other Treatment

Another advantage of evaluating combination treatments is that potential drawbacks associated with either treatment may be offset by the other. For example, the provision of support through psychotherapy may reduce the potential negative impact of side effects arising from most pharma-cotherapies. Behavioral therapies (e.g., contingency management) may be used to reinforce medication compliance for those pharmacotherapies where compliance is poor. On the other hand, stabilization or instillation of hope through administration of a drug may support continuing participation in treatment during the early stages when a developing therapeutic alliance may be fragile. In some cases, stabilization of substance abusers through the use of maintenance treatments such as methadone is necessary to provide the conditions under which effective psychotherapy may be undertaken.

PHARMACOTHERAPY OF ALCOHOL DEPENDENCE

Disulfiram

The most commonly used pharmacologic adjunct for the treatment of alcohol dependence and abuse is disulfiram (Antabuse). Disulfiram interferes with the normal metabolism of alcohol, which results in an accumulation of acetaldehyde, and hence drinking following ingestion of disulfiram results in an intense physiological reaction, characterized by flushing, rapid or irregular heartbeat, dizziness, nausea, and headache (Fuller, 1989). Thus, disulfiram treatment is intended to work as a deterrent to drinking.

Despite the sustained popularity and widespread use of disulfiram, a large-scale, well-controlled multicenter randomized clinical trial reported that disulfiram was no more effective than inactive doses of disulfiram or no medication in terms of rates of abstinence, time to first drink, unemployment, or social stability (Fuller et al., 1986). However, for subjects who did drink, disulfiram treatment was associated with significantly fewer total drinking days. Moreover, rates of compliance with disulfiram in the study were low (20% of all subjects), although abstinence rates were high (43%) among compliant subjects. This study illustrates several important problems with the use of disulfiram: (1) Compliance is a major problem, and (2) many patients are unwilling to take disulfiram, as 62% of those eligible for the study refused to participate.

Thus, several studies have evaluated the effectiveness of psychotherapy as a strategy to improve retention and compliance with disulfiram. One of the most effective strategies may be disulfiram contracts, where the patient's spouse or significant other agrees to observe the patient take disulfiram each day and reward the patient for compliance with disulfiram (O'Farrell & Bayog, 1986). Azrin, Sisson, Meyers, and Godley (1982) reported positive and durable results from a randomized clinical trial comparing unmonitored disulfiram to disulfiram contracts, where disulfiram ingestion was monitored by the patient's spouse or administered as part of a multifaceted behavioral program (CRA). The CRA, developed by Hunt and Azrin (1973), is a broad-spectrum approach (incorporating skills training, behavioral family therapy, and job-finding training) that also includes a disulfiram component. At 6-month follow-up, the traditionally treated group reported over 50% drinking days, whereas the group that received CRA was almost completely abstinent. The effectiveness of CRA illustrates how psychotherapy can be integrated with pharmacotherapy to produce better outcomes than either treatment alone.

Naltrexone

Recent clinical findings suggest the promise of naltrexone for the treatment of alcohol dependence. The application of naltrexone, an opioid antagonist, to the treatment of alcoholism derives from findings that indicate that naltrexone reduces alcohol consumption in animals (Volpicelli, Davis, & Olgin, 1986) and alcohol craving and use in humans (Volpicelli et al., 1990). In a double-blind randomized clinical trial of outpatient alcoholics, O'Malley et al. (1992) found that naltrexone was significantly better than placebo in terms of rates of abstinence, drinking days, relapse, and severity of alcohol-related problems. However, it is important to note that naltrexone effects differed with respect to the type of psychotherapy the patient received: Overall, highest rates of abstinence were found when the patient received naltrexone plus a supportive clinical management psychotherapy condition that encouraged complete abstinence from alcohol and other substances. However, for patients who drank, the combination of a cognitive-behavioral coping skills approach and naltrexone was superior in terms of rates of relapse and drinks per occasion. This study illustrates not only the promise of naltrexone in the treatment of alcohol dependence but also that the psychotherapeutic context in which medications are delivered can have a powerful impact on treatment outcomes.

PHARMACOTHERAPY OF OPIOID DEPENDENCE

Methadone Maintenance

The inception of methadone maintenance treatment revolutionized the treatment of opioid addiction as it displayed the previously unseen ability to keep addicts in treatment and to reduce their illicit opioid use, outcomes with which nonpharmacologic treatments had fared comparatively poorly (Brill, 1977; Nyswander, Winick, Bernstein, Brill, & Kaufer, 1958; O'Malley, Anderson, & Lazare, 1972). Beyond its ability to retain opioid addicts in treatment and help control opioid use, methadone maintenance also may reduce risk of HIV infection by reducing intravenous drug use (Ball, Lange, Myers, & Friedman, 1988), and provide the opportunity to evaluate and treat concurrent disorders including medical problems, family, and psychiatric problems (Lowinson et al., 1992). The bulk of the large body of literature on the effectiveness of methadone maintenance points to the success of methadone maintenance in retaining opioid addicts in treatment and reducing their illicit opioid use and illegal activity

(Ball & Ross, 1991). However, there is a great deal of variability in the success across different methadone maintenance programs, which is likely to be the result of variability in delivery of adequate dosing of methadone as well as variability in provision and quality of psychosocial services (Ball & Ross, 1991; Corty & Ball, 1987). As Kleber (1977) has pointed out, "Methadone is a drug, not a treatment."

Moreover, there are several problems with methadone maintenance, including illicit diversion of take-home methadone doses, difficulties with detoxification from methadone maintenance to a drug-free state, and the abuse of other substances, particularly alcohol and cocaine, among methadone-maintained subjects (Kosten, 1992a). Thus, psychosocial treatments have been evaluated for their ability to address these drawbacks of methadone maintenance, as well as to enhance and extend the benefits of methadone maintenance. Two major types of psychosocial treatments, behavioral treatments and psychotherapy or counseling, have been evaluated as strategies to enhance and extend the benefits of methadone maintenance treatment.

Behavioral Strategies

McLellan, Childress, and colleagues (Childress, McLellan, & O'Brien, 1984; McLellan, Childress, Ehrman, & O'Brien, 1986) have evaluated the effectiveness of a procedure intended to reduce conditioned responses to stimuli associated with drugs through repeated exposure to such stimuli. Fifty-six methadone-maintained addicts were randomly assigned to one of three groups: a combination group, which received cognitive-behavioral therapy, extinction, and relaxation training (CE); a group that received cognitive-behavioral therapy and relaxation training without extinction (CT); and a group that received drug counseling alone. The group that received extinction (CE) evidenced reduction in subjective craving for opiates with repeated extinction sections. However, although both groups that received psychotherapy (CE and CT) had significantly better 6-month outcomes than the group that received drug counseling alone, the two psychotherapy groups were not significantly different from each other, suggesting that the extinction procedure added no greater relative benefit over the cognitive therapy plus relaxation training. The authors suggested a number of factors that may have undercut the power of the outpatient extinction procedure, including the need for use of individualized stimuli and to consider modifying variables such as affect or cognitive set, and further concluded that the extinction procedure is best suited to drug-free patients.

Several studies have evaluated the use of contingency management to reduce the use of illicit drugs in addicts who are maintained on methadone. Stitzer, McCaul, Bigelow, and Liebson (1984) evaluated the use of methadone dose increases as reinforcement for drug-free urines by comparing the effect of methadone dose increases that were contingent upon drug-free urines to blind dose increases in seven methadone-maintained patients who evidenced persistent illicit opiate use while on methadone maintenance. Over an 8-week period, both groups reduced opiate use from baseline levels; however, the contingent dose increase was significantly superior to the blind dose increase in producing drug-free urines (74% vs. 48% opiate-free urines). This finding could not be attributed to the effect of dose increases producing methadone satiation, which could reduce use of illicit opiates, as subjects in the blind dose condition actually received higher doses of methadone than those in the contingent dose condition. Similarly, Noliman and Crowley (1988) reported in an uncontrolled study that contingency management of methadone dose in 14 "especially problematic" patients resulted in fewer drug-positive urine samples, although the effectiveness of contingency management appeared to diminish with time. Stitzer, Bickel, Bigelow, and Liebson (1986) have also directly compared the effects of positive versus negative contingency management in methadone maintenance treatment. Twenty polydrug-abusing methadone-maintained addicts were randomly assigned to either positive incentives (increased methadone dose for drug-free urines) or negative incentives (decreased dose for positive urines). With respect to baseline levels (87% drug-positive urines), subjects in both incentive groups showed marked improvement in percentage of drug-free urines (40–50% drug-free) which as sustained during the 18 weeks the incentive program was in effect. Although significant differences between the positive and negative contingency conditions were not found, and in both conditions about half the subjects were identified as successes and the other half as failures, subjects identified as failures in the negative contingency condition were much more likely to leave treatment than were the failures of the positive contingency condition.

In a similar design, Iguchi, Stitzer, Bigelow, and Liebson (1988) recently reported on a controlled study in which 16 polydrug-abusing methadone maintenance patients were randomly assigned to either a group with positive contingencies only (medication take-home privileges for drug-free urines) or a combined positive–aversive contingency group (addition to the former condition of reduction in methadone dose for two or more drug-positive urines in a single week). Over a 20-week intervention period, both groups evidenced significant improvement over baseline levels in number of drug-free urines, but differences between the two treatment groups were not found. However, subjects in the combined positive–aversive treatment group were more likely to drop out of treatment than those in the positive contingency group.

Glosser (1983) evaluated use of a token economy system within a methadone maintenance program, which combined both positive reinforcement (methadone dose increases) and aversive consequences (dose decreases) to reduce illicit drug use among methadone maintenance clients. In an uncontrolled study, 31 subjects in a standard full-service methadone maintenance program were compared to 97 in the token economy system. Subjects in the experimental group could receive a maximum daily methadone dose by redemption of a token. Tokens were earned through clean urines, attendance at counseling sessions, and promptness for daily methadone dose. Subjects could raise their doses by earning extra tokens. If tokens were not received, methadone dose would drop, with dosages fluctuating by a maximum of 4 mg per day. Comparison after 6 months of treatment revealed less attrition and significantly lower rates of drug-positive urines for subjects in the token economy system with respect to subjects in the regular full-service methadone program.

Dolan, Black, Penk, Robinowitz, and DeFord, (1985) reported on an uncontrolled study of 21 methadone-maintained addicts who were identified as treatment failures on the basis of their producing opiate-positive urines at least 50% of the time during a 60-day baseline period. These subjects were given treatment contracts that stipulated immediate detoxification for a single drug-positive urine. Mixed results were obtained: half the subjects (11/21) abstained from illicit drug use during the 30-day contract, with increases to 17% drug-positive urines during a 60-day follow-up. The remainder of the subjects (10/21) showed no marked decrease in drug use while the contract was in effect and were detoxified. The authors noted that the 10 "violators" of the contract had significantly more drug-positive urines during baseline than did the subjects who were able to comply, possibly indicating greater pretreatment ability of the "compliers" to control their use of illicit substances.

Negative contingency contracts, in which addicts who continue to use drugs are detoxified and withdrawn from treatment, are often criticized on the basis that they are countertherapeutic, denying treatment to addicts who are not helped by methadone to reduce their drug use and are therefore in greatest need of treatment. In response to such criticisms, McCarthy and Borders (1985) evaluated a more flexible negative contingency program which limited the number of positive urines methadone-maintained addicts could produce before they would be detoxified. Sixty-nine consecutive admissions to a full-service methadone maintenance program were randomly assigned to either a structured or an unstructured treatment program. In the structured program, subjects were told they would be detoxified from methadone if they had 4 consecutive months during which they used drugs at any point, which required the patient to be drug-free for at least 1 out of every 4 months. In the unstructured treatment, subjects were not informed of any limit on illicit drug use. Outcomes included program retention and results of urinalyses, emotional state (assessed by the General Well-Being Scale), and the Social Adjustment Scale. Results were assessed over a 12-month period. The structured group achieved significantly more drug-free months than did the unstructured group, even after correcting for the six subjects in the structured condition who were discharged for drug use. In addition, the structured condition had significantly better retention for the full 12 months than did the unstructured treatment (53% vs. 30%), and significant improvements for the structured group over the unstructured group were also obtained for the General Well-Being Scale and the Social Adjustment Scale. McCarthy and Borders (1985) suggested that this study provides evidence that limit setting and use of flexible negative contingencies do not necessarily lead to poor retention.

Although contingency management procedures seem promising in modifying traditionally intractable and difficult problems in methadone maintenance programs, particularly continued illicit drug use among clients, there are indications that the positive effects of contingency management procedures may diminish over time and sometimes return to baseline levels when the behavioral intervention is no longer in effect (Stitzer et al., 1984; Noliman & Crowley, 1988). This may suggest that in methadone maintenance treatment, specific reinforcers may grow weaker with time and/or be replaced by other reinforcers. Studies evaluating the change in strength or preference of reinforcers over time within methadone maintenance programs are needed. For example, for clients entering a methadone program from the street, contingency payments or dose increases may be highly motivating, whereas for clients who have been stabilized and are working and who may have less free time, other reinforcers, such as take-home doses or permission to omit counseling sessions, may be more attractive later in treatment. Although contingency management procedures may prove effective only over short periods, they may still be valuable in that they may provide an interruption in illicit drug use (or other undesirable behaviors), which may serve as an opportunity for other interventions to take effect.

Another important issue is that the existing studies evaluating behavioral interventions in the context of methadone maintenance programs tend not to provide data on whether behavioral interventions affect other, more broadly defined, indicators of outcome (e.g., criminality and psychiatric symptomatology). Indeed, the narrow focus of behavioral interventions suggests that broader improvements would not occur. Nor do the studies reviewed provide information on which types of clients may respond maximally to behavioral interventions, although a number of studies reviewed noted that there was evidence of substantial interindividual variability in response to behavioral interventions (Grabowski et al., 1979; Stitzer et al., 1986). This type of research is particularly critical as these studies usually involved small numbers of refractory clients who had not responded well to traditional methadone maintenance programs.

Psychotherapeutic Strategies

Two major outcome studies have been carried out using largely parallel study designs to evaluate the addition of professional psychotherapy services in a methadone maintenance program. One of the studies was carried out jointly by the University of Pennsylvania and the Veterans Administration Medical Center of Philadelphia (Woody et al., 1983), and the other was conducted at the Yale University Department of Psychiatry Substance Abuse Treatment Unit in New Haven (Rounsaville, Glazer, Wilber, Weissman, & Kleber, 1983). Although the studies were conducted separately, their largely parallel designs, the sophistication of the research techniques, and their contrasting findings point to issues that may be important in maximizing psychotherapy services in methadone maintenance programs. Both studies included the following desirable research standards, many of which were absent in previous studies evaluating psychotherapy in the context of methadone maintenance programs: (1) adequate control groups; (2) randomized treatment assignment; (3) adequate sample size; (4) use of independent evaluaters who were blind to the treatment received; (5) use of well-defined, relevant, and adequately encompassing outcome measures; (6) homogeneous client groups; and (7) specification of the treatment being offered.

Philadelphia Study. An opportunity to receive a 6-month course of professional psychotherapy in addition to paraprofessional counseling was offered to opiate addicts who were beginning a new treatment episode on a methadone maintenance program (Woody et al., 1983). The treatments offered were drug counseling alone (DC), counseling plus supportive–expressive psychotherapy (SE), or counseling plus cognitive-behavioral psychotherapy (CB). Sixty percent of patients meeting the study criteria expressed an interest in the psychotherapy program and 60% of these actually became engaged. One hundred ten subjects completed the study intake procedure, were randomly assigned to one of the three treatment conditions, and kept three or more appointments within the first 6 weeks of the project.

A variety of outcome measures showed that patients in all three treatment groups improved. Patients receiving the additional psychotherapies improved in more areas and to a greater degree than those who received counseling alone. The specific improvements seen appear to be related to the focus of the therapy used, although the two psychotherapy groups did not differ from each other. Patients with antisocial personality disorder did not benefit significantly from therapy, but those with depression did (Woody, McLellan, Luborsky, & O'Brien, 1985). Patients with high levels of psychiatric symptoms made many significant gains if they received additional therapy but improved only in drug use if they received counseling alone. Patients in all three treatment groups having low levels of psychiatric symptoms improved significantly in many areas (Woody et al., 1984). Results from a 12-month follow-up of 93 (78% of the original sample of 120) subjects in this study found that the two psychotherapy groups showed sustained and continued improvements over the group that received drug counseling alone, with the drug-counseling group evidencing some attrition in gains (Woody, McLellan, Luborsky, & O'Brien, 1987).

New Haven Study. The New Haven study (Rounsaville et al., 1983) was a clinical trial designed to evaluate the efficacy of short-term interpersonal psychotherapy (IPT) as treatment for psychiatric disorders in methadone-maintained opiate addicts who had been maintained on methadone for a minimum of 3 months and who were found to have a current psychiatric disorder (e.g., depression). Seventy-two subjects were randomly assigned to one of two treatment conditions, both of which lasted 6 months: (1) IPT, consisting of 1 hour per week of individual psychotherapy with a psychiatrist or psychologist, and (2) low-contact treatment, consisting of one 20-minute meeting per month in which symptoms and social functioning were reviewed.

The first major finding was the difficulty in recruiting and engaging subjects in the study. Despite high rates of psychopathology such as depression among treated opiate addicts, less than 5% of the methadone clinic population participated in the study at any given time. Besides the low recruitment rate, there was a high dropout rate, with only 38% completing 6 months of treatment in the IPT condition and 54% completing the low-contact condition. The second major finding was the similarity of outcomes in addicts receiving the two study treatments. Out of 12 major outcome measures, significant differences between IPT and low-contact groups were detected on only two scales; however, in many of the outcome areas, subjects in both treatment conditions were shown to have attained significant clinical improvement during the 6-month period. The lack of difference in treatment outcomes did not change if the samples were divided into those with high and low levels of depressive symptoms.

Comparison of differences in the effectiveness of psychotherapy between the New Haven and Philadelphia studies also suggests several strategies for effectively integrating psychotherapy into methadone maintenance programs. These include (1) making sure the therapists are well integrated and are seen as part of the staff of the methadone program, (2) closely attending to patient compliance with psychotherapy sessions, (3) initiating psychotherapy soon after program entry and soon after problems arise, rather than waiting until patients become refractory and continued illicit drug use in entrenched, and (4) offering psychotherapy primarily to patients with comparatively severe psychological problems and who are more likely to benefit from it (Rounsaville et al., 1983).

The Importance of Psychosocial Services in Methadone Maintenance Programs

The New Haven and Philadelphia studies indicate that outcomes from methadone maintenance treatment can be enhanced and extended by integrating the treatment with psycotherapy. More recently, the importance of psychosocial treatments in the context of methadone was impressively demonstrated by McLellan, Arndt, Metzger, Woody, and O'Brien (1993). Ninety-two opiate addicts were randomly assigned to receive (1) methadone maintenance alone, without psychosocial services, (2) methadone maintenance with standard services, which included regular meetings with a counselor, and (3) enhanced methadone maintenance, which included regular counseling plus on-site medical/psychiatric, employment, and family therapy, in a 24-week trial. Although some patients did reasonably well in the methadone-alone condition, 69% of this group had to be transferred out of this condition within 3 months of the study's inception because their substance use did not improve or even worsened, or because they experienced significant medical or psychiatric problems, which required a more intensive level of care. In terms of drug use and psychosocial outcomes, best outcomes were seen in the enhanced methadone maintenance condition, with intermediate outcomes for the standard methadone services condition and poorest outcomes for the methadone-alone condition. Results from this study suggest that although (1) methadone maintenance treatment has powerful effects in terms of keeping addicts in treatment and making them available for psychosocial treatments, and (2) minimal pharmacologic treatment may be sufficient for a small subgroup of substance abusers, the large majority of patients will not benefit from a pharmacologic approach alone and better outcomes are closely associated with higher levels of psychosocial treatments.

Naltrexone/Antagonist Treatment

Opioid antagonist treatment (naltrexone) offers many advantages over methadone maintenance: (1) It is nonaddicting and can be prescribed without concerns about diversion, (2) it has a benign side effect profile, and (3) it may be less costly, in terms of demands on professional time and of patient time, than the daily or near-daily clinic visits required for methadone maintenance (Rounsaville, 1995). Most important are behavioral aspects of the treatment, as unreinforced opiate use allows extinction of relationships between cues and drug use. Although naltrexone treatment is likely to be attractive only to a minority of opioid addicts (Greenstein, Arndt, McClellan, O'Brien, & Evans, 1984), naltrexone's unique properties make it an important alternative to methadone maintenance.

However, naltrexone has not, despite its many advantages, fulfilled its promise. Naltrexone treatment programs remain comparatively rare and underutilized in comparison to methadone maintenance programs (Rounsaville, 1995). This is in large part due to problems with retention, particularly during the induction phase, where on average 40% of patients drop out during the first month of treatment and 60% drop out by 3 months (Greenstein, Fudala, & O'Brien, 1992). Naltrexone treatment has other disadvantages compared with methadone, including (1) discomfort associated with detoxification and protracted withdrawal symptoms, (2) lack of negative consequences for abrupt discontinuation, and (3) no reinforcement for ingestion, all of which may lead to inconsistent compliance with naltrexone treatment and high rates of attrition.

Preliminary evaluations of behavioral and psychotherapeutic interventions targeted to address naltrexone's weaknesses were encouraging. Meyer, Mirin, Altman, and McNamee (1976), evaluated contingency payments as reinforcements for naltrexone consumption in addicts completing an inpatient detoxification program. In an uncontrolled study, subjects were paid $1 each day for ingesting naltrexone. After 1 month, the paid addicts had a 72% success rate.

In another uncontrolled study, Grabowski et al. (1979) evaluated the use of a variety of schedules of contingency payments to encourage naltrexone ingestion in nine subjects. In contrast to 126 patients who were paid for procedures not contingent upon adherence to naltrexone treatment, the nine subjects receiving contingent payments showed improved treatment retention. Clinic attendance, as well as naltrexone ingestion, was significantly improved when payment was response-based (payments for naltrexone ingestion) rather than time-based (payments for clinic attendance only). Although continuous reinforcement schedules (payments for each naltrexone ingestion) resulted in fewer complaints by subjects than variable reinforcement (VR) schedules (in which payments for naltrexone ingestion were irregularly spaced), the VR payment schedule generated consistent program attendance and naltrexone ingestion and was less cumbersome and difficult to implement programmatically. Furthermore, the effectiveness of the contingency payments diminished over the 20-week course of treatment. Grabowski et al. (1979) also found considerable variability in program attendance, even among subjects on same schedule of reinforcement, suggesting there may be substantial interindividual variability in treatment response among subjects in behavioral programs.

Callahan and colleagues (1980) reported on the evaluation of naltrexone alone or with behavior therapy. One hundred sixty-seven clients were randomly assigned to one of three treatments: naltrexone alone, naltrexone plus behavioral therapy, or behavioral therapy alone. Attrition was substantial in the behavioral-therapy-alone cell and this was discontinued. Only 37 of 104 (36%) patients initially assigned to either naltrexone or naltrexone plus behavioral therapy completed a pretreatment period during which they were detoxified and "earned" active status in the program, suggesting that substantial self-selection took place during this period. Behavioral therapy included contingency contracting, relaxation training, covert sensitization, self-monitoring, role playing, and social skills training. Outcomes included treatment retention, naltrexone ingestion, and urinalysis results and were analyzed for three phases: (1) inception (months 1–7), (2) intermediate (months 8–14), and (3) maintenance (months 15–21). Naltrexone ingestion and treatment retention were significantly higher for clients in the behavioral therapy group during the induction phase, but these differences did not obtain for the intermediate or maintenance phases. Subjects in the naltrexone-alone group reported significantly more naltrexone side effects than did subjects in the behavioral therapy group. The percentage of clean urines did not differ between groups during the 21-month protocol. However, the greater treatment attrition during the earlier phases of treatment in the naltrexone-alone group could produce bias against finding continued superiority in the behavioral therapy group, as only "good prognosis" patients in each group remained in treatment beyond the induction phase.

Citing that few addicts test naltrexone by injecting heroin (Kleber, 1973; Kleber et al., 1974), O'Brien, Greenstein, Ternes, McLellan, and Grabowski (1980) postulated that many addicts may relapse following cessation of naltrexone therapy through exposure to cues previously paired with drug use, particularly self-injection rituals. In an attempt to extinguish conditioned cues associated with drug preparation and self-injection rituals in addicts taking naltrexone, O'Brien et al. (1980) found that subjects who underwent an extinction procedure in which subjects' self-injections were followed by hydromorphine had slightly better outcome at 6 months, as measured by treatment retention, employment, arrest, and positive urines, than did subjects who did not undergo an extinction procedure. Subjects whose self-injections were followed by saline, however, found this procedure aversive and had poorer outcomes than did subjects who did not undergo the extinction procedure.

Family therapy and counseling have also been used to enhance retention in naltrexone programs. For example, in a nonrandomized study of multiple family therapy, Anton, Hogan, Jalali, Riordan, and Kleber (1981) demonstrated that during the first month of naltrexone therapy, addicts in family therapy had a much significantly lower dropout rate compared to those not in family therapy (92% vs. 62%).

To evaluate the value of counseling in naltrexone induction and stabilization, Resnick, Washton, and Stone-Washton (1981) randomly assigned addicts to intensive weekly individual counseling (described as supportive and insight-oriented techniques) or to low-intervention "case management" before outpatient detoxification. Within their sample, addicts were stratified into street addicts and post-methadone maintenance groups. Sixty-three percent of the addicts completed induction with counseling as compared to 48% without counseling, a nonsignificant difference. However, when the sample was analyzed by subjects' treatment history, the street addicts clearly benefited from the counseling—45% successful versus 12% in the noncounseled group, whereas among the postmethadone patients the counseled group showed no increased success on naltrexone. Thus, counseling appears to be helpful for the street addict but not for the post-methadone client. At 1 month, 77% were still in treatment in the counseling group, significantly more than the 33% of those in the noncounseled group who remained in treatment. Again, when the addicts were stratified by street versus postmethadone, overall program retention was significantly better for the street addicts with counseling than for those without, but presence or absence of counseling was not significant for retention in postmethadone addicts.

PHARMACOTHERAPY OF COCAINE DEPENDENCE

Compared with the long history of treatment outcome research for alcohol and opioid dependence, the treatment of cocaine dependence is in its infancy. Although a wide variety of pharmacologic approaches have recently been tried as treatment for cocaine abuse (Kosten, 1992a), none, as yet, have consistently demonstrated their effectiveness relative to placebo in keeping cocaine abusers in treatment or reducing their cocaine use (Meyer, 1992). Thus, the literature on the effectiveness of integrating pharmacologic and psychotherapeutic treatments for cocaine dependence is extremely limited.

Two major types of pharmacologic approaches have been evaluated for cocaine abusers. First, one set of approaches assumes a neurochemical basis for periods of high-intensity cocaine use "binges" and the "crashes" that follow periods of high-intensity use, which are thought to be primarily mediated by dopaminergic systems. This has led to the evaluation of dopaminergic agents (e.g., amantadine, bromocriptine, mazindol, and pergolide) as strategies to reduce cocaine craving and cocaine withdrawal symptoms (Kosten, 1992b). Second, antidepressants (particularly desipramine) have been evaluated because they may reverse cocaine-induced supersensitivity of dopamine receptors, and hence cocaine craving and use, in the general populations of cocaine abusers (Gawin et al., 1989). In addition, antidepressants have also been used as a strategy to treat the minority of cocaine abusers who may be primary depressives attempting to self-medicate their depressive symptoms with cocaine (Gawin & Kleber, 1986a; Ziedonis & Kosten, 1991).

There are very few data on the effectiveness of integrating psychotherapy and pharmacotherapy as treatment for cocaine abuse. Moreover, because the efficacy of pharmacologic aspects of treatments has not been of primary interest in studies evaluating pharamcologic approaches, psychosocial components of treatment have not been specified or implemented according to current standards of psychotherapy research. That is, little attention is usually given to treatment manuals, training and selection of appropriate therapists, monitoring therapist delivery of treatment, or patient compliance with psychosocial aspects of treatment. Lack of specification of pharmacologic aspects of treatment in pharmacotherapy trials with cocaine abusers has several implications. First, the role or effectiveness of psychosocial treatments in enhancing treatment retention, medication compliance, or reduction of drug use cannot be examined in such studies. Second, because variations in the "psychosocial ground" against which pharmacologic agents are evaluated may result in variations in their effectiveness (Klerman, 1975) across different studies, lack of specification of psychosocial treatments in pharmacologic treatments of cocaine dependence may impede meaningful comparison of pharmacologic effects across studies (Carroll, 1993). Third, specification of psychosocial treatments, which requires training of appropriate therapists and monitoring their delivery of treatment, may enhance their effectiveness (Rounsaville, Foley, & Weissman, 1988). Thus, studies that have not done so may underestimate the potential effectiveness of psychosocial treatments for cocaine abusers.

One study has attempted to evaluate the effects of pharmacotherapy and psychotherapy, alone and in combination, as treatment for cocaine abusers. We conducted a randomized controlled clinical trial of psychotherapy (cognitive-behavioral relapse prevention) and pharmacotherapy (desipramine), in a 2 × 2 design, for ambulatory cocaine abusers (Carroll et al., 1994). After a 12-week course of psychotherapy and pharmacotherapy, all groups showed significant reduction in cocaine use and improvements in psychosocial functioning. Desipramine reduced cocaine use significantly during the first month of treatment but did not have an effect on cocaine use over the full 12-week trial (Carroll, Rounsaville, Nich, Gordon, & Gawin, 1995). There was no evidence for the superiority of the desipramine plus relapse prevention combination in most outcomes. However, significant interactions for psychotherapy by cocaine severity were found, where relapse prevention treatment was associated with improved outcomes for higher-severity cocaine users as measured by retention, longer periods of consecutive abstinence, and a higher percentage of cocaine-free urines compared with clinical management. Preliminary results also indicate that desipramine appeared to be an effective antidepressant in this sample in that depressed subjects treated with desipramine experienced a significant reduction in depressive symptoms compared to placebo-treated depressed subjects. However, desipramine was not associated with significant improvements in cocaine use among either the depressed or the euthymic subsamples. There were, however, consistent significant interactions for depression and psychotherapy, in that depressed subjects treated with relapse prevention remained in treatment significantly longer than did depressed subjects treated with clinical management and maintained longer periods of consecutive abstinence during treatment (Carroll, Nich, & Rounsaville, 1995).

Findings from this study underline the significance of heterogeneity among cocaine abusers, which will require development of specialized treatments for clinically distinct subgroups of cocaine abusers rather than one simple pharmacologic or psychotherapeutic approach for all patients. For example, "state" aspects of cocaine dependence may indicate a need for specialized pharmacologic adjuncts, such as antidepressant treatments for depressed cocaine abusers, disulfiram treatment for alcoholic cocaine abusers (Carroll et al., 1993), methylphenidate treatment for cocaine abusers with residual attention deficit disorder (Khantzian et al., 1984), and so on. Similarly, while low-intensity psychotherapies may be sufficient for less severe cocaine abusers, specialized psychotherapies might be evaluated for cocaine abusers with distinct characteristics that would not be amenable to pharmacologic approaches. These might include motivational approaches (Miller & Rollnick, 1991) for patients who are ambivalent around renouncing substance use, community reinforcement (Azrin, 1976) or 12-Step (Nowinski, Chapter 2, this volume) approaches for patients low in social supports and resources, or cue extinction approaches (O'Brien et al., 1990) for those patients for whom continued conditioned craving for cocaine is problematic (Carroll et al., 1995).

CONCLUSIONS

Even for those classes of substance abuse for which there are powerful and effective pharmacotherapies, the availability of methadone, naltrexone, and disulfiram have by no means cured substance abuse. These very powerful agents tend to work primarily on the symptoms of substance abuse that are time-limited and autonomous but have little impact on the enduring behavioral characteristics of substance use. Moreover, pharmacotherapies work only if substance abusers see the value of stopping substance use, and substance abusers have consistently found ways to circumvent these pharmacologic interventions. It is unlikely that we will develop a pharmacologic intervention that gives addicts the motivation to stop using drugs, helps them see the value in renouncing substance use, improves their ability to cope with the day-to-day frustrations in living, or provides alternatives to the reinforcements drugs and drug-using lifestyles provide. The bulk of the evidence suggests that pharmacotherapies can be very effective treatment adjuncts, but in most cases the effects of pharmacotherapies can be broadened, enhanced, and extended by the addition of psychotherapy (Carroll & Rounsaville, 1993).

Psychotherapy and pharmacotherapies work through different mechanisms and address different problems, and neither is completely effective by itself. As the bulk of the evidence in the treatment of substance abuse suggests that the two forms of treatment tend to work better together than apart, integrated treatments, carefully matching to the particular needs of particular patients, may provide our best hope for helping patients whose lives have been devastated by substance abuse.

ACKNOWLEDGMENT

Support was provided by the National Institute on Drug Abuse grants RO1-DA04299, KO2-DA00248, and R18-DA06963, and National Institute of Alcoholism and Alcohol Abuse cooperative agreeement U10 AA08430.

NOTE

1. In this chapter, psychotherapy is used as a general term for all forms of psychosocial treatment, including individual and group counseling, psychotherapy, and behavior therapy.

REFERENCES

Alling, F. A. (1992). Detoxification and treatment of acute sequelae. In J. H. Lowinsohn, P. Ruiz, & R. B. Millman (Eds.), *Comprehensive textbook of substance abuse* (2nd ed., pp. 402–415). New York: Williams & Wilkins.

Anthony, J. C., & Helzer, J. (1990). Syndromes of drug abuse and dependence. In L. N. Robins & D. A. Regier (Eds.), *Psychiatric disorders in America*. New York: Free Press.

Anton, R. F., Hogan, I., Jalali, B., Riordan, C. E., & Kleber, H. D. (1981). Multiple family therapy and naltrexone in the treatment of opiate dependence. *Drug and Alcohol Dependence, 8,* 157–168.

Azrin, N. H. (1976). Improvements in the community-reinforcement approach to alcoholism. *Behaviour Research and Therapy, 14,* 39–348.

Azrin, N. H., Sisson, R. W., Meyers, R., & Godley, M. (1982). Alcoholism treatment by disulfiram and community reinforcement therapy. *Journal of Behavior Therapy and Experimental Psychiatry, 13,* 105–112.

Ball, J. C., Lange, W. R., Myers, C. P., & Friedman, S. R. (1988). Reducing the risk of AIDS through methadone maintenance treatment. *Journal of Health and Social Behavior, 29,* 214–216.

Ball, J. C., & Ross, A. (1991). *The effectiveness of methadone maintenance treatment.* New York: Springer-Verlag.

Beutler, L. E. (1991). Have all won and must all have prizes? Revisiting Luborsky et al.'s verdict. *Journal of Consulting and Clinical Psychology, 59,* 226–232.

Brill, L. (1977). The treatment of drug abuse: Evolution of a perspective. *American Journal of Psychiatry, 134,* 157–160.

Callahan, E. J., and Colleagues. (1980). The treatment of heroin addiction: Naltrexone alone and with behavior therapy. *International Journal of the Addictions, 15,* 795–807.

Carroll, K. M. (1993). Psychotherapeutic treatment of cocaine abuse: Models for its evaluation alone and in combination with pharmacotherapy. In F. M. Tims & C. G. Leukefeld (Eds.), *Cocaine treatment: Research and clinical perspectives* (NIDA Research Monograph Series No. 135, pp. 116–132). Rockville, MD: National Institute on Drug Abuse.

Carroll, K. M., Nich, C., & Rounsaville, B. J. (1995). Differential symptom reduction in depressed cocaine abusers treated with psychotherapy and pharmacotherapy. *Journal of Nervous and Mental Disease, 183,* 251–259.

Carroll, K. M., & Rounsaville, B. J. (1993). Implications of recent research on psychotherapy for drug abuse. In G. Edwards, J. Strang, & J. H. Jaffe (Eds.), *Drugs, alcohol, and tobacco: Making the science and policy connections* (pp. 211–221). New York: Oxford University Press.

Carroll, K. M., Rounsaville, B. J., & Gawin, F. H. (1991). A comparative trial of psychotherapies for ambulatory cocaine abusers: Relapse prevention and interpersonal psychotherapy. *American Journal of Drug and Alcohol Abuse, 17,* 229–247.

Carroll, K. M., Rounsaville, B. J., Gordon, L. T., Jatlow, P. M., Nich, C., Bisighini, R. M., & Gawin, F. H. (1994). Psychotherapy and pharmacotherapy for ambulatory cocaine abusers. *Archives of General Psychiatry, 51,* 177–187.

Carroll, K. M., Rounsaville, B. J., & Keller, D. S. (1991). Relapse prevention strategies in the treatment of cocaine abuse. *American Journal of Drug and Alcohol Abuse, 17,* 249–265.

Carroll, K. M., Rounsaville, B. J., Nich, C., Gordon, L. T., Gawin, F. H. (1995). Integrating psychotherapy and pharmacotherapy for cocaine dependence: Results of a randomized clinical trial. In L. Onken & J. Blaine (Eds.), *Potentiating the efficacy of medications: Integrating psychosocial therapies with pharmacotherapies in the treatment of drug dependence* (NIDA Research Monograph Series No. 150). Rockville, MD: National Institute on Drug Abuse.

Carroll, K. M., Ziedonis, D., O'Malley, S. S., McCance-Katz, E., Gordon, L., & Rounsaville, B. J. (1993). Pharmacologic interventions for abusers of alcohol and cocaine: A pilot study of disulfiram versus naltrexone. *American Journal on Addictions, 2,* 77–79.

Charney, D. S., Heninger, G. R., Kleber, H. D. (1986). The combined use of clonidine and naltrexone as a rapid, safe, and effective treatment of abrupt withdrawal from methadone. *American Journal of Psychiatry, 143,* 831–837.

Childress, A. R., McLellan, A. T., & O'Brien, C. P. (1984). Assessment and extinction of conditioned withdrawal-like responses in an integrated treatment for opiate dependence. In L. S. Harris (Ed.), *Problems of Drug*

Dependence, 1984 (NIDA Research Monograph Series No. 55, pp. 202–210). Rockville, MD: National Institute on Drug Abuse.

Corty, E., & Ball, J. C. (1987). Admissions to methadone maintenance: Comparisons between programs and implications for treatment. *Journal of Substance Abuse Treatment, 4,* 181–187.

Docherty, J. P., Marder, S. R., Van Kammen, D. P., & Siris, S. G. (1977). Psychotherapy and pharmacotherapy: Conceptual issues. *American Journal of Psychiatry, 134,* 529–533.

Dolan, M. P., Black, J. L., Penk, W. E., Robinowitz, R., & DeFord, H. A. (1985). Contracting for treatment termination to reduce illicit drug use among methadone maintenance treatment failures. *Journal of Consulting and Clinical Psychology, 53,* 549–551.

Elkin, I., Pilkonis, P. A., Docherty, J. P., & Sotsky, S. M. (1988a). Conceptual and methodological issues in comparative studies of psychotherapy and pharmacotherapy, I: Active ingredients and mechanisms of change. *American Journal of Psychiatry, 145,* 909–917.

Elkin, I., Pilkonis, P. A., Docherty, J. P., & Sotsky, S. M. (1988b). Conceptual and methodological issues in comparative studies of psychotherapy and pharmacotherapy, II: Nature and timing of treatment effects. *American Journal of Psychiatry, 145,* 1070–1076.

Extein, I., & Bowers, M. B. (1979). State and trait in psychiatric practice. *American Journal of Psychiatry, 136,* 690–693.

Finney, J. W., & Moos, R. H. (1986). Matching patients with treatments: Conceptual and issues. *Journal of Studies on Alcohol, 47,* 122–134.

Fuller, R. K. (1989). Antidipsotropic medications. In W. R. Miller & R. K. Hester (Eds.), *Handbook of alcoholism treatment approaches: Effective alternatives* (pp. 117–127). New York: Pergamon Press.

Fuller, R. K., Branchey, L., Brightwell, D. R., Derman, R. M., Emrick, C. D., Iber, F. L., James, K. E., Lacoursiere, R. B., Lee, K. K., Lowenstam, I., Maany, I., Neiderhiser, D., Nocks, J. J., & Shaw, S. (1986). Disulfiram treatment for alcoholism: A veterans administration cooperative study. *Journal of the American Medical Association, 256,* 1449–1455.

Galanter, M. (1993). *Network therapy for alcohol and drug abuse: A new approach in practice.* New York: Basic Books.

Gawin, F. H., & Kleber, H. D. (1986a). Abstinence symptomatology and psychiatric diagnosis in cocaine abusers. *Archives of General Psychiatry, 43,* 107–113.

Gawin, F. H., & Kleber, H. D. (1986b). Pharmacologic treatments of cocaine abuse. *Psychiatric Clinics of North America, 9,* 573–583.

Gawin, F. H., Kleber, H. D., Byck, R., Rounsaville, B. J., Kosten, T. R., Jatlow, P. I., & Morgan, C. B. (1989). Desipramine facilitation of initial cocaine abstinence. *Archives of General Psychiatry, 46,* 117–121.

Glosser, D. S. (1983). The use of a token economy to reduce illicit drug use among methadone maintenance clients. *Addictive Behaviors, 8,* 93–104.

Grabowski, J., O'Brien, C. P., Greenstein, R., Ternes, T., Long, M., & Steinberg-Donato, S. (1979). Effects of contingency payment on compliance with a naltrexone regimen. *American Journal of Drug and Alcohol Abuse, 6,* 355–365.

Greenstein, R. A., Arndt, I. C., McLellan, A. T., O'Brien, C. P., & Evans, B. (1984). Naltrexone: A clinical perspective. *Journal of Clinical Psychiatry, 45,* 25–28.

Greenstein, R. A., Fudala, P. J., & O'Brien, C. P. (1992). Alternative pharmacotherapies for opiate addiction. In J. H. Lowinsohn, P. Ruiz, & R. B. Millman (Eds.), *Comprehensive textbook of substance abuse* (2nd ed., pp. 562–573). New York: Williams & Wilkins.

Holder, H. D., Longabaugh, R., Miller, W. R., & Rubonis, A. V. (1991). The cost effectiveness of treatment for alcohol problems: A first approximation. *Journal of Studies on Alcohol, 52,* 517–540.

Hunt, G. M., & Azrin, N. H. (1973). A community- reinforcement approach to alcoholism. *Behaviour Research and Therapy, 11,* 91–104.

Iguchi, M. Y., Stitzer, M. L., Bigelow, G. E., & Liebson, I. A. (1988). Contingency management in methadone maintenance: Effects of reinforcing and aversive consequences on illicit polydrug use. *Drug and Alcohol Dependence, 22,* 1–7.

Kadden, R., Carroll, K. M., Donovan, D., Cooney, N., Monti, P., Abrams, D., Litt, M., & Hester, R. (1992). *Cognitive-behavioral coping skills therapy manual: A clinical research guide for therapists treating individuals with alcohol abuse and dependence* (NIAAA Project MATCH Monograph Series, Vol. 3, DHHS Publication No. ADM 92–1895). Rockville, MD: National Institute on Alcohol Abuse and Alcoholism.

Karasu, T. B. (1990). Toward a clinical model of psychotherapy for depression, II: An integrative and selective treatment approach. *American Journal of Psychiatry, 147,* 269–278.

Keller, D. S., Carroll, K. M., Nich, C., & Rounsaville, B. J. (in press). Differential treatment response in alexithymic cocaine abusers: Findings from a randomized clinical trial of psychotherapy and pharmacotherapy. *American Journal on Addictions.*

Khantzian, E. J. (1975). Self-selection and progression in drug dependence. *Psychiatry Digest, 10,* 19–22.

Khantzian, E. J., Gawin, F. H., Kleber, H. D., & Riordan, C. E. (1984). Methylphenidate treatment of cocaine dependence: A preliminary report. *Journal of Substance Abuse Treatment, 1,* 107–112.

Kleber, H. D. (1973). Clinical experiences with narcotic antagonists. In S. Fisher & A. M. Freedman (Eds.), *Opiate addiction: Origins and treatment.* New York: Winston.

Kleber, H. D. (1977). Methadone maintenance treatment—A reply. *American Journal of Drug and Alcohol Abuse, 4,* 267–272.

Kleber, H. D., Kinsella, J. K., Riordan, C., Greaves, S., & Sweeney, D. (1974). The use of cyclazocine in treating narcotic addicts in a low-intervention setting. *Archives of General Psychiatry, 30,* 37–42.

Kleber, H. D., Weissman, M. M., Rounsaville, B. J., Prusoff, B. A., Wilber, C. H. (1983). Imipramine as treatment for depression in opiate addicts. *Archives of General Psychiatry, 40,* 649–653.

Klerman, G. L. (1963). Assessing the influence of the hospital milieu upon the effectiveness of psychiatric drug therapy: Problems of conceptualization and of research methodology. *Journal of Nervous and Mental Disease, 137,* 143–154.

Klerman, G. L. (1975). Combining drugs and psychotherapy in the treatment of depression. In M. Greenblatt (Ed.), *Drugs in combination with other therapies* (pp. 67–81). New York: Grune & Stratton.

Kosten, T. R. (1992a). Pharmacotherapies. In T. R. Kosten & H. D. Kleber (Eds.), *Clinician's guide to cocaine addiction: Theory, research, and treatment* (pp. 273–289). New York: Guilford Press.

Kosten, T. R. (1992b). *Pharmacotherapy of drug dependence.* Fourth Triennial Report to Congress.

Kosten, T. R., & Kleber, H. D. (1986). Buprenorphine detoxification from opioid dependence: A pilot study. *Life Sciences, 42,* 635–641.

Longabaugh, R., Beattie, M., Noel, R., Stout, R., & Malloy, P. (1993). The effect of social support on treatment outcome. *Journal of Studies on Alcohol, 54,* 465–478.

Lowinson, J. H., Marion, I. J., Joseph, H., & Dole, V. P. (1992). Methadone maintenance. In J. H. Lowinsohn, P. Ruiz, & R. B. Millman (Eds.), *Comprehensive textbook of substance abuse* (2nd ed., pp. 550–561). New York: Williams & Wilkins.

Luborsky, L., Singer, B., & Luborsky, L. (1975). Comparative studies of psychotherapies: Is it true that "everyone has won and all must have prizes"? *Archives of General Psychiatry, 32,* 995–1007.

Marlatt, G. A., & Gordon, J. R. (Eds.). (1985). *Relapse prevention: Maintenance strategies in the treatment of addictive behaviors.* New York: Guilford Press.

McCarthy, J. J., & Borders, O. T. (1985). Limit setting on drug abuse in methadone maintenance treatment. *American Journal of Psychiatry, 142,* 1419–1423.

McLellan, A. T., Arndt, I. O., Metzger, D. S., Woody, G. E., & O'Brien, C. P. (1993). The effects of psychosocial services in substance abuse treatment. *Journal of the American Medical Association, 269,* 1953–1959.

McLellan, A. T., Childress, A. R., Ehrman, R., & O'Brien, C. P. (1986). Extinguishing conditioned responses during opiate dependence treatment: Turning laboratory findings into clinical procedures. *Journal of Substance Abuse Treatment, 3,* 33–40.

Meyer, R. E. (1992). New pharmacotherapies for cocaine dependence—Revisited. *Archives of General Psychiatry, 49,* 900–904.

Meyer, R. E. (Ed.). (1986). *Psychopathology and addictive disorders.* New York: Guilford Press.

Meyer, R. E., Mirin, S. M., Altman, J. L., & McNamee, B. (1976). A behavioral paradigm for the evaluation of narcotic antagonists. *Archives of General Psychiatry, 33,* 371–377.

Miller, W. R., & Hester, R. K. (1986). The effectiveness of alcoholism treatment: What research reveals. In W. R. Miller & R. K. Hester (Eds.), *Treating addictive behaviors: Processes of change* (pp. 121–174). New York: Plenum Press.

Miller, W. R., & Rollnick, S. (1991). *Motivational interviewing: Preparing people to change addictive behavior.* New York: Guilford Press.

Miller, W. R., Zweben, A., DiClemente, C. C., & Rychtarik, R. G. (1992). *Motivational enhancement therapy manual: A clinical research guide for therapists treating individuals with alcohol abuse and dependence* (NIAAA Project MATCH Monograph Series, Vol. 2, DHHS Publication No. ADM 92-1894). Rockville, MD: National Institute on Alcohol Abuse and Alcoholism.

Monti, P. M., Abrams, D. B., Kadden, R. M., & Cooney, N. L. (1989). *Treating alcohol dependence: A coping skills training guide.* New York: Guilford Press.

Noliman, D., & Crowley, T. (1988). Difficulties in a clinical application of methadone dose contingency contracting. In L. S. Harris (Ed.), *Problems of drug dependence, 1988* (NIDA Research Monograph Series No. 90, p. 69). Rockville, MD: National Institute on Drug Abuse.

Nunes, E. V., Quitkin, F. M., Brady, R., Stewart, J. W. (1991). Imipramine treatment of methadone maintenance patients with affective disorder and illicit drug use. *American Journal of Psychiatry, 148,* 667–669.

Nyswander, M., Winick, C., Bernstein, A., Brill, I., & Kaufer, G. (1958). The treatment of drug addicts as voluntary outpatients: A progress report. *American Journal of Orthopsychiatry, 28,* 714–727.

O'Brien, C. P., Greenstein, R., Ternes, J., McLellan A. T., & Grabowski, J. (1980). Unreinforced self-injections: Effects on rituals and outcome in heroin addicts. In L. S. Harris (Ed.), *Problems of drug dependence, 1979* (NIDA Research Monograph Series No. 27, pp. 275–281). Rockville, MD: National Institute on Drug Abuse.

O'Brien, C. P., Childress, A. R., McLellan, A. T., Ehrman, R. (1990). Integrating systematic cue exposure with standard treatment in recovering drug dependent patients. *Addictive Behaviors, 15,* 355–365.

O'Farrell, T. J., & Bayog, R. D. (1986). Antabuse contracts for married alcoholics and their spouses: A method to insure Antabuse taking and decrease conflict about alcohol. *Journal of Substance Abuse Treatment, 3,* 1–8.

O'Malley, J. E., Anderson, W. H., & Lazare, A. (1972). Failure of outpatient treatment of drug abuse. I. Heroin. *American Journal of Psychiatry, 128,* 865–868.

O'Malley, S. S., Jaffe, A. J., Chang, G., Schottenfeld, R. S., Meyer, R. E., & Rounsaville, B. J. (1992). Naltrexone and coping skills therapy for alcohol dependence: A controlled study. *Archives of General Psychiatry, 49,* 881–887.

Onken, L. S., & Blaine, J. D. (1990). Psychotherapy and counseling research in drug abuse treatment: Questions, problems, and solutions. In L. S. Onken & J. D. Blaine (Eds.), *Psychotherapy and counseling in the treatment of drug abuse* (NIDA Research Monograph Series No. 104, pp. 1–8). Rockville, MD: National Institute on Drug Abuse.

Rawson, R. A., Obert, J. L., McCann, M. J., & Mann, A. J. (1986). Cocaine treatment outcome: Cocaine use following inpatient, outpatient, and no treatment. In L. S. Harris (Ed.), *Problems of drug dependence, 1985* (NIDA

Research Monograph Series No. 67, pp. 271–277). Rockville, MD: National Institute on Drug Abuse.

Regier, D. A., Farmer, M. E., Rae, D. S., Locke, B. Z., Keith, S. J., Judd, L. L., & Goodwin, F. K. (1990). Comorbidity of mental disorders with alcohol and other drug use. *Journal of the American Medical Association, 264,* 2511–2518.

Resnick, R. B., Washton, A. M., & Stone-Washton, N. (1981). Psychotherapy and naltrexone in opioid dependence. In L. S. Harris (Ed.), *Problems of drug dependence, 1980* (NIDA Research Monograph Series No. 34, pp. 109–115). Rockville, MD: National Institute on Drug Abuse.

Rounsaville, B. J. (1995). Can psychotherapy rescue naltrexone treatment of opioid addiction? In L. Onken & J. Blaine (Eds.), *Potentiating the efficacy of medications: Integrating psychosocial therapies with pharmacotherapies in the treatment of drug dependence* (NIDA Research Monograph Series No. 150, pp. 37–52.) Rockville, MD: National Institution on Drug Abuse.

Rounsaville, B. J., Anton, S. F., Carroll, K. M., Budde, D., Prusoff, B. A., & Gawin, F.I. (1991). Psychiatric diagnosis of treatment seeking cocaine abusers. *Archives of General Psychiatry, 48,* 43–51.

Rounsaville, B. J., & Carroll, K. M. (1992). Individual psychotherapy for drug abusers. In J. H. Lowinson, P. Ruiz, & R. B. Millman (Eds.), *Comprehensive textbook of substance abuse* (2nd ed., pp. 496–508). New York: Williams & Wilkins.

Rounsaville, B. J., Gawin, F. H., & Kleber, H. D. (1985). Interpersonal psychotherapy adapted for ambulatory cocaine abusers. *American Journal of Drug and Alcohol Abuse, 11,* 171–191.

Rounsaville, B. J., Glazer, W., Wilber, C. H., Weissman, M. M., & Kleber, H. D. (1983). Short-term interpersonal psychotherapy in methadone maintained opiate addicts. *Archives of General Psychiatry, 40,* 629–636.

Rounsaville, B. J., & Kleber, H. D. (1985). Psychotherapy/counseling for opiate addicts: Strategies for use in different treatment settings. *International Journal of the Addictions, 20,* 869–896.

Rounsaville, B. J., O'Malley, S., Foley, S., & Weissman, M. M. (1988). Role of manual-guided training in the conduct and efficacy of interpersonal psychotherapy for depression. *Journal of Consulting and Clinical Psychology, 56,* 681–688.

Rounsaville, B. J., Weissman, M. M., Kleber, H. D., & Wilber, C. W. (1982). Heterogeneity of psychiatric diagnosis in treated opiate addicts. *Archives of General Psychiatry, 39,* 161–166.

Shaw, J. A., Donley, P., Morgan, D. W., & Robinson, J. A. (1975). Treatment of depression in alcoholics. *American Journal of Psychiatry, 132,* 641–644.

Smith, M. L., Glass, G. V., & Miller, T. I. (1980). *The benefits of psychotherapy.* Baltimore: Johns Hopkins University Press.

Stitzer, M. L., Bickel, W. K., Bigelow, G. E., & Liebson, I. A. (1986). Effect of methadone dose on urinalysis test results of polydrug-abusing methadone maintenance patients. *Drug and Alcohol Dependence, 18,* 341–348.

Stitzer, M. L., McCaul, M. E., Bigelow, G. E., & Liebson, I. A. (1984). Comparison of a behavioral and a pharmacological treatment for reduction of illicit opiate use. In L. S. Harris (Ed.), *Problems of drug dependence, 1983* (NIDA Research Monograph Series No. 49, pp. 255–261). Rockville, MD: National Institute on Drug Abuse.

Taylor, G. J., Parker, J. D., & Bagby, R. M. (1990). A preliminary investigation of alexithymia in men with psychoactive substance dependence. *American Journal of Psychiatry, 147,* 1228–1230.

Uhlenhuth, E. H., Lipman, R. S., & Covi, L. (1969). Combined pharmacotherapy and psychotherapy: Controlled studies. *Journal of Nervous and Mental Disease, 148,* 52–64.

Volpicelli, J. R., Davis, M. A., & Olgin, J. E. (1986). Naltrexone blocks the post-shock increase of ethanol consumption. *Life Sciences, 38,* 841–847.

Volpicelli, J. R., O'Brien, C. P., Alterman, A. I., & Hayshida, M. (1990). Naltrexone and the treatment of alcohol dependence. In L. D. Reid (Ed.), *Opioids, bulimia, and alcohol abuse and alcoholism.* New York: Springer-Verlag.

Woody, G. E., Luborsky, L., McLellan, A. T., O'Brien, C. P., Beck, A. T., Blaine, J., Herman, I., & Hole, A. (1983). Psychotherapy for opiate addicts: Does it help? *Archives of General Psychiatry, 40,* 639–645.

Woody, G. E., McLellan, A. T., Luborsky, L., & O'Brien, C. P. (1985). Sociopathy and psychotherapy outcome. *Archives of General Psychiatry, 42,* 1081–1086.

Woody, G. E., McLellan, A. T., Luborsky, L., & O'Brien, C. P. (1987). Twelve-month follow-up of psychotherapy for opiate dependence. *American Journal of Psychiatry, 144,* 590–596.

Woody, G. E., McLellan, A. T., Luborsky, L., O'Brien, C. P., Blaine, J., Fox, S., Herman, I., & Beck, A. T. (1984). Severity of psychiatric symptoms as a predictor of benefits from psychotherapy: The Veterans Administration–Penn Study. *American Journal of Psychiatry, 141,* 1172–1177.

Wurmser, L. (1978). *The hidden dimension.* New York: Jason Aronson.

Ziedonis, D. M., & Kosten, T. R. (1991). Depression as a prognostic factor for pharmacological treatment of cocaine dependency. *Psychopharmacology Bulletin, 27,* 337–343.

Index